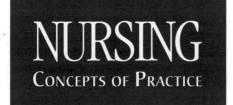

NURSING
CONCEPTS OF PRACTICE

Visit our website at **www.mosby.com**

NURSING
CONCEPTS OF PRACTICE

Dorothea E. Orem
Savannah, Georgia

with a contributed chapter by

Susan G. Taylor
Columbia, Missouri

and

Kathie McLaughlin Renpenning
White Rock, British Columbia, Canada

Sixth Edition

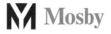 Mosby

A Harcourt Health Sciences Company

St. Louis   London   Philadelphia   Sydney   Toronto

PJC PENSACOLA CAMPUS LRC

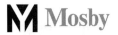
Mosby

A Harcourt Health Sciences Company

Vice President, Nursing Editorial Director: Sally Schrefer
Editor: Yvonne Alexopoulos
Developmental Editor: Kimberly A. Netterville
Project Manager: Deborah L. Vogel
Project Specialist: Mary Drone
Design Manager: Bill Drone
Cover Designer: Teresa Breckwoldt

SIXTH EDITION

Mosby, Inc.
A Harcourt Health Sciences Company
11830 Westline Industrial Drive
St. Louis, Missouri 63146

Printed in the United States of America

Library of Congress Cataloging-in-Publication Data

Orem, Dorothea E. (Dorothea Elizabeth)
   Nursing: concepts of practice / Dorothea E. Orem, with a contributed chapter by Susan
     G. Taylor and Kathie McLaughline Renpenning—6th ed.
     p. cm.
   Includes bibliographical references and index.
   ISBN 0-323-00864-X
   1. Nursing—Philosophy. I. Taylor, Susan G. II. Renpenning, Kathie
     McLaughlin. III.
   Title.
   RT84.5 .O73 .2001
   610.73—dc21   00-049614

01 02 03 04 05 GW/MVY 9 8 7 6 5 4 3 2 1

Foreword

Self-care Deficit Nursing Theory was chosen by the Faculty of the School of Nursing, University of Missouri—Columbia, in 1975 to provide the conceptual framework for the undergraduate curriculum and the substantive base for instruction. The faculty, challenged by the thoughtful insights and clear view of nursing presented by Orem, restructured the programs of instruction to emphasize nursing and nurse's role in aiding patients to reach the goal of promoting and or maintaining health and well-being through self-care. Dr. Orem's work is a core of the curriculum and is an important component in the success of our graduates.

Nursing: Concepts of Practice has undergone five revisions since our students began using it as a text. Each edition has brought new knowledge and insights into nursing. The changes that have been made through the years have made the book more useful. The text is much more than a book on nursing theory. It is a basic nursing text that initiates the student of nursing into a scholarly view of nursing, one that enables the student to understand that nursing is more than tasks. The book is an important part of the socialization of the students to nursing as a profession requiring a liberal arts and science knowledge base. The graduates of our program understand that nursing has a unique disciplinary perspective that is complementary to other health professions in providing service to persons who need assistance. The focus on the agency of persons is empowering to students of nursing.

This edition is structured to move from the general to the particular, from the abstract to the concrete, from the theoretic to the practical. The inclusion of a prologue to understanding nursing provides a bridge from the liberal arts and sciences to the practical science of nursing. The focus of nursing as human service is especially important in a contemporary society that places high value on technology and tends to isolate us from each other. The enhanced emphasis on the interpersonal aspects of nursing provides students with an appreciation of the importance of the substantial unity of the person as they interact with others. The inclusion of material on positive mental health makes the importance of Orem's work to health promotion and to the field of mental health more apparent. The action perspective, formalized in the concepts of therapeutic self-care demand and self-care and nursing agency, provides a basis for selection of nursing interventions that encourages the participation of the patient and others. Finally, the focus on the many units of service of the nurse, from

v

individual to community, establishes the appropriateness of using Orem's theory and insights in a full array of nursing situations.

Nursing: Concepts of Practice is an important work for undergraduate students, but it is also very important for graduate students. It provides the much-needed foundation for theoretic and empiric inquiry that will lead the field into the future. Individuals who are already nurses also benefit from this work. They gain new insights into their experiences as nurses. They are able to understand and interpret events in ways previously unknown to them. They gain their voice as nurse. Nurses who know and understand nursing value themselves and their contributions. They can explain and interpret their work from a coherent, congruent nursing perspective.

We, the faculty and students at the Sinclair School of Nursing, University of Missouri—Columbia, are privileged to have had a long relationship with Dr. Orem. The full value of Orem's work is yet to be realized.

Susan G. Taylor, PhD, RN, FAAN
Elizabeth A. Geden, PhD, RN, FAAN
On behalf of the Faculty,
Sinclair School of Nursing,
University of Missouri-Columbia,
Columbia, MO

Preface

This sixth edition of *Nursing: Concepts of Practice* continues the development and organization of the essential features of nursing considered as a field of knowledge and a field of practice. The edition begins with new content in the form of a Prologue that examines nursing in its most general nature as a direct human health service, including nursing's commonalities with other health services. To ignore the service features of nursing is to ignore why nursing continues to be maintained in or introduced into human groups. The distinguishing features of nursing are further developed or revised in accord with themes introduced in prior editions. The themes provide both structure and content for the text.

The first theme that flows throughout the text is the reason why persons need and can be helped through nursing. This theme, developed as the self-care deficit theory of nursing with its supporting theories, establishes the proper object of nursing, defines nursing's domain and boundaries as a field of knowledge and a field of practice and specifies the results sought through nursing. The conceptual elements of the theory and the substantive structure of each concept provide the subject matter of nursing science and point to the concrete features of persons in their life situations to which nurses should attend. Associated with the self-care deficit theory of nursing is the insight and the knowledge that humanely produced systems of care of self and care of dependents are enduring realities in societies. They are enduring in the sense that they are constant features of the daily life of individuals of all ages. Their enduring presence rests in their continual production by individuals, not in the lasting presence of the deliberately performed actions and action sequences that form systems of self-care and dependent-care. Without the continual production of these care systems and without their adequacy in meeting individuals' functional and developmental requisites, the lives, health, and well-being of individuals are at risk.

This first and major theme is associated with the second theme of the tridimensional relationship between persons who need nursing and persons who produce it—a societal relationship, an interpersonal relationship, and a technologic or clinical relationship. Both of these themes are permeated by a third theme that expresses the unitary nature of human beings who function as persons in their life situations. Each person has developing or developed powers and capabilities, personal dispositions, talents, interests, and values.

Mature and maturing individuals have requirements and responsibilities for self-maintenance, self-management, care of dependents, and the fulfillment of their human potential. Associated with this and the prior themes is the fourth theme of deliberate action—actions that are deliberately selected and deliberately performed by persons to achieve a foreseen and desired result or condition that does not presently exist. Deliberate action carries with it, regardless of the result or condition sought, requirements for engagement in investigative, judgment making, decision making, and production operations. These are the process operations of self-care, dependent-care, and nursing.

A fifth theme is that of the methods that one person can use in the process of assisting or helping a person or persons do what should be done but which the person is unable to do because of limited powers or capabilities for engaging in some or all of the process operations of deliberate action. Methods of helping or assisting provide the foundations for identifying valid systems of nursing when certain configurations of action limitations exist in persons who need nursing.

The sixth theme is that of nursing as practical science with theoretically practical and practically practical content components. To formalize the nursing sciences, including the organization of knowledge that has known validity and reliability in nursing practice, nurses require models of practical science and nursing in the form of a valid general theory of what nursing is and what it should be. The text includes the formalization and naming of three nursing practice sciences and three foundational nursing sciences.

These themes do not exhaust the content of the sixth edition. They provide the means that weaves the content together to form a unified meaningful whole. The themes may elicit interest on part of nurses to engage in their further investigation and development.

Nursing: Concepts of Practice has been used by nurses and nursing students in many countries of the world. Its use attests to its value in expressing the meaning of nursing and its identification and explication of the theoretically practical components of nursing that direct nurses to attend to the essential features of all nursing practice situations, including nursing specialization situations. Its place in nursing literature is that of a general and comprehensive introduction to the nature of nursing as a socially institutionalized direct human health service and to the nature of the nursing sciences that support it. Members of societies vary in cultural orientation, but all of them require self-care, and all may be subject to limitations for its provision for themselves or their dependents.

The continued use of the text and its value to nurses in the practice of nursing also rests on the deliberate integration of the conceptual elements of self-care deficit nursing theory with the process operations of nursing practice—nursing diagnosis, nursing prescription, nursing design, and nursing treatment or regulation. Without this integration self-care deficit nursing theory would retain the status of a *theory*, and nursing process operations would be *types of operations* without identified human and environmental foci and without designation of nursing outcomes sought. It can be said that the content of the sixth edition of *Nursing: Concepts of Practice* supports the judgment that self-care deficit nursing theory has served to give direction, meaning, and structure to nursing practice, as well as to emerging theoretic nursing sciences.

Dorothea Orem

Philosophic Foundations
of Orem's Work

Before my introduction to nursing theory in general, and to Orem's self-care deficit nursing theory, I had worked as a staff nurse for 10 years. During those years I often experienced difficulty expressing to others what it was that I, as a nurse, contributed to the care of the patient. As I became acquainted with Orem's theory, I recognized that this conceptualization of nursing was consistent with my nursing practice experiences. It provided me with the language and structure to explain what it was that was unique about nursing—what nurses contributed when they nursed patients. Throughout my master's program, I used the self-care deficit nursing theory for the conceptualization of clinical problems as well as my research.

As I entered doctoral studies, I began to hear comments regarding the mechanistic or reductionistic nature of the self-care deficit nursing theory from my fellow doctoral students. Some commented that the theory focused on human beings as the sum of parts. These views were incompatible with my understanding of Orem's work.

The disparity between my understanding of Orem's theory and the claims made by others about her theory revolved around the philosophic assumptions and beliefs on which the theory rests. Orem's work has been criticized for lack of clarity with regard to the philosophic foundations of the theory (Smith, Uys). Her work has focused on the human requirements for nursing and the processes for the production of nursing. She has addressed topics from a nursing perspective, not from an abstract philosophic perspective. In addition, she has put forth a position regarding the form of nursing as a science, identifying it as a practical science and a set of applied sciences.

Characterizations of Orem's theory that were not consistent with my understanding have appeared in the nursing literature. For example, Hanchett (1990) identified Orem's theory as a mechanistic causal model (p. 68). Parse claimed that nursing science is characterized by two paradigms, the totality and the simultaneity. Within the totality paradigm, the paradigm to which Parse assigned the self-care deficit nursing theory, human beings are considered to be bio-psycho-sociospiritual organisms whose environments can be manipulated to maintain or promote balance (p. 32). According to Sarter, Orem's view of human beings is consistent with the philosophy of evolutionary idealism (p. 102). The claims by these authors represent diverse interpretations of Orem's theory. In fact, the interpretation of Sarter is contradictory to the interpretations of both Hanchett and Parse.

Lack of clarity regarding the philosophic foundations of the self-care deficit nursing theory has permitted divergent and inaccurate interpretations of the theory, such as those made by Hanchett, Parse, and Sarter. Rather than being based on a thorough, comprehensive understanding of Orem's theory, these claims seemed to be based on statements taken out of context.

To identify and clarify the foundational beliefs and assumptions of Orem's theory, I conducted a philosophic inquiry of her work that was reported in a dissertation entitled *A Philosophical Inquiry of Orem's Self-Care Deficit Nursing Theory,* completed in 1997.

PHILOSOPHIC INQUIRY

Philosophizing involves engaging in intellectual activities to answer philosophic questions. These intellectual activities, which include such things as the identification of assumptions, the analysis of positions, the construction of interpretations, and the evaluation of forms of reasoning, can be construed as forms of argument (Edgerton, p. 171). Philosophizing is not limited to those who consider themselves to be philosophers. Rather, philosophic inquiry is the approach to be taken when attempting to answer philosophic questions.

Considered as a discipline, philosophy consists of four major branches or divisions: metaphysics, which deals with being; epistemology, which deals with knowing; ethics, which deals with right and wrong; and logic, which deals with proper forms of reasoning. The phrase "philosophic system" is used to refer to the work of a philosopher or group of philosophers that addresses questions related to these various branches.

For my dissertation, I addressed questions pertaining to the metaphysical and epistemological foundations of Orem's self-care deficit nursing theory. Three main topics were examined: (1) the nature of human beings, (2) the knowledge necessary for the development of the practical science of nursing, and (3) the appropriateness of various research methods for development of the needed knowledge. The inquiry process used for this study involved an in-depth examination and analysis of Orem's work, as well as the work of those authors whom Orem cites. Through this process the philosophic assumptions and beliefs foundational to Orem's work were explicated.

FINDINGS

Although not specifically addressed, the philosophic foundations of the self-care deficit nursing theory are embedded in Orem's discussions of various topics. The examination and analysis of her work, as well as the work of authors whom she cites, revealed that Orem's theory is based on a coherent philosophic foundation. The assumptions and beliefs underlying the self-care deficit nursing theory are based on the philosophic system of moderate realism. This type of realism, which is just one of many types of realism, is generally associated with the work of St. Thomas Aquinas. Orem's views on the nature of reality, the nature of human beings, and nursing as a practical science reflect the philosophy of moderate realism.

Nature of Reality

With regard to the nature of reality, moderate realism supports the view that there is a world that exists independent of thought, a world that is the way it is, regardless of what people think about it. This position can be contrasted with idealism, which supports the position that the nature of the world depends on or is relative to the thoughts of the knower. Sarter's position that the self-care deficit nursing theory fits with evolutionary idealism is clearly mistaken; Orem's work is based on a realist view of reality. Statements by Orem, such as "function within a veridical (reality) frame of reference" (p. 198) and "dispositions and orientations that result in perceptions, meanings, and appraisals of situations that are not in accord with reality" (p. 237), reflect the position of moderate realism. In addition to the position that the world exists independent of thought, moderate realism also maintains that it is possible to gain knowledge of this world.

Nature of Human Beings*

In relation to the nature of human beings, the following statement describes the philosophic view of human beings underlying the self-care deficit nursing theory:

> Human beings are unitary beings who exist in their environments, influencing the world as well as being influenced by the world. Unitary humans are beings in process, striving to achieve their human potential and self-ideal through developmental processes. Human beings possess free will; are capable of maintaining an awareness of self and environment, attaching meaning to what is experienced, and reflecting upon their experiences; and possess the ability to engage in deliberate action. In addition to freedom, other essential qualities of human beings include bonding together with others through human love, the unrestricted desire to know, the appreciation of beauty and goodness, the joy of creative endeavor, the love of God, and the desire for happiness. (Banfield, p. 51).

This description, which represents a synthesis of Orem's views, is based on Orem's work, as well as on the work of authors whom she cites.

The view of the nature of human beings that is foundational to Orem's self-care deficit nursing theory reflects the moderate realist conception of humans. This view is certainly not in keeping with the characterizations of

---

*From Banfield BE: Philosophical inquiry of Orem's self-care deficit nursing theory (Doctoral dissertation, Wayne State University, 1997), *Dissertation Abstr Int* 58(02): 5885B, 1997. Reprinted with permission of Barbara E. Banfield, Farmington Hills, MI.

Orem's theory as put forth by Hanchet, Parse, and Sarter. Their interpretations are based on misunderstandings of the beliefs and assumptions on which Orem's work rests.

To gain an in-depth understanding of Orem's views, a thorough reading of her work is needed. It is possible to read certain sections of Orem's text and, based on those sections, misinterpret the philosophic position underlying her theory. For example, Orem has identified five views of humans that may be taken for some practical purpose. The view of humans as persons reflects the philosophic position on the nature of human beings that is foundational to Orem's work. The views of human beings as agents, as symbolizers, organisms, and objects subject to physical force offer perspectives that may be helpful in understanding the self-care deficit nursing theory, as well as designing nursing care. Another example can be found in the section pertaining to health. In this section Orem discusses the view of humans as structural and functional differentiations. It is important to recognize that she does not claim that human beings are structural and functional differentiations, but rather that they have these differentiations. The reader is cautioned to avoid making judgments about the philosophic foundations of Orem's work based on selective readings from her text.

Not only has Orem's position on the nature of human beings been incorrectly interpreted, the nature of the nurse-patient relationship has also been incorrectly characterized. It is often insinuated that nurses who use the self-care deficit nursing theory to guide their practice do not relate on a human-to-human basis when providing nursing care. This is a misrepresentation of Orem's ideas regarding nursing. She states that nurses "cannot function therapeutically for their patients unless they seek to know and believe in the humanness of themselves and the persons for whom they provide care" (Orem, p. 77).

Knowledge Development

In the dissertation two areas related to knowledge development were addressed: the knowledge needed to develop the practical science of nursing and the research methods appropriate for this knowledge development.

Orem's position regarding nursing science as a practical science is based on the philosophy of moderate realism. In practical sciences knowledge is developed for the sake of the work to be done. For the practical science of nursing, the goal is to develop substantive knowledge that will enable nurses to achieve nursing results for people. The self-care deficit nursing theory provides a descriptive explanation of the elements and relationships that are common to all instances of nursing. To provide direction for nursing practice, knowledge regarding these conceptual elements and relationships must be developed. Orem has identified five stages of knowledge development and offered direction in terms of what is needed at each of these stages.

The suggestions for knowledge development offered by Orem relate to knowledge that will be useful to nurses in designing and producing nursing for persons. For Orem the priority for research is to build a body of knowledge useful for nursing practice, not to test her theory.

Orem has not identified the research methods that she considers appropriate for the development of knowledge related to the self-care deficit nursing theory. However, Parse (1987) claims that the qualitative methods are appropriate for theory testing of nursing theories within the totality paradigm (p. 33). As described by Parse, the totality paradigm does not reflect the beliefs foundational to the self-care deficit nursing theory. For Orem the emphasis is not on the testing of the theory; it is on the development of knowledge useful to nursing practice.

In terms of the research methods useful for the generation of this knowledge, a variety of methods are needed to develop practical nursing science. In designing a study, the researcher needs to consider the compatibility between Orem's theory and the philosophic assumptions underlying a particular research method. In my dissertation the relationship between the philosophic foundations of Orem's theory and the philosophic foundations of the empiricism, interpretive, and critical theory research paradigms was examined. The appropriate research method(s) to be used for a particular study depends on the questions being addressed. What is important is that there is compatibility between the beliefs regarding the phenomenon being investigated and the research method selected. A couple of examples are provided to illustrate the relationship between Orem's suggestions for knowledge development and the appropriateness of research methods.

Knowledge regarding the self-care practices of persons with specific types and values of self-care requisites needs to be developed. In designing a study to investigate self-care, it is essential that the researcher thoroughly understand this concept. For a behavior to be considered self-care, it must be a behavior engaged in for the purpose of meeting some self-care requisite. Therefore the research must be designed in such a way as to incorporate the intention or purpose for the particular behavior. Another issue that needs to be considered is that self-care is not caused behavior; it is behavior that is deliberately engaged in by persons who possess free will. Studies must be carefully designed so that self-care is not treated as a dependent variable that is caused by the independent variables.

Descriptive studies may be used to investigate the self-care practices related to particular self-care requisites—universal, developmental, or health-deviation—or to the total self-care system. Areas to explore include the creation, use, and effectiveness of various self-care practices (Orem, p. 214).

Another research method that may be used to generate knowledge about self-care is mini-ethnography. Such a study could explore the self-care practices engaged in by people of various cultures. According to Orem, "the activities of self-care are learned according to the beliefs, habits, and practices that characterize the cultural way of life of the group to which the individual belongs" (p. 226). An ethnographic method could also be used to develop knowledge about the influence of culture on therapeutic self-care demand and self-care agency.

Phenomenological methods may be useful in exploring the experiences of persons living with certain health problems. Human beings create meaning based on their experiences. Understanding of persons' perspectives and experiences can contribute to the practical science of nursing.

As useful as phenomenological methods might be for the investigation of human experiences, they would not be appropriate for the investigation of some of the concepts of the self-care deficit nursing theory, such as therapeutic self-care demand. "A therapeutic self-care demand is a humanly constructed entity, with an objective basis in information that describes an individual structurally, functionally, and developmentally" (Orem, p. 111). The therapeutic self-care demand represents the totality of actions required to meet the self-care requisites. These requisites are regarded as objective requirements. Therefore a phenomenological method would be an inappropriate approach to the investigation of this concept.

CONCLUSION

Through the process of philosophic inquiry, the philosophic foundations of the self-care deficit nursing theory were identified. Orem's theory rests on a coherent philosophic system. Her views regarding the nature of reality, the nature of human beings, and nursing as a practical science all reflect the philosophic system of moderate realism. Before making judgments about the beliefs and assumptions underlying the self-care deficit nursing theory, it is necessary to have a thorough, comprehensive understanding of Orem's work.

Barbara E. Banfield, RN, PhD
Farmington Hills, Michigan

References

Banfield BE: A philosophical inquiry of Orem's self-care deficit nursing theory (Doctoral dissertation, Wayne State University, 1997), *Dissertation Abstr Int* 58(02):5885B, 1997.

Edgerton, SG: Philosophical analysis. In Sarter B, editor: *Paths to knowledge: Innovative research methods for nursing,* New York, 1988, NLN.

Hanchett, ES: Nursing models and community as client, *Nurs Sci Q* 3:67-72, 1990.

Orem, DE: *Nursing concepts of practice,* ed 4, St Louis, 1991, Mosby.

Orem, DE: *Nursing concepts of practice,* ed 5, St Louis, 1995, Mosby.

Parse, RR: *Nursing science major paradigms, theories, and critiques,* Philadelphia, 1987, WB Saunders.

Sarter, B: *The stream of becoming: A study of Martha Rogers's theory,* New York, 1988, NLN.

Smith, MJ: A critique of Orem's theory. In Parse RR, editor: *Nursing science major paradigms, theories, and critiques,* Philadelphia, 1987, WB Saunders.

Uys, LR: Foundational studies in nursing, *J Adv Nurs* 12:275-280, 1987.

Contents

Prologue

CHAPTER 1

A Prologue to Understanding Nursing: The Human Service Features of Nursing

Outline

Common Features of Direct Human
Health Services

Knowledge of Professionals in Human
Health Services

Key Items

Domains of Health Service
Intellectual Virtues
Interpersonal Relationship
Legitimacy of Relations
Moral Virtues
Production of the Needed
Health Service

Professionals in Health Services
Prudence
Seekers of Health Service
Sciences
Service
Social Features

Nursing is one of the services that societies make publicly available to persons who need and seek it. **Service** refers to work done to meet some general need, a need characteristic of some or all persons who constitute a society. Nursing belongs to the *family of health services* that are organized to provide *direct care to persons* who have legitimate needs for different forms of direct care because of their health states or the nature of their health care requirements. Direct care services stand in contrast to health services that control the quality and safety of food and water, environmental conditions, or other features of community living.

Direct health services differ from one another by the nature of the health care requirements of the people that they are organized to meet; because requirements differ, they must be expressed in terms of *what is needed* and *why* it is needed, *who* provides it, and *how* it is provided. Each specific **domain of health service** sets requirements for knowledge, skills, and educational preparation and training of persons who learn to effectively design and produce health service within that specific domain. Time and place requirements of people for direct health service also differ; for example, requirements for care during a heart attack and during recovery from a heart attack. Needs of persons for different health services may occur concurrently; requirements for nursing care and medical care often are concurrent. They may also occur sequentially.

Direct human health care services have common features as well as features that distinguish them one from another. This chapter develops the general features that nursing has in common with other direct health services. These general features, when understood by nurses, help nurses accept that nursing has a specific domain of service and that nurses have the responsibility to function within it and to develop it as a field of practice and a field of knowledge. Subsequent chapters develop the features that nursing has in common with other direct health services.

The prologue also addresses the required forms of knowledge of persons who provide direct human health services. All knowledge has form and content. In the various direct human health services, the forms of knowledge are more or less similar, but the content differs. Producers of services seek to determine the relevant human and environmental conditions that are associated with each individual's need for a specific service. They make judgments and decisions about what can and what should be done to regulate or control existent conditions in the interest of each individual's life, health, and well-being. This is a practical endeavor. The knowledge requirements of persons who engage in the practical endeavor of providing health services are extensive, complex, and often oversimplified and misunderstood by academics. Furthermore, the knowledge demands on *professionals* in the human health service *nursing* have too often been minimized, or they have been recognized and taught as tasks rather than as bodies of structured knowledge that provide the rationales for both the tasks and the outcomes sought.

COMMON FEATURES OF DIRECT HUMAN HEALTH SERVICES

All direct human health services that are publicly available to individuals, families, or groups within a society have three common characterizing features. Figure 1-1 shows that persons who need a service and persons who provide the service are independently related to the society and independently fulfill conditions that legitimize their seeking and provision of health service. They are related to one another as *independent persons* who come together to be provided

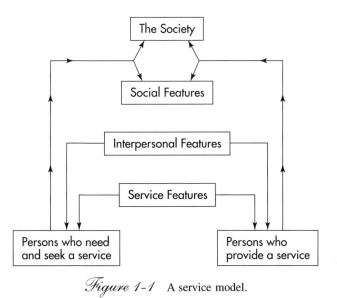

Figure 1-1   A service model.

with a needed health service and to provide the needed service. Each person has to fulfill requirements for communication and collaboration. As previously stated, each domain of *service* is defined in terms of persons with care requirements that are associated with their health states or the nature of their health care requirements.

Social Features

Developed and developing societies have as one focus of organized community effort the protection of the lives and health of their members. Societies therefore are concerned with the institution and development of health services and with their legitimacy, availability, and quality of services. Health service agencies and institutions must have approved charters or be incorporated within the governmental jurisdiction where they operate. Providers of specific services must be certified or licensed by socially designated bodies as qualified and capable. Providers of health services also belong to professional and occupational groups that may impose, for example, qualifications and career movement. Societies also have socioeconomic concerns about the continuing availability of direct human health services. The financing of services and their distribution to persons in need are major economic considerations. Table 1-1 is a summary of identified **social features.**

Person-to-Person Relations

The interpersonal features of direct human health care services come about when seekers and providers of services are in contact and communication with one another. Such contact presumes the social legitimacy of their positions and responsibilities within health service situations and their willingness to negotiate

Table 1-1   Selected Social Features of Direct Human Services

Types of Features	Focus	Considerations
Social control of services	Approval of the nature, institution, and operation of services in the community	Incorporating organizations and practice groups that provide health services; certifications or licensing of health service providers; regulating the operation of incorporated organizations through annual licensure or other means
Socioeconomic features	Continuing the availability of services in a community	Distribution and production of services in accord with human needs and availability of service; costs and financing of services; payment for services by receivers of services; payment to providers
Organized professional groups	Standard setting for the education and career movement of persons who function at a professional level of practice	Jurisdictional boundaries of service and levels of practice; form and content of initial and continuing education; promotion of efforts for the formalization and validation of the knowledge foundations for the service; research and development; certification for levels of practice
Organized occupational groups	Standard setting for workers who function in settings where required techniques of service are reliable and validated—technical level of practice, high- or low-level technical	Wages and benefits; areas and limits of responsibility in service situations; requirements for additional education for continued licensure or for movement to an advanced level of work

about what is to be done. If persons in need of a specific service are unable to communicate, providers must communicate with family members or other responsible persons.

Initial person-to-person contacts may result in decisions of mutual acceptance of the relationship or in decisions on the part of providers or seekers of the health service to withdraw from it because of personal or professional reasons. When contact continues, the development of an interpersonal relationship demands continuing communication. Any developing relationship is affected by the personalities of the related individuals; by their attitudes, beliefs, and values; by their maturity as persons; and by their states of health.

The nature of the health service that is to be provided sets the minimum requirements for contact and communication. These minimum requirements may be increased by factors that affect the ability of the persons in need of services to actively participate with providers. Such factors include, for example, age and developmental state, language, emotional state, overwhelming interests and concerns, and life experiences. Persons seek specific health services because in their own judgment or that of families or friends they need health care that they cannot provide for themselves. As a generality, it can be said that they are in need of *help*. Thus providers of direct health care services can be seen as helpers to those in need. This helping relationship becomes a feature of both the **interpersonal relationship** and the *service-providing relationship*. This comes about through the ways or methods of helping selected for the provision of service. For example, if persons in need of a health service are unconscious or in the developmental stage of infancy, the method of helping is that of *taking care of the other* and *doing for the other*. The ways of helping selected should not only conform to what persons cannot at present do for themselves, but should also take into consideration what it is they need to do now or in the future. Such considerations justify the use of the helping methods of *giving guidance, direction, and teaching*. See Chapter 3 for descriptions of helping methods and helping relationships in the "Understanding Nursing as a Helping Service."

Both individuals who need a direct health service and those who provide it in specific concrete health service situations meet and relate to one another as thinking, feeling persons. This relating as *persons* differs from the relating of the same individuals as **seekers of health service** and *providers* of needed health services. The social roles (seekers and providers) are opposite roles that are fulfilled by performing different kinds of activities. The coming together of persons as persons is unifying, forming a "we," not an opposition. It arises from within the "wealth and abundance of the [human] spirit."[1] Ideally, it is an intersubjective communication, an intimate personal contact exemplified, for example, by one's presence to the other, by gestures of personal respect, and by respect for the freedom of the other; and it is in no sense a fostering of dependency.

Such personal giving and receiving can permeate the activities of daily living as well as the receiving and the giving of a direct health service. In health service situations, it is important to know that a person can conceal self from others and appear different from what he or she is. Persons can treat others as objects, humiliate others, disregard others' feelings, avoid contact, and refuse dialogue. These are failures in interpersonal giving and receiving that can frustrate both the giving and the receiving of a health service.

The interpersonal contact of persons with the opposite roles of seekers and providers of a health service within a legitimate social contract may be brief or prolonged. Contact may be sustained over time, or it may be within a single service episode. Regardless of duration, it is the openness of thinking, feeling persons to one another in a giving and receiving relationship that fosters the well-being of each and is enabling for the **production of the needed health**

service. These ideas about the intersubjective relationship of seekers and providers of health services are adopted in part from M.G. Plattel.[1]

Service Features

The social and interpersonal features of direct human health services are brought about and continued by persons, the seekers and providers of services, so that existent needs of persons seeking health service can become known and met. The production of needed health service is totally dependent on (1) the willingness, the knowing, and the actions of persons who are legitimate producers of specific services—for example, qualified and experienced nurses and physicians; and (2) the willingness and the reasoned knowing of persons with health care needs to cooperate and participate. There are common process features that service providers, regardless of their specific health services, must perform. These include the providers' development and maintenance of functional, cooperative engagement of persons with health care needs; establishment of these persons' existent and changing needs for the specific health service; making judgments on the basis of knowledge (scientific and experiential) about what can and should be done to meet established needs; informing persons with health care needs about these judgments and about factors that will affect the actions taken and results sought; reaching mutual decisions about what will be done; designing of a plan of procedure; and producing and managing of health care services for individuals.

These process features of health service production may differ in the extent and depth of their performance by providers of health services. In limited episodic health service situations, such as care of minor wounds or immunizations specified by age, circumstances, or environment, effective health service providers perform all the process features but coalesce them into short time periods. In rendering specific health services for persons who are critically ill, severely injured, or suffering from chronic disabling conditions, performance of each process feature may be separated in time from the others; some may be repeated throughout the total period of the rendering of the health service, some may be performed continuously throughout the period of service, and some may be performed in collaboration with providers from one or more related health services.

The provision of direct health services is dependent on actions of providers and the cooperation and participation of recipients. However, health services can be positively or negatively affected by types of prevailing factors and circumstances that condition the needs and actions of seekers and the actions of providers. These include, for example, accessibility of a service to persons with specific needs, the time available to providers to give services, the availability and accessibility of required resources of equipment and supplies, safe physical environmental conditions, and a social environment that promotes the exercise of freedom and responsibility and affords respect to the rights and needs of both seekers and providers of service. Each of the named factors that negatively affect the availability and provision of a health service constitutes an obstacle that providers and seekers of service must contend with and find ways to overcome. This requires time and effort. When desirable conditions prevail, the provision of health services is facilitated.

In each specific direct human health service, it is persons who are prepared to function and persons who do function at the level of professional practice who must know and master the form and content of knowledge specific to their field. If their field of service is to endure, they must contribute to the extension and validation of the field through professional practice, scholarly endeavor, and research. It is the professionals in each field who must organize; structure validated knowledge into specific named **sciences;** and develop, validate, and establish the reliability of practice technologies. The number of organized and named sciences in any specific direct human health service, the continuing development of these sciences, and the introduction of new sciences or areas of a science are entirely dependent on the scientific endeavors of professionals in the field and on the work of scientists in supportive basic fields. Supportive fields include both biologic and behavioral fields.

KNOWLEDGE OF PROFESSIONALS IN HUMAN HEALTH SERVICES

Five areas of knowing are suggested. The *first area* describes persons who are experienced **professionals in health services** who know their specific field of service in a firm and stable way. Their knowing is capable of advancing with experience toward certitude and the human power of applying their knowledge critically and practically.[2] This movement of individuals toward the wisdom that characterizes the expert professional requires the exercise of scholarship to master the basic sciences as well as the sciences that (1) describe and *explain* the enduring realities to be dealt with in the **domain of a health service** and (2) guide and lead the professional practitioner to accomplish each of the process features of the service. This form of knowing involves association and integration of antecedent knowledge (what is already known) and information about reality situations with awareness of meaning of different realities and configurations of knowledge.

This area of knowing begins when individuals prepared within the professional form of education and training for practice understand their domain of health service, and have mastered the nature and purpose of the validated and reliable technologies through which the health service is produced. These individuals progress to develop the action capabilities and the skills required for the safe and effective use of these technologies in normal—that is, commonly recurring—types of health service situations within the domain. They learn from practical experience how to be themselves and manage themselves in health service situations. They learn the dynamic interpersonal features of providing service and develop the skills necessary for the practice of the interpersonal arts associated with communication and with the maintenance of interpersonal unity, including cooperation and coordination of effort toward goal achievement.

The *second area* of knowing is knowledge of the sciences specific to the service. The provision of health service is a practical endeavor; there is some practical objective to be done. The provider moves through a number of stages that characterize any practical endeavor: from insight about some existent human or environmental condition(s) that should be regulated or controlled and finally to a decision about *what to do* to achieve the foreseen result and to *engagement in action* to achieve the result. Health service sciences thus are sciences of the practical. They are referred to by some philosophers as *practical sciences* with speculatively practical and practically practical form and content. The idea and descriptions of practical sciences by Maritain[3] and Wallace[4,5] provide guides for understanding and incentives for scholarly movement to develop underdeveloped service sciences such as nursing and are illustrated by the form and content of developed health service sciences such as those of medicine. Practical science is a more productive and appropriate view than simply referring to the health service sciences as applied sciences, as do some academics. The health services are highly complex and demanding in terms of both knowledge and practice. Development of specific practical sciences is a prolonged endeavor, prolonged to initially establish form and content, with continued development over time.

A *third area* of knowing of professionals in the direct human health services relates to themselves and to those they serve as persons with bonds to families, communities, and larger societies. A developing bond between seekers and providers of health services must be seen by them as legitimate. **Legitimacy of relations** relates to the validity of the social contract into which they have entered and to awarding legitimacy to the relationship by the interactive persons. Such personally conferred legitimacy is marked by deference of one to the other and by effectiveness in developing systems of communication. Ways of relating, interacting, and communicating must be both culturally appropriate and effective if a health service is to be both understood by and produced for individuals in accord with their existent needs for it.

In addition, providers of human health services should have knowledge of themselves as persons who not only relate to other persons in health services situations but also make judgments and decisions and deliberately do things that should do good but may inadvertently do harm to persons they serve. This knowledge of providers concerns their own understanding and possession of the intellectual and moral virtues or dispositions that are enabling for the habitual control of their deliberate actions and in making judgments of good and bad, right and wrong in concrete situations where they provide health services to specific individuals in need. **Intellectual virtues** are habits or enduring dispositions that mentally dispose persons to act so that they can make right judgments and choices in concrete situations, considering existent features, conditions, and surrounding circumstances. **Moral virtues** dispose persons to judge and do what is good and avoid what is wrong or harmful to themselves or other persons in concrete situations of human living.

A *fourth area* of knowledge, associated with the prior area, relates to the integrity of persons who provide direct health services. Integrity is associated with life experiences, with experiences in specific health services, and with efforts to develop ways of reasoning and decision making that reflect the acquired disposition or virtue or habit of **prudence.** The habit of prudence disposes persons to make right choices and decisions about what to do in specific concrete life situations where existent conditions and surrounding circumstances may be extensive and complex. *Prudence* is usually expressed as *right reason about things to be done.* Acting prudently may require acting in accord with what is *just.* It involves acting with courage and with *moderation, in control* of one's *instincts and desires.*

Some distinguishing characteristics of persons who behave prudently in single, specific health service situations are listed in the following box. These characteristics are adopted from notes from lectures of William A. Wallace at the Catholic University of America, 1966. The characteristics noted conform to those expressed in St. Thomas Aquinas's treatise on prudence.[6]

A *fifth area* of knowledge necessary for all providers of human health services relates to their understanding of *voluntary action, deliberate action* engaged in to achieve some foreseen end or goal or result. This includes the ability to investigate, analyze, and synthesize. Understanding the nature of deliberate action is essential background knowledge for understanding the process features of providing a health service, as well as knowing actions involved in the everyday pursuits of persons as they work, care for others, recreate, and take care of themselves.

Indicators That Reveal the Exercise of Prudence by Human Health Service Providers

Action-Related Indicators

Experience in specific situations within a field where actions with specific forms, content, and outcomes were taken

Memory of these situations and results of the action taken; comparing features of particular situations and extracting relevant items

Facility in judging concrete situations in a field that (1) exhibits normal or expected features and (2) exhibits extraordinary features outside the norm

Exercising foresight about possible untoward occurrences; being circumspect, taking everything that is relevant into consideration

Being cautious when making decisions about what to do but not avoiding making decisions and taking action

Personal Indications

Possession of integrity, moral soundness, and wholeness

Modified from W.A. Wallace's lecture notes, School of Nursing, the Catholic University of America, 1966.

These five areas of knowledge of professionals in specific human health services are summarized as a listing. All areas presuppose knowing the specific domain of a health service.

1. The knowing that characterizes experienced professionals in a specific health service; knowing that is complex and integrated and continues to advance and that they can apply critically and practically. This knowing has a base in professional-level education and initial practice.

2. Professionals' knowing of the speculatively practical sciences that describe and explain their field of service and the practically practical sciences that guide in the production of the health service, along with basic sciences that support these practical sciences.

3. Professionals' knowing of humankind and the features of the legitimacy of the relationship of seekers to providers of health service personally conferred by them.

4. Professionals' self-knowing—integrity, experience, and prudence in reasoning, judging, and deciding what should be done for persons in specific concrete health service situations.

5. Professionals' knowing of the nature and features of deliberate action and how to construct the steps to be taken in movement from knowledge of an end to be sought to the achievement of the end.

The service, interpersonal, and social features of nursing are developed in subsequent chapters. Chapter 2 introduces the knowledge requirements for nursing in terms of the need for nurses to define and understand the nature and purpose of this human health service. These requirements continue to be developed throughout the book.

References

1. Plattel MG: *Social philosophy,* Pittsburgh, 1965, Duquesne University Press, pp 64-67.
2. Maritain J: *Science and wisdom,* translated by Bernard Wall, London, 1944, Centenary Press, p 4.
3. Maritain J: *The degrees of knowledge,* translated under the supervision of Gerald Q. Phelan, New York, 1959, Charles Scribner's Sons, pp. 456-464, especially pp 458-459.
4. Wallace WA: *The modeling of nature, philosophy of science and philosophy of nature in synthesis,* Washington, DC, 1996, Catholic University of America Press, pp 174, 180-189.
5. Wallace WA: Essay XIII: Being scientific in a practice discipline. From *In a realist point of view: essays on the philosophy of science,* ed 2, Lanham, Md, 1988, University Press of America.
6. Aquinas, St. Thomas: Prudence, *Summa theologiae,* vol. 36, translated by Thomas Gilby, Cambridge, 1974, Blackfriars; and New York, 1974, McGraw-Hill.

PART I

The Service, Societal, and Interpersonal Features of Nursing

CHAPTER 2

Understanding Nursing

A realistic starting point for nurses and nursing students who seek understanding of nursing is their acceptance that *nursing is a direct human health service.* This statement, when accepted as a *premise,* as true, leads nurses to identify two questions that must be answered: What human conditions and circumstances are associated with persons' requirements for the service of nursing? and What is the nature and structure of the service, the product that nurses make for persons who have requirements for nursing? Implicit in the first question is another question that forms a bridge to the second question: What brings the human conditions and circumstances associated with requirements for nursing outside the domain of personal and family responsibilities and into the domain of a publicly available service, nursing? Adequate definitions and descriptive explanations of nursing address and answer the three questions and explicate the relations among them.

This chapter considers these questions and, in so doing, introduces definitions, descriptions, and explanations of the specific *service features of nursing.* (See the section "Developing insights about nursing.") This chapter also discusses nurses' need for insights about the nature of persons' requirements for nursing and the nature of its production in order to attach nursing meaning to the persons, objects, places, and events that make up their world. In the section "Nursing and caring," the meaning and use of the terms *care* and *caring* are discussed. The chapter concludes with accounts of the ways nurses have viewed and should view nursing and with a view of the critical element in the production of the health service of nursing, the nurse as agent.

THE WORLD OF THE NURSE

The **world of the nurse** is manifested to each nurse as a system of "qualitatively differentiable and separately locatable"[1] persons and things. It is a world of experiences with people, of information seeking, of making judgments and decisions, and of acting to achieve foreseen results that fulfill existent or projected requirements of people for nursing. It is also a world of knowledge seeking and knowledge building. Nursing students initially show concern about what they will be expected to do when confronted with persons or groups of persons in need of nursing. They have concerns about whether they will have requisite knowledge and skill. To reassure themselves, they at times seek to learn the details of how to do this or that, things that nurses traditionally do.

The reality that is the world of the nurse must be accepted as a world mediated by meaning. The notion of meaning embraces a great variety of things. In nursing, however, meaning must be attached to persons, things, events, conditions, and circumstances in terms of how they affect the actions nurses perform in designing and producing nursing care. Nurses require knowledge (1) that affords meaning to specific individuals seeking nursing and to their conditions and circumstances that are nursing relevant and (2) that indicates what can and should be done for them through nursing. Nurses' application of this knowledge in nursing practice situations is always a *personal* application, an existential application, and one that is done with *professional judgment and integrity*. Nurses must not only master such knowledge—that is, make the knowing their own—but also master its application in practice situations.

Young children attach meaning to actors and objects introduced into the play situations they create. They set protocols for action and specify relations between and among players and objects, thereby establishing order. Children draw on their own experiences, on stories they have heard or read, and on their imaginations in creating play situations. Children (as well as men and women), when confronted with concrete life situations of types that are disliked or not before encountered, may turn away or may elect to enter into them as actors or as participant observers motivated by a desire to know, to experience, or to make events occur.

Concrete situations of human living are complex and are more often lived than understood. There are constituent elements or parts, persons or objects, or environmental conditions. Persons and objects have attributes or properties. Environmental conditions are of various types, physical, social, or biologic; and each type can vary over a range of values. The connections among elements and their properties determine the existent and changing order among situational elements. Because situations of human living are dynamic, changes in elements or relations among them are possible and are predictable. Persons acquire experiential knowledge from concrete life situations and can draw on this knowledge to attach meaning to similar, recurring situations.

Some life situations are outside the usual day-to-day experiences of persons who live together in community. These are situations in which specialized knowledge and abilities are required for observing, for attaching meaning and value to judgments about what is, and for developing insights about what can be changed and what should be changed. Nursing situations as described and explained in *Nursing: Concepts of Practice* require specialized knowledge and skills on the part of persons who elect to become able to take action in them, that is, to be nurses with developed capabilities and powers to provide nursing to persons who require it.

When nurses approach and enter into concrete **situations of nursing practice,** they are confronted with needs to ask and answer certain questions: What does this situation that involves me with others in this time-place localization mean to me, not just as a person but as a person who is Nurse? Why am I here? As Nurse, what must I know? What do I inquire about? What questions do I need to ask? What meaning do I attach to the information obtained, to the judgments I make? What conclusions are valid? Do I have a language to express what I know so what I know is communicated meaningfully to persons I nurse, to other nurses, and to other health workers? Do I have knowledge of what can be changed through deliberately designed action and what cannot be changed? These questions identify the kinds of specialized, theoretical knowledge that nurses should have as they investigate the nursing-relevant details of concrete nursing practice situations. Without such structured nursing knowledge, nurses rely on their common-sense knowledge that is uninformed by nursing science.

Nurses function in community with other nurses, with other health workers, and with persons and families who require and can benefit from nursing. The sector of reality that is the world of the nurse must become known to nursing students and nurses if they are to function as effective practitioners of the health service nursing. The world of the nurse includes elements in common with the worlds of other health workers, for example, the persons and families served, but the world of the nurse has a defined domain within boundaries. The domain and boundaries of nursing practice are defined by what nurses are concerned with as nurses within their world and by the way in which they are concerned. Nurses' productive efforts to identify, understand, conceptualize, and express what nurses are concerned within their world and the ways in which they are concerned lead to the beginning formalization of the content and structure of nursing as systematized and validated knowledge (i.e., as nursing science).

DEVELOPING INSIGHTS ABOUT NURSING

Nurses must be knowledgable, insightful, and skilled enough to know what events, conditions, and circumstances characterizing persons in health care situations are within the domain of clinical nursing practice. A first step in the process of reaching understanding of nursing can be one of identifying the connotations of the word **nursing.** Connotation signifies the things to which a word can be correctly applied. Identification can proceed from analysis of dictionary *definitions of nursing* to analysis of definitions formulated by nursing scholars. A second step can begin with inquiry about what is recognized as the *proper object of nursing,* nursing's objective focus in society. This step should then proceed to a development of nursing models and theories.

The Word *Nursing*

Nursing is an English-language word. It is used as a noun, as an adjective, and as a verbal auxiliary derived from the verb *to nurse.* Used as a noun and an adjective, *nursing* signifies the kind of care or service that nurses provide. It is the work that persons who are nurses do. The word *nursing* as used in the statement *I am nursing* is a verbal auxiliary, a participle. *To nurse* literally means (1) to attend to and serve and (2) to provide close care of a person, an infant or a sick or disabled person, unable to care for self, with the goal of helping the person become sound in health and "self-sufficient."* This nominal (lexicographic) definition of nursing identifies that engagement in nursing signifies that persons are:

• Attending to and serving others
• Providing close care of other persons unable to care for themselves
• Helping such persons become sound in health and self-sufficient

This definition describes nursing in that it signifies the proper use of the word in its broadest sense, but it is not an adequate definition of the *specialized health service nursing.* It does not differentiate persons who require the specialized health service nursing from persons who require nursing in other forms, such as the close care required by and provided for infants.

Orem's 1956 definition of nursing[2] is a more precise identification of what properly can be referred to as nursing.

> Nursing is an art through which the nurse, the practitioner of nursing, gives specialized assistance to persons with disabilities of such a character that more than ordinary assistance is necessary to meet daily needs for self-care and to intelligently participate in the medical care they are receiving from the physician. The art of nursing is practiced by "doing for" the person with the disability, by "helping him to do for himself" and/or by "helping him to learn how to do for himself." Nursing is also practiced by helping a capable person from the patient's family or a friend of the patient to learn how "to do for" the patient. Nursing the patient is thus a practical and a didactic art.

In this definition the definitive structure of nursing begins to emerge. In any field of inquiry *structure* refers to relatively fixed relationships between elements

*From *Webster's dictionary of synonyms,* ed 1, Springfield, Mass, 1951, G & C Merriam Co, p. 577.

Broad Work Operations of Nurses in Clinical Nursing Practice

Entering into and maintaining interactive relationships with persons seeking nursing for themselves or their dependents as individuals or as members of social units such as families or households in their time-place localizations.

Establishing the kind and amount of the immediate and continuing care (care demand) required to regulate these persons' functioning and development at this time and in subsequent time periods; determining the action capabilities and limitations of these persons to know and to meet the care demand.

Designing, planning for, instituting, and managing systems of nursing care with identified nurse and patient roles valid during specific time periods to ensure that the established care demand is met, that persons' exercise or development of powers to care for self or dependents is regulated, and that these powers are protected. Controlling the quality of systems of nursing care in terms of results sought and achieved.

Responding to these persons' requests for help and to their overt or covert needs for nurse contact and assistance.

Coordinating the nursing provided to these persons by different nurses within and over time periods.

Coordinating components of the systems of care produced by nurses with persons in other services who provide help and care for these persons, including, for example, medical care or social services.

Discharging these persons from the care of nurses when they demonstrate ability to follow and meet a prescribed care demand, and to make needed adjustments in it, doing this alone or with help from family members or others and with or without continuing consultation from nurses.

From *Validated lists of work operations of nurses in seven areas of endeavor in nursing.* Created by Dear M, Orem D: Washington, DC, 1976, Georgetown University School of Nursing. Revised by Orem D, 1982 and 1994.

or parts with characterizing features. The beginning emergence of the definitive structure of nursing results from addition of detail about persons who attend to and serve others and persons who are attended to and served. Details include:

- Naming the attending person as nurse.
- Identification of what the nurse does as practical art, including didactic (instructional) features.
- Identification of persons provided with care as having disabilities of such a character that specialized assistance is required. This is in distinction to assistance from untrained persons.
- Identification of the reasons why assistance is required, that is, to meet daily needs for self-care and needs for intelligent participation in medical care received.
- Naming the methods of helping that nurses use, methods that relate nurses and patients according to the roles of each in the provision of care.

This definition adds detail to and sets limits on the lexicographic definition of nursing, but it falls short of being an adequate descriptive explanation of nursing.

Formalization of Nursing's Proper Object

Scholars and theorists in various fields have found that the most productive beginning approach to explain descriptively their specialized fields of knowledge or practice is to identify the proper object of the field. *Object* means that toward which or because of which action is taken. *Proper* means that which belongs to the field. Object is used in the philosophic or scientific sense as that which is studied or observed, that to which action is directed to obtain information about it or to bring about some new condition. Object is not used in the sense of something tangible.

The whole reality of human beings—men, women, and children—cared for either singly or as social units, constitute (in the philosophic sense) "the material object" of the activities of nurses, physicians, clinical psychologists, social workers, and others who provide direct care for persons in need. Each of the named human services has its own proper object, which identifies with what and why men, women, or children require each specific service and can be helped through its provision.

A 1958 expression by Orem[3] of the **proper object of nursing** answered the following question: What condition exists in a person when judgments are made that a nurse(s) should be brought into the situation (i.e., that persons should be under nursing care)? The answer was expressed in this fashion: The condition is the inability of persons to provide continuously for themselves the amount and quality of required self-care because of situations of personal health. With children it is the inability of parents or guardians to provide the amount and quality of care required by their child because of their child's health situation. **Self-care** is the personal care that individuals require each day to regulate their own functioning and development. Provision of this care emerges as a system of care actions, a self-care system. Requirements of persons for this day-to-day regulatory care will be affected by, among other factors, age, developmental stage, health state, environmental conditions, and effects of medical care. **Dependent-care** is the continuing health-related personal regulatory and developmental care provided by responsible adults for infants and children or persons with disabling conditions, forming systems of dependent-care.

This specification of the proper object of nursing makes it possible to conceptualize and express characterizing features of the *specialized health service nursing*. Persons identified in the nominal definition of nursing as "unable to care for self" are now limited to persons who are in this state of inability because of the activity-limiting effects of their states of health or because of the nature and complexity of their day-to-day self-care requirements that contribute to regulation of their functioning and development. The specialized health service nursing is differentiated not only from other specialized human services, such as medicine, but also from the care of infants and young children and the continuing care of children or adults with illnesses or

Exercise

Exercise to Assist in the Development of a Concept of Self-Care

1. Select an individual (a relative, friend, or associate or an inpatient or outpatient at a hospital) who has a chronic disease, has sustained an injury, has experienced an acute illness, or is pregnant for the first time.
2. In accordance with the individual's ability, interest, and willingness to comply with your request for information, ask the following questions (rephrase if desired) and record the answers.
   a. Since the occurrence of (name the conditioning factor, disease, injury, etc.), do you have to care for yourself differently than you did before its occurrence?
   b. What are some of your new activities or tasks? How did you learn about the need to engage in them?
   c. How do you fit the new tasks into the schedule of your daily activities?
   d. Can you do all of these new tasks by yourself? If not, who helps you?
   e. Did you know how to do these new tasks before the occurrence of (same as in *a*, above)?
   f. How did you feel about learning to do the new tasks? How do you feel about doing them now?
   g. Of all the things that you know you should do, are there some things that you tend to forget or deliberately decide not to do? If so, why?

disabilities by family members. The expressed proper object of the specialized health service nursing is identified as a *subclass* of the *class of persons who are unable to care for themselves.*

Experienced nurses recognize life situations in which persons require the specialized health service nursing. Experienced, efficient nurses know when their work of nursing others, caring for others, or helping others care for themselves, produces beneficial results. However, as previously stated, it is essential for nurses to know and be able to express and thereby communicate what they do, why and how they do it, and the results of what they do.

Orem's insights, formulations, and expressions of the proper object of nursing in 1958 provided the conceptual foundations that enabled her to begin to formulate, organize, classify, and structure her knowing of nursing from her years in nursing education and nursing practice. The project in which she was engaged in 1958 was one of "upgrading the training of practical nurses" by inclusion of nursing content in distinction to a simple listing of tasks performed by practical nurses. This project was the reason for her asking the question: What condition exists in a person when judgments are made . . . that a person should be under nursing care? She required an answer to the question because the work of the project demanded that she know in explicit terms the **domain and boundaries of nursing** as a human health service in order to select areas of nursing knowledge appropriate for practical nurse education. The 1959 publication[4] developed for curriculum designers and teachers resulting from this project includes the beginning structuring of nursing content.

Orem continued work to further define and structure the domain and boundaries of nursing as a field of knowledge and a field of practice. One result of this work was a description of nursing that was published in 1971 in the first edition of *Nursing: Concepts of Practice.*[5]

A Description of Nursing

The following description of nursing is formed from three expressed generalizations about the persons, elements, and features that are common to nursing practice situations.

> Nursing has as its special concern man's need for self-care action and the provision and maintenance of it on a continuous basis in order to sustain life and health, recover from disease and injury, and cope with their effects (pp. 1-2).[5]
>
> The condition that validates the existence of a requirement for nursing in an adult is the absence of the ability to maintain for himself continuously that amount and quality of self-care which is therapeutic in sustaining life and health, in recovering from disease or injury, or in coping with their effects. With children, the condition is the inability of the parent (or guardian) to maintain continuously for the child that amount and quality of care which is therapeutic (p. 2).[5]

Actions in the domain of nursing must be consciously selected and directed by nurses toward accomplishing nursing goals within health care situations.

> On this basis, the results nurses achieve through their nursing (actions) are beneficial to patients to the degree that (1) the patient's therapeutic self-care is accomplished; (2) the nursing actions are helpful in moving the patient toward responsible action in matters of self-care (the patient may move toward steadily increasing independence or adapt to interruptions in the exercise of his capacities or to steadily declining capacities for self-care action); or (3) members of the patient's family or a non-nurse who attends the patient becomes increasingly competent in making decisions relative to the continuing daily, personalized care of the patient or in providing and managing the patient's care using nurse supervision and consultation as required. One or all of these general goals of nursing action may be appropriate in specific nursing situations (p. 156).[5]

This description of nursing is comprehensive but not complete in that relations among features of seekers and providers of nursing are not adequately developed .and expressed. The description is wordy because insights about the expressed nursing-relevant features and actions in nursing practice situations had not been formalized and conceptualized, and appropriate terms had not been selected with which to express the concepts.

Conceptualization of insights about identified elements and features of nursing practice situations proceeded during the 1960s. This allowed for the development and expression of conceptual frameworks, models, and theories of nursing. A pictorial model of nursing, showing relationships among the conceptual elements specific to nurses and nurses' patients, is shown in Appendix B, Figure B-1. A theory of nursing is presented in the following section.

A General Theory of Nursing

The explanation of nursing offered here has the form of a general theory—one that is descriptively explanatory of nursing in all types of practice situations. The theory expresses a picture or a model of nursing, what it is, what it should be. The theory encompasses both nurses and persons nursed, including the relations between them as persons, the relevant powers and capabilities of each, action processes produced as powers are activated both by nurses and persons nursed, and the types of results sought. The proper object of nursing as described in a preceding section, Formalization of nursing's proper object, was the essential reality base for theory formulation.

The theory, named the **self-care deficit theory of nursing,** is expressed here in three sets of sentences (p. 35).[1] The sets identified numerically include: (I) facts, occurrences, and circumstances observed or observable in society in concrete situations of human living for which the theory was devised; (II) the central idea of the theory (the expressed model); and (III) a summary of the materials and models on which the central idea is based. Set I is expressed in three parts.

Set IA

Adult persons, all things being equal, have developed powers and capabilities to meet their own requirements for continuing care that is regulatory of their own functioning and development (self-care) and that of their dependents (dependent-care). The power and capability to engage in self-care are named self-care agency. The power and capability to engage in dependent-care are named dependent-care agency. The totality of required regulatory care measures is named therapeutic self-care demand.

There are individuals in various sectors of society in time-place localizations whose developed and operative powers and capabilities for self-care or dependent-care because of health-associated factors are not equal to engaging in the kinds of action necessary to know and meet their own or their dependents' therapeutic self-care demands. This imbalance between powers to produce care and the care demand is referred to as a self-care or dependent-care deficit. Such deficit relationships can range from partial to complete.

Individuals with discernible types of health-associated action limitations for knowing and meeting their own or their dependents' therapeutic self-care demands may exhibit intact capabilities and undeveloped powers for knowing or meeting their own or their dependents' regulatory care demands.

Set IB

There are individuals in various sectors of society who, as nurses, legitimately design, produce, and manage systems of nursing for persons who need and can benefit from it.

Set IC

There are means within various sectors of society to bring persons in need of nursing into legitimate relations with nurses who can design, produce, and manage nursing care according to individuals' existent and emerging needs for it.

Set II

All systems of care in societies identifiable as nursing are designed and produced by nurses for and with persons with health-associated action limitations for knowing and meeting their own or their dependents' self-care requisites by performing the care measure components of their therapeutic self-care demands. Nurses activate their own developed powers and capabilities to nurse (their nursing agency) as they meet, interact with, attend to, and seek information from persons with health-associated self-care or dependent-care deficits. Through nurses' actions and, when possible, in collaboration with persons for whom nursing is provided, action systems (care systems) are designed, produced, and managed to ensure the following: (1) requirements of persons for self-maintenance and self-regulation of their human functioning and development (or those of their dependents) are known and continuously met in time; (2) selected methods of helping and care measures for self-maintenance and self-regulation are adequate and safe in enabling persons with requisite assistance from nurses to participate in care and to regulate the exercise and development of their powers for self-care or dependent-care; (3) the totality of care provided by nurses at specific times and over a duration of time contributes to the effective living and the health and well-being of persons provided with care, without harm to them as persons physically or psychologically or spiritually or socially.

Set III

The self-care deficit theory of nursing is based on a model of practical science with theoretic and practical components, models of human assistance in societies, practical insight into situations as a necessary basis for creativity and change, models of result-producing practical endeavor and deliberate human action, knowledge of human functioning and human development, and models of human behavior in interpersonal and multiperson situations.

The self-care deficit theory of nursing is recognized in the text (and by numbers of nurses in nursing practice, nursing research, and nursing education) as descriptively explanatory of what nursing is and what nursing should be. It is used by nurses to give direction to nursing practice and to other areas of endeavor such as nursing research. It is useful to beginning nursing students in their efforts to learn to focus on the nursing-relevant and the nursing-specific features of health care situations.

In a subsequent chapter, this general theory of nursing is more fully expressed in the form of a *theory of nursing system* that articulates with a *theory of self-care deficit* and a *theory of self-care.*

The self-care deficit theory of nursing is complex because it is a theory that encompasses human requirements of people for nursing as well as processes for its production. Nursing from the perspective of science is considered a practical science or a practice discipline with theoretical and practical components. The self-care deficit theory of nursing, while theoretical in origin and form, expresses the structure of the practical endeavors involved in the production of nursing in reality situations.

Theoretical terms are used in the expression of the self-care deficit theory of nursing. These terms signify ideas and conceptualizations about elements and relationships that the theory proposes to be the structure of nursing. Each term derives its meaning from the content of the idea or concept for which it stands. These concepts are defined and developed in subsequent chapters. Some terms signify elements or relationships that are common to humankind; others signify elements common only to those individuals who require nursing.

Terms such as *nurse* and *patient* have concrete referents, namely, the persons who fulfill these roles. The terms *nursing, self-care,* and *dependent-care* signify behavioral processes. *Self-care agency, dependent-care agency,* and *nursing agency* stand for abstractions about the nature of powers and capabilities of persons to engage in these named forms of care. *Self-care requisite* is a term that signifies a specific need for regulation of human functioning and development. Therapeutic self-care demand signifies all the care measures necessary to meet existent and emerging self-care requisites of individuals at particular times. Self-care deficit or dependent-care deficit signifies that the nature of a therapeutic self-care demand of individuals exceeds the powers and capabilities that constitute individuals' self-care agency or dependent-care agency.

Nursing students and nurses sometimes reject the use of theoretical terms. Their importance in precise communication among nurses and in achieving the development of the practical science of nursing should not be minimized.

NURSING AND CARING

Care is a word used to signify different things in different contexts. In the health professions, care is commonly used in the sense *to take care of. Take care of* means to watch over, to be responsible for, to make provision for, to look after some person or some thing.[6] The critical feature is one person's responsibility for another person or for an artifact, a house, a piece of land, or the like. The person or thing to be taken care of has distinguishing characteristics that are relevant to how it can and should be provided for and looked after. These characteristics must be known to the person who bears and fulfills responsibilities for taking care of persons or things.

Persons who are in positions of responsibility to take care of other persons are referred to as *care agents, care givers,* or by more specific terms. Parents are care agents for their children; adult children are often care agents for elderly parents. *Care agent* is a general term. In the health profession, persons qualified to take care of others in limited ways under specific conditions and circumstances bear names specific to each profession, for example, nurse, physician, social worker, physiotherapist. Persons looked after, cared for, provided for, have relationships to their care agents. These relationships are understood in terms of the nature and the degree of persons' existent social dependency for care of a specific kind(s) from other persons and in terms of the familial or contractual character of the relationship.

Nursing as Care

Nursing is accepted as one form of care within the health professions. Nursing and other forms of professional care are often referred to in a general fashion as patient care or health care. Such designations do not signify the nature of and specifications for the care or the producer of care. The totality of the kinds of care provided by health professionals for individuals or groups is commonly designated as health care. The specific kinds of health care provided for individuals or groups and the *relationships* between the *kinds of care* provided and the *producers of care* are referred to in their totality as a *health care system.*

Care is a general term commonly used to designate what health professionals do for others. It does not specify why persons need care or the specifications for the care needed or the kinds of actions to be performed or resources required. Nursing care, for example, is necessarily understood within the frame of reference of when and why individuals singly or in groups need and can be helped through nursing and the kinds of actions that are valid and reliable in meeting such needs. The question that has been answered in a prior section of this chapter is: What is the nature of the type of **social dependency** that sets up requirements for nursing? This same question can be asked for each health profession.

All members of the health professions (as well as parents and other care givers) should understand that there are *common demands* on persons charged with taking care of others. The common demands arise from the fact that both care givers and individuals cared for are human beings at some stage of human growth and development. Each one has achieved or will be achieving some measure of personal maturity, and each individual will have a potential for further development, and may be helped or harmed by factors in care situations.

Some of the features common to all types of care situations include the following:

1. Care, regardless of type, is for a person(s) in some place(s) and for some amount of time.
2. Care requires a care agent whose responsibility is to watch over, provide for, and look after another person(s).
3. Care of others demands an interpersonal situation(s); care givers must have access to and foster communication with persons whom they take care of and with persons legally responsible for them in the case of dependents.
4. Care includes the care agent's bringing about and maintaining environmental conditions conducive to the personal development of the other for the duration of care.
5. Care demands recognition by the care agent of the essential freedom of the other as a developing person to grasp possible courses of action, to reflect, and to decide, including decisions to function cooperatively with the care agent.
6. Care demands that the care agent view the person being taken care of *objectively* to determine presenting conditions and needs. The objective approach to the other prevails when the focus is on collaboration and

understanding with one another with respect to some objectively discernible reality.

7. Care demands that the care agent view the *person being taken care of* as *subject* who lives, experiences, has awareness of self and environment, attaches meaning to what is experienced, and may be accepting or not accepting of the care agent's presence and actions.

8. Care demands that the care agent *respect* and *accept* the person being taken care of as *subject* who has more and more to do with his or her own becoming or developing.

9. Care demands that the care agent view self as subject who lives through the care situation, experiences events and conditions, attaches meaning to them, is accepting or not accepting of the actions of the other, and is able in self-management.

10. Care demands that care agents have sufficient theoretical and experiential knowledge to provide care. They must know the persons to be taken care of and why care is instituted, as well as information about events and conditions in the concrete care situation to make judgments and decisions that will be protective of others as persons living and developing within their social units.

These common features of care as previously mentioned do not specify why the providing for or looking after is required. Nor do they indicate the kinds of actions or resources required to fulfill the responsibility. It is evident that the general *characteristics of care* have their origins in *persons who are to be cared for* and in *persons who are care agents*. Specific characteristics of care, however, are associated with the reasons why care is required. For example, infant care differs from the care required by older children because specifications for care arise from children's care needs at different stages of growth and development.

Fulfillment of responsibilities of persons "to take care of" other persons requires freedom to obtain care-relevant information about others in their time-place localizations and to have access to them, as well as knowing how to look after and provide for them. The responsibility can be fulfilled when the care agent—the provider of care—understands what is included under care and can perform actions and use resources to ensure for others a state of being looked after and provided for. The care agent also must be able to manage self and care for self.

A care responsibility for another person includes the provision of "help" when the person is confronted with specific things to be done that he or she is unable or unwilling to do. Nurses must be able to differentiate between the broad dimensions of *taking care of patients* and *helping them meet an immediate need for action*. In some types of nursing practice situations, these features come together within the responsibility of nurses; in others, one feature predominates.

Concrete situations where nurses or other care agents provide care are complex and dynamic and often are energy depleting and stress producing for all persons involved. The extent of the need to be with the other, to provide for the other, to protect the other, to promote the other's personal development, and to meet the other's needs for help, as well as the amount of concern and anxiety generated within the care situation, determine, in part, the demand on the care agent. The availability and adequacy of the resources of daily living also affect what the care agent can do in a situation. Taking care of others during long or short time periods may be exhausting for the care agent and may be a strain and trial as well as exhausting for persons being taken care of. Mutual respect and loving regard of the care agent and the one cared for may ease the burden of the care situation but do not eliminate the need to attend to and provide for the welfare and well-being of the care agent, as well as the person under care.

Some nurses forget or have never recognized that nursing is provided for persons. These nurses tend to focus on action sequences or tasks that they have learned to perform in nursing situations or on things that persons under care should or should not do. A nurse's task orientation to nursing often disallows a person focus. A person focus will never be explicated if the uniquely human qualities of men, women, and children are ignored and not recognized as operative in nursing practice situations.

Situations in which persons take care of others give rise to a number of common questions that require answers because of professional or legal implications for the care agent, as well as for persons needing care. The first question frequently asked is: Can I positively and effectively contribute to providing for or looking after this person(s) under these circumstances? Other questions

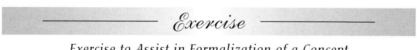

Exercise

Exercise to Assist in Formalization of a Concept of Being the Recipient of Care

Part A

A Personal Experience. Reflect on experiences when you were taken care of on a particular occasion by a family member or friend or by a health care professional.
1. Select one of these occasions.
2. Identify and describe why you required care or were judged by others to be in need of it.
3. Describe the events that occurred, including:
   a. How contact was effected between you and the care provider
   b. Events following contact
   c. Characteristics of the care provided
   d. The feelings you experienced
   e. Your judgments about the relationship between your perceptions of what you needed and how you were taken care of
4. Describe what you now perceive as short- and long-term results of the experience.

Part B

Experience of Another. Use the instructions in Part A to elicit from a family member or a friend his or her observations and judgments about a care experience.

include: Is it legitimate for me to serve as care agent in this situation? What is the source of my right to be here and to serve? What is the duration of my responsibility? Does my responsibility extend to all aspects of life situations of others or to specific aspects? Nursing students and nurses must be aware of and deal with such questions in each situation of nursing practice. These same questions need to be asked in all helping situations.

The ten named general features of care are as relevant to self-care and dependent-care as they are to nursing. The three forms of care differ in that two, dependent-care and nursing care, involve interpersonal relationships between care agents and persons in need of care. Self-care, on the other hand, demands that each person take on the role of care agent for self to regulate his or her own functioning and development. Self-care can be as exhausting and stressful as dependent-care or nursing care.

Insights About Caring in Nursing

There is a growing body of literature on **caring** in nursing and in other fields where there are demands for contact, interaction, communication, and coordination among individuals. This literature represents caring both as an attribute, a quality of humankind, and as a way of behaving in interpersonal and group situations. Roach[7] in her monograph *Caring: The Human Mode of Being, Implications for Nursing,* states that "caring is not unique to nursing and it does not distinguish nursing from other occupations or professions." However, some nurses identify nursing as the "caring profession" and indicate that caring is the *core of nursing* or the *unique focus of nursing.* The word *caring* is also used at times as a substitute for the term *nursing.*

In the nursing literature, the word *caring* is used to signify an innate human capacity foundational to moral consciousness, a desire that expresses for individuals their mode of being human, or a response to others that affirms held values.[7] *Caring* is also used to signify, among other things, a mode of living and a goal to be achieved.

The question for nursing students is: Does *caring* add something (and if so what?) to the prior sections of this chapter that expressed the proper object of nursing and the elements of nursing and the general description of nursing? It is suggested for consideration that caring brings into focus persons who are nurses and persons who are nurses' patients or clients, as well as the behaviors that express their person-to-person responsiveness. The literature on caring in nursing usually *assumes* the ongoing existence of a legitimate nurse-patient relationship. This is a relationship that is based on the presence of an individual(s) with existent or projected needs for nursing who is willing to be a patient or a client of a nurse(s). Second, it is based on the presence of a nurse(s) who is able and willing to work with and for the person who is patient or client. This work is ordered to knowing and meeting a patient's existent and developing requirements for care of self and dependents, care that will overcome or surmount health-associated action limitations for knowing and providing the required self-care.

The nursing literature on *caring* raises questions for investigation. One question is: What is a valid and reliable conceptualization of caring within the context of interpersonal situations? Pondering and investigating the question leads to another question. Given described experiences of caring on the part of individual nurses and persons nursed, what is the model(s) used to organize and identify what is observed as *caring?* Continued investigation leads to two conclusions. First, the experiential *referents of caring* (cited as evidence) as set forth in the nursing literature are subsumed under conceptualizations of *human love* as expressed by psychologists, theologians, and some psychotherapists. *Care and concern for others* is an *element of human love,* mature love. Second, mature love with its element of care and concern for others develops and is expressed when individuals live in or seek communion with one another in fundamental unity as *persons in community.*

Descriptive explanations of mature love and true community may be of aid to students of nursing in sorting out ideas about *caring* found in the nursing literature. This process can contribute to their developing insights about nursing and conceptualizations of self-as-nurse.

Human Love

Love is identified as a positive human emotion, positive because it moves people toward rather than away from persons, objects, situations. Arnold,[8,9] in her classic two-volume work, *Emotion and Personality,* describes emotion as a tendency that "prepares for and urges for action" (p. 281).[8] Human emotions aroused by objects or persons or situations are preceded by persons' reflective or value judgments that something is "good or bad for me here and now" (p. 310).[8] The development of love from infancy onward is described as movement from "casual liking" of things and people to "enduring love and interest." This is development from "episodic emotion" to an enduring tendency to react with love when opportunities prevail.[9]

Human love is understood as more than liking or sexual desire. The movement of a person to others in the world that is expressive of mature love is enabling for relating self to others with admiration, sympathy, some degree of understanding, urging toward cooperative action with others, and concern and care for them.

Fromm,[10] in his work *The Art of Loving,* develops the idea that *mature love* is an *attitude,* an *orientation of character* of a person, which determines the relatedness of that person to the world as a whole, not toward one object of love (p. 46). Brotherly love is identified as the most fundamental kind of love, which underlies all forms of love. It is love between equals even though one may be in a transitory state of helplessness (pp. 47-48).[10] The active character of mature love is represented as *giving.* Giving includes giving of material things, but its most important sphere is the giving of oneself—one's joy, interest, understanding, knowledge, humor, sadness. In giving, the other person is enriched, and that which is brought to life in the other reflects back on the giver (p. 24).[10]

Although the active character of love is giving, love always implies four mutually interdependent basic elements, namely, *care, responsibility, respect,* and *knowledge* (p. 26).[10] These elements are identified as a characteristic set of *attitudes* that are to be found in *mature persons* (p. 32).[10] Love viewed as a moving out to others eliminates separateness. Each basic element when exercised contributes to this elimination. *Active concern* and *provision of care* help to ensure life and growth and personal development of the other. Readiness and ability to respond to others to meet their needs is the exercise of *responsibility*. *Respect* is a person's reaching awareness of the unique individuality of the other person with the desire that the person develop and unfold in his or her individuality. *Knowledge* is described by Fromm as "layered" knowledge moving from what is visible—for example, anger or fear—to what is less visible, such as anxiety or worry, and finally to insight about the suffering being experienced by the person. The need to know the other person as well as oneself objectively is emphasized as necessary to see the reality of the other person and to overcome illusions about the other (pp. 26-31).[10]

The element *knowledge* is identified as related to and essential for the giving that is *care, responsibility,* and *respect*. To respect a person is impossible without knowing the person, and care and responsibility are blind when not guided by knowledge (p. 29).[10]

The foregoing statements describe brotherly love as a set of characteristics of mature persons. These characteristics or qualities of persons affect their being in the world with others and their giving to others, giving of self that eliminates separateness from them. The giving that is the active element of mature love enables professionals, nurses, and others to achieve unity with persons who are their patients or clients. Unity is enabling for the reaching of mutual understanding of specific life situations and for each person becoming active in the resolution and the solution of problem situations.

Caring and Community

Some social philosophers and anthropologists associate caring for or about other persons with men, women, and children living and developing together in their worlds. Their essentially human attributes distinguish them and are enabling for them to develop themselves as *persons in community*. Plattel[11] states that "being-a-person" is revealed to the developing child or adult as "being-together-with-my-fellowmen" (p. 23). The developing child, man, or woman comes to understand his or her relationships to others as conjoined with *person-hood,* leading to a fundamental unity of persons within their world. This, according to Plattel, is a "personalist conception" of community with a base in "phenomenological anthropology." Its focus is the "entire mystery of the intersubjectivity" of men, women, and children and "interhuman communication." This "personalist conception" of community is in accord with the idea that persons who take care of and care for and help others within or outside family units are interested in the welfare of others in their world—that they function to do good for others. Such persons often are viewed as benevolent, as possessing a native kindliness, as persons who act with love and compassion for others.

In the course of everyday life in families, in other social units, and in work situations, persons encounter one another. The quality of their responsiveness to one another depends on how well they have learned the lesson of love (Gannon,[12] pp. 12-13). Child abuse and spouse abuse in families are evidence of absence of community and of mutual love, with its giving elements of care, responsibility, respect, and knowledge. Abuse in families is evidence that members have not achieved personal maturity and positive mental health. Excessive emotion such as blinding anger or chronic emotion such as chronic worry or chronic resentment may be operative in intrafamilial violence.

Absence of true community and mature love is expressed in failure to attend to persons in need and in lack of social harmony. Rejection or lack of consideration of patients as persons by members of the health service professions and lack of mutual consideration on the part of members or organizations also express these absences. Obstacles to the development of true community are attitudes of negation and rejection of persons because of differences of race, color, occupation, religion, culture elements, location of residence, social position, or other factors.

Communities of persons, small or large, must be created and maintained through focused human effort. Groups formed by men and women can be transformed into communities when community is understood as a desirable form of life, even though community life may be lived differently by different culture groups. De Montcheuil[13] (pp. 21-23) identifies characteristics of true *community* as follows:

1. Persons are united by the search for the same goal.
2. The union of persons is for the good of all, not for the interest of a few with others serving as production instruments.
3. There can be diversity of functions and a hierarchy, but there must be fundamental equality in virtue of which each can give and receive and be enriched by others in "being" as well as in "having."
4. Each member is treated as a person. Individuals help one another but also unite as they enter into contact with one another to enrich themselves and achieve communion; these are manifestations of "true love."
5. Individual persons must freely join a community; membership cannot be forced. This is in distinction to groups to which a person may belong whether the person wishes to or not.
6. There is integration of all members in a community, but a particular community must never be closed within itself; each limited community must be integrated into a broader community in which it has a particular role.

Two obstacles to community are identified: *individual egoism,* which serves to divide members, and *group egoism,* resultant from the contentment of members being together so that they refuse to "broaden."

Nursing students can help themselves by a search for insights about community. In the personal and professional aspects of their living, nurses seek for community not only in their families and in their work groups but also within the profession of nursing, relating all to the "broadest community," humanity itself (p. 23).[13]

VIEWS OF NURSING

Nursing has been described in prior sections of the chapter as the specialized work of nurses with its own domain and boundaries that distinguish it from other human health services. A summary of views of nursing is now presented from an historical perspective.

Four Views

The word *nursing* in the 1911 historical work *Reminiscences of Linda Richards, America's First Trained Nurse*[14] is used in four different but related ways. In the following three cited quotations from these reminiscences, the word *nursing* signifies *care of patients by nurses.*

> Only a small portion of time was given to the care of patients; the household duties were considered of far greater importance than nursing (p. 57).
> Previous to this date, September 1, 1872, nurses had received instructions in the care of obstetrical cases only. Now the work was regularly organized for the definite training of young women in general nursing (pp. 9-10).
> The course was for only one year and embraced training in medical, surgical and obstetrical nursing, but the kind and amount of instruction was very limited (p. 11).

Modifications of the noun *nursing* by the adjectives *obstetrical, medical,* and *surgical* signify specialization of nursing because of the clinical conditions of patients and the kinds of medical care received. In the context of the quotations, the term *general nursing* is interpreted as signifying all forms of nursing.

The word *nursing* in Linda Richards' description of her year of formal preparation for nursing, from 1872 to 1873 at the New England Hospital for Women and Children, signifies a particular kind of knowledge that some persons had, knowledge that could be imparted to others.

> It does not seem quite loyal to my school to tell how little training we received, for everyone in authority gave us of her best nursing knowledge. (p. 14)

Linda Richards visited Florence Nightingale at her home in England in 1877. In the reminiscences about the visit, the phrase "my nursing years" (p. 38) appears. Implicit in the phrase is the idea of vocation or field of work or occupation or profession.

> The one dream of my nursing years was being fulfilled: I was indeed talking with the one woman whose name and the record of whose good works were known throughout the civilized world. (p. 38) (See Stewart and Austin for an account of these "nursing years.")[15]

At the beginning of her reminiscences, Linda Richards used *nursing* in a fourth sense. She wrote about her search for a place, a hospital where she could prepare for her "desired vocation," a place where she "could really learn the art of nursing" (pp. 5-6).[14] Because art is a human quality, the reference to nursing as a *particular art* signifies Linda Richards' desire for personal development as a nurse with respect to those qualities of mind required in using practical intelligence in designing and producing nursing for those in need.

Some or all of the senses in which the word *nursing* was used by Linda Richards in reminiscing about her "nursing years" are identified in earlier as well as in later works by nurses and others concerned with the condition of or with the advancement of nurses and nursing.

In Florence Nightingale's *Notes on Nursing,* printed in 1859, *nursing* signifies the *care of "sick and well persons"* in their homes or in hospitals by "nurses professional and non-professional."[16] Nursing is "good" or "poor." "Symptoms" and "suffering" result from poor nursing or lack of nursing. Nursing is *knowledge.* There are laws, "canons," or basic rules of nursing. "Laws of health" and "laws of nursing" are said to be the same laws. These laws hold for both the well and the sick. There are "elements" of what constitutes good nursing, and these elements are little understood in relation to nursing the sick or the well. *Notes on Nursing* also specifies nursing as "art" and as a "calling."

The meanings attached to the word *nursing* in the historical material cited are considered to be four different ways of viewing nursing, points of view from which nursing can be examined.

The four expressed points of view are summarized.

1. Nursing is a form of *care provided by nurses* to individuals in their homes or in hospitals, care that varies with the clinical conditions of individuals, care that is good or poor, care that has elements, care designed and produced according to nursing laws.

2. Nursing is a *particular kind of knowledge,* including knowledge of elements of what constitutes good nursing for the well or the sick, and knowledge of the laws or canons of nursing.

3. Nursing is the *particular art,* the *quality of a nurse,* that is enabling for both designing and producing nursing for others.

4. Nursing is a *field of work,* a vocation, occupation, or profession.

The four positions from which nursing can be examined serve the investigations of nurses as well as those of persons from other disciplines.

Examining nursing from a *particular point of view* limits what one must attend to and study and provides organizers for what is said or written. For example, in describing the body of writings about nursing available to nurses in the United States in the early part of the twentieth century, Lavinia Dock and Isabel Stewart's *A Short History of Nursing* says that "our nursing literature" consists chiefly of manuals on the practice of nursing with "some interesting historical material" (p. 173).[17] The focus here is on the available *body of writings* about nursing with reference to kinds of content. ·

Practice manuals referred to by Dock and Stewart present accumulated knowledge of what nurses should and should not do in their practice of nursing. This knowledge is properly referred to as *nursing knowledge*—that is, *knowledge of nursing* essential for use in the practice of nursing. Historical material highlights how nurses and nursing came to be what they are at particular times and over some duration of time. Nursing is attended to in historical material from all four points of view.

Some scholars organize information around one point of view. The social scientist Esther Lucille Brown in the 1930s studied the occupation of nursing with a view toward determining its status as a profession in the United States. Her monograph *Nursing as a Profession* was one of the Russell Sage Foundation's series of monographs on "established" or "emerging" professions.[18]

Nursing as art is a point of view that is recognized in the often-repeated statements "Nursing is an art and a science" and "Nursing is an art but not a science." *Nursing as art* encompasses the point of view of *nursing as care provided by nurses.* Its primary focus, however, is the skilled use by nurses of their practical intelligence in the *creative designing* of care for individuals or groups living under unique and prevailing or changing conditions and circumstances (of which they can have greater or lesser degrees of knowledge) and in the *creative production* of care. The point of view of nursing as art has implicit in it the idea of the nurse as the creator, the maker of nursing under prevailing conditions and circumstances that are or are not subject to regulation or control through nursing.

Nurses as well as others—for example, lawyers in malpractice suits—raise questions at certain times about the *state of the art and the science* of nursing. The reference here is to developing or developed nursing technologies and knowledge for use by nurses in attaining nursing results, the qualifications and capabilities of nurses using the knowledge and the technologies, and to the extent of their use by nurses in geographic areas.

POINTS OF VIEW IN NURSING PRACTICE

The four described points of view are of importance in *nursing practice* where nurses necessarily take and operate from each of them with respect to different matters. The central and enduring point of view in each nursing practice situation, however, is that of *nursing as care provided by nurses.* Nurses take the other three points of view as needed because as nurses they are the essential knowing and skilled human elements of nursing situations with socially designated statuses and roles.

In taking the second point of view, nurses identify in each situation of practice the adequacy of their own nursing *knowledge and skills,* the availability to them of additional knowledge in works of nursing, and the availability to them of nursing consultants, knowledgeable and skilled nursing experts. Nurses who examine and evaluate not only their own capabilities, including their mastery of nursing science and techniques of practice, but also their own creative approaches to the design and production of nursing under conditions prevailing in specific situations of practice take the third point of view. Finally, nurses who examine their legitimate roles in the *occupation of nursing* as these roles relate to what nurses can legitimately do in particular situations of practice take the fourth point of view.

Nurses who consistently take these points of view in nursing situations meet two basic requirements. First, they accept the nursing point of view as central and enduring in each practice situation. Second, these nurses accept themselves as responsible, knowing, and skilled designers and providers of nursing in specific situations of practice with understanding of their legitimate roles in the occupation and the extent and limits of their nursing capabilities.

Capable and effective nurses understand that their taking the described points of view is a general but necessary way for ensuring their patients' welfare as well as their own. However, the taking by a nurse of any one or all of the points of view, with both discrimination and effectiveness, is not in itself productive of nursing. It is a means used by nurses for *directing and holding their attention* on their patients, on environmental conditions, and on themselves as responsible practitioners of nursing within an occupational field. Appropriate focusing and holding of attention is necessary if nurses are to inquire into the questions associated with each point of view in nursing practice situations. Some questions relevant to each point of view are identified in subsequent paragraphs.

Taking the point of view of *nursing as care provided by nurses* directs nurses' attention to persons under care with concern for questions such as the following:
• Is nursing a needed service? If it is, with what human and environmental conditions is the need associated?
• What can and what should be accomplished through nursing?
• What kind and amount of nursing will be required and for what time duration?
• If this kind and amount of nursing are to be provided, what capabilities must nurses have, and how many nurses will be needed?

Exercise

Exercise to Assist in Developing the Habit of Identifying Expressed Points of View About Nursing

Select an article about nursing in a national or international nursing journal.
Identify the author(s) by name, country, and expressed credentials for writing about nursing.
Read the article and reflect about what you read.
Identify the point of view or the combinations of points of view about nursing taken by the author(s).
Is nursing written about as care, as knowledge, as art, as a field of work, or as combination thereof?
Was the point(s) of view expressed by the author in introductory material? If so, how was it phrased?
Did the content of the article describe points of view about nursing in a general fashion or in relation to specifics of place, time, persons, et cetera?
Was the article helpful to you in understanding the four points of view about nursing? If so, in what way was it helpful?

Taking the point of view of *nursing as knowledge* directs the nurse's attention from *self* to *others* who are at more advanced levels of knowing nursing, and to *written works.* The nurse has concern for answering a number of questions, for example:
- Is my nursing knowledge sufficient for the demands for application of particular kinds of knowledge in this situation?
- What are authoritative sources for obtaining knowledge that I lack?
- In what way is my nursing knowledge developing as I work with this person or these persons under nursing care? Have I arrived at new understandings? Should my developing knowledge of elements of nursing and my insights be discussed with nurse colleagues? Should steps be taken toward verification and formalization of this knowledge?

Taking the point of view of *nursing as art* directs a nurse's attention to *self* considered in relationship to the *kind of nursing that should be produced* for each individual under the nurse's care. Inexperienced nurses and nursing students naturally tend to focus on themselves in relationship to isolated tasks that are constituent elements of care. However, experienced nurses can see the dimensions of and a design for the immediate work of nursing this or that individual or group of individuals with understanding of how the work can and should be done creatively and effectively. The question in the art point of view is whether a nurse's mastery of *science* and *technique* is equal to his or her understanding of the work of nursing to be done; for example, can nurses creatively design nursing in light of prevailing conditions and circumstances and produce effective care through which nursing results are obtained? Because the art of nursing subsumes a number of basic arts, nurses must ask questions about their mastery of knowledge and technique with respect to the following *basic arts:*

The art of talking to reveal what is known by the nurse about the presenting situation and thereby provoke questions about things the nurse has overlooked and to which attention should be given

The art of relating person-to-person to others with recognition of the functions and responsibilities of each in the situation and the kind of experiences each brings to it

The art of coordinating one's actions with those of others whenever the actions of each contribute to or will affect the achievement of some desired result

The art of eliciting cooperation from others in the achievement of a desired outcome

The art of representing facts, positions, needs, desired outcomes, types of action, and results of action to others who are involved in a situation

The arts of discussion and persuasion

These basic arts contribute to the production of nursing because nursing is *care* of some persons by other persons. But the art of nursing is the nurse's quality or habit of reasoning and judging correctly about the design and production of the kind and amount of nursing needed according to the principles or laws of nursing itself. Science and technique are "the first necessary conditions for honest art" (p. 188).[19] The point of view of nursing as art therefore encompasses the point of view of *nursing as knowledge.*

In taking the point of view of *nursing as a field of work, occupation, or profession,* the nurse's attention is directed to self and to society. The nurse attends to and reflects on self as having a field of work and an occupational status within society and as one among many with the same status or with different but related statuses. The nurse attends to his or her legally and occupationally defined roles and responsibilities and to proscribed types of contractual relationships to persons under nursing care and whenever relevant to an employing institution. Roles and responsibilities may extend to persons nursed, to their next of kin or legal guardian, as well as to an employer or an associate and to persons who serve as helpers to nurses.

From the fourth point of view nurses seek answers to questions such as the following:

- Am I legally and occupationally qualified to take on the roles and responsibilities of nurse in this practice situation?
- Am I personally *capable* and *willing* to be related to this person (or these persons) as nurse and bear and fulfill the nursing responsibility? Now? When predicted changes occur? For what time duration?
- Is this person (or these persons) or the next of kin or legal guardian willing to have me as nurse and enter into a *nurse–patient* or a *nurse–legally responsible person* relationship with me?
- Who are the *nurses* available to me and to persons under my care as *nursing consultants* in the event that nursing matters requiring consultation arise?
- With what other persons participating in the health care or the residential care of this person (or these persons) must I cooperate?
- What are the nature and degree of coordination of nursing with other care providers that are likely to be needed? What are my role responsibilities related to these care providers?

Some nurses from time to time also ask a much broader question that is of deep concern to them. The question is: Can I, on a day-to-day basis, live the occupational aspects of my life with a style that yields good performance, recognition and respect from others, and at times affection (p. 188)[19] and also move within the occupation of nursing in accord with my interests and talents?

Nurses who ask this question more likely than not have a *career orientation to nursing* as their field of work, their profession.

THE NURSE AS AGENT

In the nineteenth century and earlier, the formal education and training of women and in some settings men was recognized by concerned individuals as essential for making nursing available to those who need it. Nursing came to be viewed as an endeavor of women and men who were educated and trained as *nurses.* The educated nurse was recognized as essential for nursing because the *nurse* is the **agent** whose actions are productive of nursing care.

Nineteenth-century advances toward providing nursing were associated with increasing social awareness and concern on the part of individuals and groups for the poor, the homeless, orphans and neglected children, the insane, prisoners, the sick poor, and the hospitalized sick. During this period, the word *nursing* gradually took on the meaning of *care provided by "trained nurses" or by "pupil nurses" in training.*[20]

In the United States in the nineteenth century and into the twentieth century, persons with formal preparation for nursing were referred to as "trained nurses." However, training programs varied so in length and in the quality of the experiences provided to "pupil nurses" that Isabel A. Hampton in 1893, speaking to the topic "the standards of education for nurses," remarked that "a trained nurse may mean anything, everything, or next to nothing" (pp. 1-12).[20]

Trained nurses stood in contrast to uneducated and untrained workers assigned or employed to care for the sick in hospitals or in households in a community (pp. 6-7).[14] They also stood in contrast to "born nurses," women described by Linda Richards as having earned the *title nurse* for themselves through "kindness of heart," "cheerful service," "experience," and the "instruction of older women and of the family doctor." These women went outside their homes to provide care to neighbors or others in the community (pp. 3-4).[14]

During the nineteenth century and into the twentieth century, nursing was a field to be discovered by those who aspired to its practice. Linda Richards noted that:

> We pioneer nurses entered the school with a strong desire to learn; we were well and strong, we were on the watch for stray bits of knowledge, and were quick to grasp any that came within our reach. What we learned we learned thoroughly, and it has proved a good foundation for the building of subsequent years (p. 14).[14]

The concerned women and men who instituted training schools for nurses and thoughtful graduates of those schools saw nursing as a specific field of practice, however unclear its domain and its boundaries might be. Nursing was being differentiated from the work of untrained and uneducated workers assigned or employed to care for the sick, the suffering, and the helpless. Nursing also was differentiated from housekeeping, welfare services, and medical practice.

Hospital nurses had both housekeeping and nursing responsibilities. These two functions of nurses were distinguished. Housekeeping or household duties were not called nursing (p. 57).[14] District or instructive visiting nurses were not to engage in almsgiving, a welfare service. They were to restrict their work in households to nursing. This included nursing sick members of a household, care of women after childbirth and their infants, and instructing members of households in healthful personal care practices and home nursing and in household sanitation (pp. 127-133).[20]

That nursing was a form of care different from medical care was recognized in the eighteenth and nineteenth centuries by men and women who were concerned about meeting the unmet needs of the sick and injured in hospitals and in their homes. It was known that being under the care of a physician did not meet the continuing care requirements of such persons. Nor did the presence of obstetricians and "sanitary officers" in communities meet the needs of adult household members for instruction about how to care for themselves, their dependents, and their household to prevent death and sickness and maintain the well-being of household members.

In the first quarter of the twentieth century, the meaning of the word *nursing* thus became associated with the word *nurse* in the sense of one who *knows nursing* and *can and does produce it*. Additionally, the *action* that is properly named *nursing* was distinguished from action that is not nursing, including actions of untrained persons who attend the sick, housekeeping, welfare service, and medical care.

However, as the twentieth century progressed with an increase in the number of educated nurses and an extension of nursing to more and more people, nurses became burdened not just with housekeeping but with work from other domains. Nursing in its uniqueness as a required human service was overshadowed by the array of duties and tasks from other fields that were showered on nurses. Then nurses began to seek answers to the question: What is nursing? How can one distinguish nursing from other forms of care and service?

SUMMARY

This chapter presents nurses as agents in societies who ensure the continuing availability of the health service nursing. The focus of nurses' attention and endeavors is identified as persons with health-associated self-care or dependent-care deficits. The elementary structure of nursing is explicated through analyses of definitions of nursing. The definitive characterizing structure of nursing is formalized and expressed in a general theory of nursing named the self-care deficit theory of nursing. The general features of one person's responsibility to take care of another person are presented. These features of nurses' responsibilities in practice situations are common to all situations when persons take care of others.

Caring, care, and concern, as developed in a segment of nursing literature, are represented as features of the interpersonal responsiveness of nurses, patients, and others. They are developed as expressions of mature love and community.

The four ways of viewing nursing are presented as important sources of insights to be developed by nursing students. Nurses who internalize the four views enhance their ability to maintain their personal integrity as they function in the profession and in society.

Subsequent chapters develop the foregoing generalizations about nurses and nursing by adding detail to move them into higher, more complex levels of organization.

The ways of knowing nursing presented in this chapter must be mastered and made dynamic by nurses in practice situations. The content is not to be read and memorized. It is to be read and studied to seek understanding and to become able to formalize one's own conceptualizations of these aspects of nursing. Developing understanding is aided by seeking out the reality bases for what is presented in concrete life situations.

References

1. Harre R: *The principles of scientific thinking,* Chicago, 1970, University of Chicago Press.
2. Orem DE: *Hospital nursing service, an analysis,* Indianapolis, 1956, Division of Hospital and Institutional Services, Indiana State Board of Health, p 85.
3. Orem DE: Personal knowledge of the 1958 event.
4. Orem DE: Guides for developing curricula for the education of practical nurses, *Vocational Division Bulletin* N. 274, p 18, Washington, DC, 1959, United States Government Printing Office.
5. Orem DE: *Nursing: concepts of practice,* New York, 1971, McGraw-Hill.
6. *The Random House dictionary of the English language,* unabridged edition, New York, 1973, Random House, p 223.
7. Roach Sister MS: *Caring: the human mode of being, implications for nursing,* Toronto, 1984, Faculty of Nursing, University of Toronto.
8. Arnold MB: *Neurological and physiological aspects,* vol II: *Emotion and personality,* New York, 1960, Columbia University Press, pp 281, 310.
9. Arnold MB: *Psychological aspects,* vol I: *Emotion and personality,* New York, 1960, Columbia University Press, p 212.
10. Fromm E: *The art of loving,* New York, 1962, Harper Colophon Books, pp 24, 26-32, 40-48.
11. Plattel MG: *Social philosophy,* Pittsburgh, 1965, Duquesne University Press, p 23.
12. Gannon TJ: Emotional development and spiritual growth. In O'Brien M, Steimel R, editors: *Psychological aspects of spiritual development,* Washington, DC, 1964, Catholic University of America Press, pp 12-17.
13. De Montcheuil Y: *Guide for social action,* Chicago, 1954, Fides, pp 21-25.
14. Richards LAJ: *Reminiscences of Linda Richards, America's first trained nurse,* Boston, 1911, M Barrows, pp 5-6, 9-11, 14, 38, 57.
15. Stewart IM, Austin AL: *A history of nursing,* New York, 1962, GP Putnam's Sons, pp 142-143.
16. Nightingale F: *Notes on nursing: what it is and what it is not,* London, 1859, Harrison & Sons.
17. Dock LL, Stewart IM: *A short history of nursing,* ed 3, New York, 1931, GP Putnam's Sons, p 173.
18. Brown EL: *Nursing as a profession,* ed 2, New York, 1940, Russell Sage.
19. Lonergan BJF: *Insight, a study of human understanding,* New York, 1958, Philosophical Library, p 188.
20. Hampton IA, et al: *Nursing of the sick 1893,* New York, 1949, McGraw-Hill, pp 1-12, 127-133.

CHAPTER 3

The Human Condition and Nursing Requirements of Individuals

Nurses and individuals for whom they produce nursing are embodied persons. Nurses understand that requirements of individuals for nursing represent needs of these persons to be met at particular times, needs specific to the continuance of life, healthful functioning, or general well-being. In this sense, requirements for nursing are *conditions to be fulfilled* for individuals. These conditions, expressed in the self-care deficit theory of nursing, are (1) knowing and continuously meeting persons' requirements for self-maintenance and self-regulation of their human functioning and development through engagement in self-care and (2) regulating the exercise or development of their powers and capabilities for engagement in self-care. However, there are other relevant kinds of human conditions, not conditions to be fulfilled but conditions that affect if and how the two conditions essential for life, health, or well-being can be fulfilled. These latter conditions are internal or external to persons. Internal conditions include health and growth and developmental states; external conditions include those associated with external environmental conditions.

Nursing requirements of individuals are the conditions to be fulfilled. The modifying or restricting human or environmental conditions determine qualitative and quantitative specifications for the condition to be fulfilled and affect how and to what degree they can be fulfilled. Maintaining an adequate intake of food (a condition to be fulfilled), for example, would have specifications of adequacy set by a person's stage of growth and development and by aspects of a person's health state. Actual intake of food would be affected by growth and development and health state factors as they condition mode of intake and form of the nutrients to be ingested, as well as by availability of food resources.

This chapter describes the nature of self-care and the nature of existent or developing requirements for such care, named *self-care requisites*. Methods of helping persons with limitations for engaging in action to do what they need to do at particular times and places are described and explained. The chapter concludes with an explication of the nature of deliberate human action to set forth the features that self-care has in common with all human practical endeavors.

SELF-CARE

Self-care is action of mature and maturing persons who have the powers and who have developed or developing capabilities to use appropriate, reliable, and valid measures to regulate their own functioning and development in stable or changing environments. Self-care is the deliberate use of valid means to control or regulate internal and external factors that affect the smooth activity of a person's own functional and developmental processes or contribute to a person's personal well-being.

Self-care has purpose. It is action that has sequence and pattern and, when performed effectively, contributes in specific ways to human structured integrity, human functioning, and human development. The term *self-care,* as used in this book, is formed from the prefix *self* and the verb *care.* In this context, self-care refers to "by oneself" and for oneself, with *self* as the subject of the verb *care.*[1]

Self-care thus carries the dual connotation of care "for oneself" and "given by onseself." The provider of self-care is referred to as a *self-care agent.* The provider of infant care, child care, or dependent adult care is referred to by the general term *dependent-care agent.* The term *agent* is used in the sense of *the person taking action.* **Self-care** is the practice of activities that individuals initiate and perform on their own behalf in maintaining life, health, and well-being. Normally, adults voluntarily care for themselves. Infants, children, the aged, the ill, and the disabled require complete care or assistance with self-care activities. Figure 3-1 illustrates features of self-care and *dependent-care.*

Infants and children require care from others because they are in the early stages of development physically, psychologically, and psychosocially. The aged person requires total care or assistance when declining physical and mental abilities limit the selection or performance of self-care actions. The ill or disabled

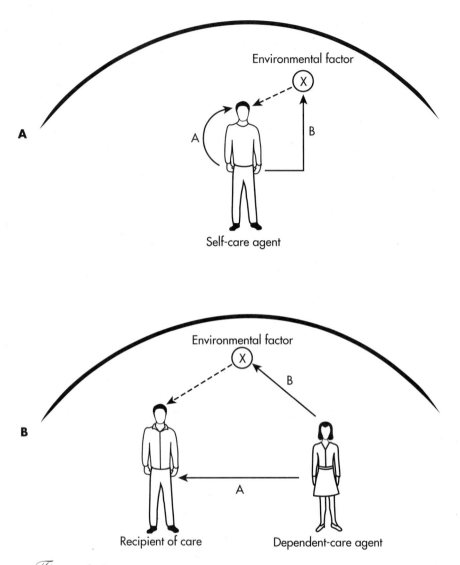

Figure 3-1 Self-care and dependent-care agents. **A,** care directed to self or to another who is the recipient of care; **B,** care directed to the regulation of environmental factors; *X,* environmental factor.

person requires partial or total care from others (or assistance in the form of teaching or guidance) depending on his or her health state and immediate or future requirements for self-care. Self-care is an adult's continuous contribution to his or her own continued existence, health, and well-being. Care of others is an adult's contribution to the health and well-being of dependent members of the adult's social group.

Self-Care, a Regulatory Function

Self-care is a human regulatory function. It differs from other regulatory functions, for example, neuroendocrine regulation, in that it is action deliberately performed by persons to regulate their own functioning and development or that of their dependents. Performed actions supply or ensure the supply of materials (air, water, food) needed for continued life, for growth and development, and for maintenance of human integrity. Performed actions also are directed to bring about or maintain internal and external conditions needed to maintain and promote health, as well as growth and development. Actions, at times, also focus on the prevention, alleviation, cure, or control of untoward human conditions that are affecting or can affect life, health, or well-being. This includes, when indicated, seeking and participating in medical care in its various modalities, as well as nursing and other forms of health care.

Formalization of the Concept Self-Care

The conceptualization of self-care used in this text (see Box above) was begun in 1956. The concept was formalized and validated in 1967 through the work of the Nursing Development Conference Group. The work of formalization is described in the first and second editions of *Concept Formalization in Nursing: Process and Product.*[2] That work included the revision and acceptance of a 1965 set of five presuppositions about self-care. It also included work to determine if the idea of self-care was useful in handling data from concrete nursing practice situations. The value of the idea in providing meaning for data was established. It was also established that the term and the conceptualization of self-care did serve as a consistent symbolization of the same conceptual and reality phenomena encountered in analysis of fictional and real nursing cases.[2]

The revised presuppositions about self-care as understood from experiences in concrete situations of daily living are as follows:

1. Self-care is understood as conduct, as voluntary behavior guided by principles that give direction to action. In terms of ego psychology, it is ego-processed behavior.
2. Self-care is understood as learned activity, learned through interpersonal relations and communication.
3. Adult persons are viewed as having the right and responsibility to care for themselves to maintain their own rational life and health, and as having such responsibilities for persons socially dependent on them.
4. Giving, assisting with, or supervising the self-care of another is a component of infant and child care, care of the aged, and care of adolescents.
5. Adult persons require assistance from persons in social services or health care services whenever they are unable to obtain needed resources and maintain conditions necessary for the preservation of life and promotion of health for themselves or their dependents; assistance may be needed for the accomplishment or supervision of care of self and care of dependents.

The 1967 work of formalization of the concept of self-care included the revision and expansion of three sets of statements (propositions) that emphasized the personal, health, and sociocultural features of self-care. The frame of reference for the expression of the statements is one of voluntary behavior of individuals in reality situations of daily living. The three sets of statements revised and accepted in 1967 are presented.

SOME STATEMENTS ABOUT SELF-CARE

Set One—Conditioning Factors
1. Self-care conduct is affected by self-concept and by the level of maturity of the individual.
2. Self-care conduct is affected by culturally derived goals and practices.
3. Self-care conduct is affected by the scientifically derived health knowledge possessed by a person.
4. Self-care conduct is affected by placement in the family constellation.
5. Self-care conduct is affected by membership in social groups exclusive of the family, for example, friendship and work groups.
6. Adults may or may not choose to engage themselves in specific self-care actions.
7. Lack of scientifically derived knowledge about self-care, disorders of health and malfunctioning, lack of self-care skills, and inadequate habits of self-care limit what a person can do with respect to his own self-care or in assisting another person in such matters.

Set Two—Self-Care in Health and Disease
1. Self-care contributes to and is necessary for a person's integrity as a psychophysiologic organism with a rational life.
2. Each person must perform or have performed for him each day a minimum of activities directed to, or performed for the sake of, himself in order to continue his existence as an organism with a rational life. If health is to be maintained and improved, he must perform additional activities. In the event of disease, injury, or mental or physical malfunctioning he must perform other activities to sustain life or improve health.
3. Self-care directed to the maintenance and promotion of health requires a scientifically derived fund of knowledge about self-care goals and practices as well as related skills and habits.
4. Disease, injury, and mental or physical malfunctioning may limit what a person can do for himself, since such states may limit his ability to reason, to make decisions, and to engage in activity to accomplish self-care goals. Disease, injury, and malfunctionings may involve structural changes as well as functional changes, which may necessitate the use of specialized self-care measures, some of which may be medically prescribed.

Set Three—Behavioral and Resource Demands of Self-Care
1. Self-care requires general knowledge of self-care goals and practices as well as specific knowledge about self, including health state, and about the physical and social environment. It also requires internalization of insights and sanctions and motivation. Acquiring specific knowledge involves making observations and judgments and leads to understanding of present self-care requirements as well as the self-care deficit; it may require contact and interactions with workers in the health services.
2. Self-care includes seeking and participating in medical care prescribed by the physician in the event of deviations or departures from health, and periodic scientific evaluations of health states.
3. Self-care requires internally oriented activities directed to the control of behavior; self-care also requires externally oriented behavior directed to the control of the environment, to establishing contact and communication with others, and to the securing and utilization of resources.

4. Self-care requires the use of resources that may include living in a healthful or a therapeutic physical and social environment; consumption of water, food, and drugs; application of physical agents and drugs to external surfaces and to those internal surfaces that communicate with the exterior; introduction of drugs into the body tissues to supply substances that the body is not producing; use of artificial devices to control the position of the body or its parts, or to aid in movement; use of prosthetic devices to facilitate functioning (pp 133-134).[2]

The foregoing statements about self-care provided the basis for subsequent work to place self-care structurally and functionally within the framework of nursing practice.

An essential part of the work of formalizing and validating the concept of self-care was establishing the boundaries of the concept. The need for this was made clear by the notion that the concept of self-care could be so rubbery, flexible, or expandable that it could encompass or subsume everything that persons did for themselves in the course of daily living. Boundaries were established and formalized through development and expression of the concept *self-care requisite* and through descriptive explanations of *types of self-care requisites.*

Naming and describing types of self-care requisites established the boundaries for self-care as a form of human endeavor. At the same time they made explicit the relation of self-care to human life, to health, and to well-being. Basic ideas about self-care requisites are presented here. Further development of the ideas appears in Chapters 7 and 10.

Self-Care Requisites

Self-care requisites are formulated and expressed insights about the kinds and sequences of action that are known to be necessary or hypothesized to have validity in individuals' regulation of aspects of their own functioning, development, or well-being as they live day to day in stable or changing environments. For example, it is universally accepted that persons must maintain an adequate intake of food in order to live and maintain health. This expression of a universally required self-care requisite does not state what is to be regulated and how the regulation is to be effected. A more precise but rough expression of this requisite would be: *maintain a total intake of food with an appropriate balance of different foods sufficient to supply the metabolic need of persons with consideration of their energy demands and environmental conditions but not so much food as to cause obesity.*[3]

This more detailed expression of the requisite maintaining an adequate intake of food gives some indication of the kinds of knowledge nurses need to properly understand the regulatory nature of the requisite, including internal regulatory mechanisms as well as persons' deliberate regulation of their food intake. Detailed, valid expressions of self-care requisites serve nurses as guiding principles for their actions. Such expressions contain two elements or features: the *nature of action* required and the *specification of the required regulation.* In the example given, the required action is *maintaining intake of a regulated amount of food.* The action is both a process of maintaining food intake continuously at intervals of time and a process of regulating the amount and kind of food consumed. The regulation to be achieved is ensuring that persons' metabolic needs are met continuously and obesity avoided. Self-care requisites express both the nature of and reasons for types of self-care.

Three types of self-care requisites are identified: *universal, developmental,* and *health-deviation.* They rest on the following assumptions:

- Human beings, by nature, have common needs for the intake of materials (air, water, food) and for bringing about and maintaining living conditions that support life processes, the formation and maintenance of structural integrity, and the maintenance and promotion of functional integrity.
- Human development, from intrauterine life to adult maturation, requires the formation and maintenance of conditions that promote known growth and developmental processes at each period of the life cycle.
- Genetic and constitutional defects and deviations from normal structural and functional integrity and well-being bring about requirements for (1) their prevention and (2) regulatory action to control their extension and to control and mitigate their effects.

The three assumptions express the *commonly known human conditions and circumstances* that set up demands for persons *to attend to and care for themselves or their dependents.* The assumptions support the following general descriptions of the three identified types of self-care requisites.

- Universal self-care requisites are common to all human beings during all stages of the life cycle, adjusted to age, developmental state, and environmental and other factors. They are associated with life processes, with the maintenance of the integrity of human structure and functioning, and with general well-being.
- Developmental self-care requisites are associated with human growth and developmental processes and with conditions and events occurring during various stages of the life cycle (e.g., prematurity, pregnancy) and events that can adversely affect development.
- Health-deviation self-care requisites are associated with genetic and constitutional defects and human structural and functional deviations and with their effects and with medical diagnostic and treatment measures and their effects.

When these three types of requisites are effectively met, they are productive of human and environmental conditions that (1) support life processes, (2) maintain human structures and human functioning within a normal range, (3) support development in accord with the human potential, (4) prevent injury and pathologic states, (5) contribute to the regulation or control of the effects of injury and pathology, (6) contribute to the cure or regulation of pathologic processes, and (7) promote general well-being. From the perspective of preventive health care, effectively meeting universal and developmental self-care requisites in healthy individuals is ideally in the nature of primary prevention of disease and ill health. Meeting health-deviation requisites may aid in the control of pathology in its early stages (secondary prevention) and in the prevention of defect and disability (tertiary prevention). Effectively meeting the universal and developmental self-care requisites is essential when there is pathology in order to maintain human structure and functioning and to promote development and thereby contribute to rehabilitation. Rehabilitation focuses on developmental and other self-care requisites associated with conditions resulting from pathology, medical diagnoses or treatment procedures, or the results of inadequate nursing or dependent care.

Self-care requisites are expressions of the purposes that individuals should have when they engage in self-care. Formalized self-care requisites that have been validated by their successful use in aiding individuals to manage their health and well-being become elements of the general culture or remain within the domains of the health care professions. Self-care requisites must be known before they can serve as the purposes of self-care. Universal self-care requisites should become known by all educable adults. Ideally, this also holds for developmental self-care requisites. For both types of requisites, however, reliable knowledge is not always effectively selected and adequately organized for public dissemination. Health-deviation self-care requisites usually become known by those who have genetic or constitutional defects or health deviations or whose family members or associates have such defects or health deviations.

Meeting Self-Care Requisites

When self-care requisites are viewed as formulated and expressed purposes of self-care, the ways and means through which these purposes can be attained are an important consideration in understanding self-care as human action. For example, an adult who is judged by herself and her physician to be edematous and in a state of fluid and electrolyte imbalance has, as one object of self-care, this prescribed health-deviation self-care requisite: to maintain fluid intake at no more than 1000 ml during each 24-hour period. This is an adjustment of the universal self-care requisite to maintain a sufficient intake of water. The actions to achieve this adjusted purpose must be known and be within the capabilities of the person with the self-care requisite (or another person who can act for the individual).

In addition to making judgments and decisions about the kinds of fluids to be ingested and the distribution of amounts over the 24 hours of the day, there are action sequences for procuring the fluids, preparing them as necessary for ingestion, measuring them into appropriate vessels, drinking them, and accounting for the fluids taken at particular times and for the entire 24-hour period. Throughout each 24-hour period there would be actions for self-restraint, self-orientation, and maintenance of awareness of the purpose of the self-care requisite. Acceptance of oneself as being in need of this kind of care (or at least willingness to attain the purpose of care) is also required.

The operations required to maintain fluid intake within a specified maximum may be thought of as a segment of a person's daily self-care. Because self-care directed to achieve a particular object is necessarily a series of actions performed in some sequence, self-care is properly referred to as an action system or a dynamic process. It is helpful for nurses and other care providers to conceptualize all self-care actions performed in sequence to meet known requisites on a day-to-day basis as constituting an individual's self-care system. Actions directed to meet particular, individual self-care requisites can be conceptualized as constituting subsystems of the total self-care system.

The ways and means for meeting particular self-care requisites can be described in terms of (1) general method and (2) required operations or actions to use the method. In the example outlined in Table 3-1, the general method is drinking, the natural method used by human beings after infancy to consume substances in a liquid state. The sets of operations in Table 3-1 identify the kinds of actions to be taken to achieve partial results toward accomplishing one particular self-care purpose, using a specified method.

Required operations vary with general method. If the general method selected for use in the example in Table 3-1 was injection of fluids into a vein (intravenous administration of fluids), the types of operations required would conform in a general way to the sets named in Table 3-1, but the specific actions would differ. When the general method and required operations for achieving a desired result have been identified, tested, and integrated into an explicit system of action, the result is a formulated process that becomes part of the technologic knowledge of particular practice disciplines, for example, the intravenous administration of fluids.

The example of specification of fluid intake in Table 3-1 represents the particularization of the requisite for an individual in accord with what was known about the person's health state, including disturbances of water concentration of body fluids. Nurses must understand that existent and emerging self-care requisites of individuals in concrete life situations cannot be effectively met unless they are both adequately formulated and expressed and then particularized

Table 3-1 **Elements of an Action System to Meet a Particularized Self-Care Requisite**

Particularized Self-Care Requisite	General Method	Sets of Required Operations
Maintain fluid intake at no more than 1000 ml every 24 h	Ingestion by mouth, drinking from a container	Seek and validate knowledge of the requisite, its meaning, its duration, and projected effects Prepare self, materials, and the environmental setting Consume measured fluids and account for the amounts consumed Monitor self for evidence of effects—desired or adverse Communicate results of monitoring to the prescribing physician

for individuals. Therefore nurses must develop the knowledge and skill needed to understand already formulated and expressed requisites and in some circumstances to formulate and express them. For example, when nurses care for persons under particular forms of medical or surgical therapy, they know that there are unexpressed self-care requisites implicit in each therapy. These requisites must be isolated and expressed. It is often the work of nurses to identify, formulate, and express such requisites and to meet them in cooperation with persons nursed. Health-deviation requisites are usually particularized by physicians, but in many instances nurse and patient in cooperation work out the unexpressed requisites and the details of the processes of meeting particularized requisites.

The sets of required operations shown in Table 3-1 express a coalescence of large numbers of required deliberate actions in the form of process configurations. Each process requires performance of numbers of deliberate actions related as sequences of a variety of actions sometimes referred to as *unit acts** or as care measures. Fifteen such action sequences or unit acts or care measures were identified as necessary to meet the self-care requisites for maintenance of an adequate intake of fluid in the 1997–1998 work of members of the Orem Study Group. One example of an action sequence or unit act was expressed as "knowing my fluid balance status." For nurses, it is easy to image all the essential actions to be performed by persons in proper sequences to reach this state of knowing when conditions dictate its necessity for them.

Each individual in his or her time and place location has an identifiable number of self-care requisites to be met consistently, continuously, or periodically. Performing the actions (engaging in self-care) to meet not one but all of the identified self-care requisites generates persons' *self-care systems* (as referred to previously). For each person, the continuously produced system of care of self (with changes over time) constitutes a continuing reality that specifies the forms of self-maintenance and self-regulation in which the person is engaging or has engaged in the past. Actions of a person are occurrences in time that do not continue in existence, but memories of performance and results of performance endure.

Another feature to be understood about self-care requisites is the occurrence of internal human and external environmental conditions that indicate that immediate attention should be given to meeting particular requisites. The conditions, when identified and expressed, are referred to as *indicative criteria* that specify that immediate or continuing attention should be given to meeting the requisite. These criteria can be identified and formulated for each universal and developmental type of requisite and for health deviation types of requisites. One example is the need for immediate attention to self to prevent heat

---

*Talcott Parsons[4,5] used this term, later changing it to *units of action,* to refer to the smallest distinct unit in the total process of doing something that makes sense, is meaningful, when it stands alone within a larger system of action.

exhaustion or heat stroke when a person is exposed to high external temperatures. This example is specific to the universal self-care requisite "maintaining normalcy" with reference in this example to "normalcy of body temperature," that is, to keep it within norms compatible with human life and normal functioning. This criterion measure must be understood in its application to persons of different ages.

Therapeutic Self-Care Demand

Therapeutic self-care demand is a conceptual construct that stands for the operations, the action sequences necessary to meet not just one formalized and particularized self-care requisite of a person but all requisites to be met by or for a person during a specific time period. The development of the concept, as well as a search for understanding the concept therapeutic self-care demand, moves from having the knowledge that persons' self-care requisites are identified to knowledge that methods and means for meeting them have been selected; the effort then proceeds to identify the action sequences, unit acts, or care measures necessary to use the selected means to meet each of the formalized, particularized requisites. The summation of the actions or care measures to meet outstanding requisites is the *self-care demand*. The adjective *therapeutic* is attached to the term *self-care demand* to indicate that the processes, the action sequences, or the care measures through which requisites are to be met have actual or presumed validity in effecting the desired regulations of human functioning or development.

In the foregoing frame of reference, the term *therapeutic self-care demand* stands for a humanly constructed concept with its basis in nurses' knowledge of what action sequences or care measures must be performed if each self-care requisite of an individual is to be met. Such a concept stands in distinction to conceptualizations of naturally existent entities, for example, the existent powers and capabilities of persons to produce self-care (self-care agency). In a sense, the formulation of a therapeutic self-care demand for an individual is a short, practical way of expressing the care measures persons should elect to perform (or have performed for them) to meet their outstanding self-care requisites. Nurses use their knowledge about individuals under nursing care to arrive at judgments about how and to what degree to involve them in the formulation of their own therapeutic self-care demands (or those of their dependents).

Self-care and care of dependents may be well intentioned but not therapeutic. It is necessary to determine the therapeutic value of practices prescribed by the general culture and even by health professionals. A single self-care practice or a whole system of self-care is therapeutic to the degree that it actually contributes to the achievement of the following results: (1) support of life processes and promotion of normal functioning; (2) maintenance of normal growth, development, and maturation; (3) prevention, control, or cure of disease processes and injuries; (4) prevention of or compensation for disability; and (5) promotion of well-being. Some of these results are required by all persons on a continuing basis during all stages of the life cycle, but others are required only in the event of disease or injury.

Self-Care Summary

Self-care is a practical response to an experienced demand to attend to oneself. The demands may originate in the individual, for example, a person experiencing a lack of energy or intense emotional reactions, or from knowledge that a care measure should be performed because it is health-promoting. Demands may originate from others, for example, the directives of parents to children or health workers to clients and patients or neighbors and friends. The demand as experienced is a stimulus to which the person responds in some manner. Demands may be met or ignored. Awareness of the demand may remain, even when the demand has been ignored. A person may identify the presence of a tumor and know he or she should seek medical assistance, but does not and yet worries about having cancer. When persons know that what they are experiencing is significant to life or health, they feel a heavy responsibility toward themselves.

The concepts *therapeutic self-care demand* and **self-care agency** stand, respectively, for what persons need to do and what their developed powers and capabilities to engage in self-care enable them to do at particular times. When persons' self-care agency is of a value that is not adequate for their performance of actions specified by their therapeutic self-care demands, there is a deficit relationship between what persons should do and what they can or will do. This type of relationship is referred to as a **self-care deficit,** an indicator that persons need help if their self-care requirements are to be met. Both dependent-care and nursing care are types of help for persons unable to meet their continuing needs for self-maintenance and self-regulation. The next section presents ideas about the nature of helping situations, ways of helping, and helping relationships.

UNDERSTANDING NURSING AS A HELPING SERVICE

Considering nursing as a helping service brings into focus the interpersonal features of nursing and some essential differences between and among individuals who need nursing and those who nurse. In helping situations, persons are cast into roles: persons in specific places with needs that must be met at specific times and persons who can help in meeting their needs, helpers. Needs for help arise at specific times under specific circumstances. Television reports of street accidents vividly represent these circumstances, as injured persons are helped by trained paramedics who have rushed to the scene.

Helping Situations

In daily living, individuals sometimes face situations in which they know that existent or emerging needs of others cannot be met without help. Neighbors become ill and are taken to the doctor's office or to the clinic or emergency room. Strangers ask for directions and persons asked try to help them. These types of situations do not require the helping person to have specialized education and training to act in such situations, but they do require knowledge about the other's need, the extent to which they can help, and what is practical and not practical in meeting another's need.

Nurses, physicians, lawyers, and social workers are educated and train themselves to be skilled in specialized types of **helping situations.** Training in first aid and disaster work represent other types of preparation for helping in specialized situations.

Helping situations are often complex, and taking action is difficult because it demands that one person (the helper) does something to supply what another person with needs should have or do but which the person does not have or cannot do, must not do, prefers not to do, or outright refuses to do. A helping situation is complicated for the helper because the need being met is a requirement of another person. It is complicated for needy persons because they are experiencing an inability to manage and care for themselves and to meet the demands that the situation places on them.

Individuals may be reluctant to accept help from other persons because the positions and the manners and abilities of persons offering help do not fit certain cultural prescriptions or do not inspire the confidence of the person in need. The process of giving and receiving help is affected by the knowledge and skills, personalities, experiences, and life situations of helpers and of persons in need of help. The failure of persons to give help where it is needed may be a function of levels of personal development and maturity. It is more difficult for some persons to engage in processes of helping than it is for others. Helping is basically a practical endeavor demanding insights about what can and should be changed in concrete life situations. Having the desire to help another does not mean that a person has the ability to help.

Persons who need help may be unable to seek it or ask for it. They may lack the necessary information or communication skills. They may be afraid. Sometimes persons believe that they do not have a right to seek and receive help. In such situations, persons need to be "helped to get help" to meet specific existent or emerging needs.

There are similarities and differences in helping situations. The similarities are enabling for understanding some of the basic characteristics of situations in which persons are helped through nursing.

Characteristics of Helping Situations

All helping situations have a similar general structure. Structure is engendered by the roles of the persons involved—a person who requires help and a person who is to give help—and by the expected behaviors (roles) of these persons. Ideally, the behavior of the person requiring help is complemented by the behavior of the helper. Consider the following situation:

> Two men have been in an accident. Their car skidded and crashed into a tree. One of the men, the owner and driver of the car, has suffered an injury to his back and hip. He cannot move without severe pain, and he realizes that he can prevent further injury by not moving. His companion, though shaken, is on his feet. He asks about his friend's condition and, recognizing his friend's injured state, extends assurance that help will come. He knows that he should not move his friend, so he stops a passing motorist and asks him to report the accident and request help in the next town. The motorist agrees; soon the police and an ambulance arrive, and the injured man is

carefully immobilized, moved onto a stretcher, and taken to the local hospital. The uninjured man, with his friend's approval, arranges through the resident physician for medical care and attends to the details of the admission. He calls the injured man's family, arranges for the removal of the wrecked car, notifies the insurance company, and confers with the police officers.

In this hypothetical situation, the behavior of the uninjured man complemented the role of his injured friend. The man with the helping role communicated with a variety of persons on behalf of his friend. His communications with the passing motorist and with the ambulance attendants, physician, nurses, hospital admitting personnel, garage attendants, insurance agent, and his friend's family contributed to meeting the needs of his friend.

Further examination of the helping activities of the injured man's companion shows that the activities were directed toward achieving four goals: (1) preventing further injury to his friend, (2) securing health services for his friend, (3) taking care of his friend's property—the car, and (4) attending to his friend's personal affairs—notifying his friend's family and insurance company of the accident. To achieve these goals, the companion had to demonstrate his awareness of his friend's injured state; of the need for immobility and medical attention; and of the legal, financial, and family implications of the accident.

In this example of a helping situation, while a helper actively tried to achieve a goal or goals for another person, he had full knowledge of his actions and his own limitations. In this situation, the helper was aware that he could not give effective health care to his injured friend but could secure such services for him. Thus, the helper first defined and limited what he would do in relation to (1) the condition for which help was required, (2) what he knew how to do and was able to do, and (3) what was considered permissible or advisable under the circumstances.

Helping Methods

As men, women, and children live together and help one another, they develop methods for overcoming or compensating for the action limitations that individuals and families have at specific times under specific circumstances to meet existent and emerging needs. Method usually signifies an orderly way of accomplishing something. A **helping method** from a nursing perspective is a sequential series of actions, which, if performed, will overcome or compensate for the health-associated limitations of persons to engage in actions to regulate their own functioning and development or that of their dependents. There are a limited number of methods that one person can use to help another person perform a task or meet a need. Helping methods are used within the human service occupations and professions and in all situations in which bonds of friendship and neighborliness prevail.

There are at least five helping methods through which one person can compensate for or overcome the limitations of others to act for themselves in day-to-day living. In concrete helping situations, the methods are often used in combination. Nurses use all the methods, selecting and combining them in

Characteristics of Helping Situations, a Summary

There are at least two persons in the situation in different statuses, the status of helper and the status of person in need of help.

The status of the person in need of help is legitimized by meeting two criteria:

There is a need for this person to act to achieve specific purposes immediately or in the future because of prevailing conditions and circumstances.

There are action limitations that make immediate or future action on the part of this person impossible or imprudent or would render action ineffective or incomplete.

The helper's status is legitimized by meeting two criteria:

The helper has identified, has knowledge of, and accepts the demand for the person in need of help to act and the person's action limitations.

The helper knows how to, is willing to, and does act for the welfare of the other in accordance with factors that limit what can and what should be done under prevailing conditions and circumstances.

The actions of the helper:

Complement (or substitute for) the actions of the person needing help in order to accomplish the specific purposes of the person needing help.

Provide and foster conditions to facilitate the development or exercise of this person's capabilities to take necessary actions for achieving specific purposes.

relation to the action demands on persons under nursing care and their health-associated action limitations. These methods are identified as follows:

1. Acting for or doing for another
2. Guiding and directing
3. Providing physical or psychologic support
4. Providing and maintaining an environment that supports personal development
5. Teaching

The named helping methods are used in all health services. Selection of helping methods for use singly or in combination rests on the health professionals' insights, judgments, and decisions about what others cannot do, or do effectively, and about what can and should be done in the interests of the life, health, and well-being of others. Each helping method has certain characterizing features. For example, some methods under some circumstances demand that helpers be in the physical presence of persons helped, or in physical contact with them, or be continuously available to them in their time and place locations. The kind and amount of communication vary. Descriptions of helping methods and criteria to validate the selection and use of each method are presented.

Acting for or Doing for Another

Acting for another is a helping method that requires the helper to use developed abilities toward achieving specific results for persons in need of help. Examples are a nurse positioning a helpless patient or a mother feeding her baby. The person being helped, if conscious, must permit the helper to act for him or her. The method, therefore, cannot be used with a conscious person unless there is a measure of cooperation. Ideally, the helper assists the person in making inquiries, decisions, and plans whenever possible and prudent. The helper should also tell the person being helped what needs to be done, what to expect, and what to report. When the person to be helped is unconscious, incompetent, or unable to participate in making decisions, the helper must act with regard for the rights of the one helped and be clear about the helper's role.

The usefulness and validity of *acting for or doing for another* is determined by the type of result sought. Acting for another is not valid when results depend on internal acts, such as control of one's own behavior. The method is valid, however, in giving care to an acutely ill person or to a physically or mentally incapacitated person according to the nature, degree, and duration of the self-care deficit. In the service professions and occupations, the method of assisting by acting for another is commonly used in situations in which scientifically derived knowledge and highly specialized techniques are required for accomplishing a result.

Acting for another is necessary in infant and child care situations, but other methods should be added as soon as the child is ready for them. In the care of the aged or the infirm, acting for another is used in compensating for declining physical and mental abilities. Acting for another often may be gradually replaced by methods of *guiding another, supporting another,* and *teaching.*

Guiding Another

Guiding another person considered as a method of assisting is valid in situations in which persons must (1) make choices—for example, choosing one course of action in preference to another—or (2) pursue a course of action, but not without direction or supervision. This method requires that the person extending guidance and the person being guided be in communication with one another. The one being guided must be motivated and able to perform the activities required. In turn, the guidance given must be appropriate, whether in the form of suggestions, instructions, directions, or supervision. For example, a nurse may suggest that an ambulatory patient take a rest from current activity, the nurse may discuss reasons for the limits on the patient's activities, or the nurse may tell the patient how to secure nursing assistance after discharge from a hospital. Guiding another often is used in conjunction with *supporting another.*

Supporting Another

To support another person means to "sustain in an effort" and thereby prevent the person from failing or from avoiding an unpleasant situation or decision. It also may enable the person in need of support to do something without undue stress because of the sustaining influence of the helper. Supportive activity is a valid way of assistance when a patient is faced with something unpleasant or painful. The patient must be capable of controlling and directing the action in the situation, once psychologic or physical support has been received. For example, a nurse may remain with and give support to a seriously ill person who is permitted to be up and to walk for a short period of time. The presence of the nurse and the nurse's words of encouragement and assurance may be needed just as much as physical help when the patient gets out of bed, maintains an erect posture, and walks. The nurse has the responsibility for judging how much the patient being helped can do or endure and when to intervene. Knowing when to step in requires wisdom and understanding. The communication between the helper and the helped (the patient) may not be in words—the helper may convey support by his or her presence, by a look or a touch, or by physical support. In other situations, speech may be necessary. A patient may need both encouragement and physical help. The action to be performed may be practicing a new skill, making a decision, or living through a stressful personal or family situation.

By giving physical and emotional support, the helper is able to encourage another person to initiate or persevere in the performance of a task, to think about a situation, or to make a decision. Support that encourages action is related to both the kind of action the person helped must make and to the stressful effects of the situation. Parents, teachers, social workers, and nurses frequently use this method. Supporting another is also used extensively in child care and other situations in which individuals are in the process of developmental change.

Providing another person with material resources differs from, but is closely related to, giving physical and psychologic support. This manner of support is used by adults with dependents, by the state with respect to deprived persons, by citizens of one country for citizens of another country in greater need, and by all persons who have concern for their less fortunate neighbors. This type of support is not the specialized work of nurses. Nonetheless, nurses often assist their patients in obtaining resources from institutions or agencies. As a method of assisting, then, supportive activity may include the securing of resources. It is related to and may be a part of providing a developmental environment.

Providing a Developmental Environment

This method of assistance requires the helper to provide or help to provide environmental conditions that motivate the person being helped to establish appropriate goals and adjust behavior to achieve results specified by the goals. The needed environmental conditions may be psychosocial or physical. It is the total environment, not any single part of it, that makes it developmental. Developmental results include the forming or changing of attitudes and values, the creative use of abilities, and the adjustment of self-concept, as well as physical development. Helpers may be required to provide opportunities for interaction and communication with themselves and with other persons, to give both guidance and support, and to use other ways of helping. The essence of this method is the continued and proper relating of selected environmental elements in light of the patient's special needs and the changes being sought in the patient's health state or manner of living.

Environmental conditions conducive to development provide opportunities for persons being helped to be with other persons or to become members of groups in which:

1. Care is offered and provided to those with needs.
2. There are opportunities for solitude and companionship.
3. Help is available with respect to personal and group interests and concerns.
4. Individual decisions and pursuits are personal matters; there is no interference, except in matters of grave consequence to the individual or others affected by the situation.
5. Respect, belief, and trust are given to others; and developmental potential is both recognized and fostered.
6. Each person expects or strives to earn respect and trust from others.
7. Each person assumes or attempts to assume responsibility for self and personal development.

Physical conditions that contribute to personal growth and development provide the necessities for daily life and for psychosocial and intellectual development. For example, when an individual is tense and frightened because of the demands of daily life, *sufficient resources*—necessities as well as luxuries— *under some circumstances* may enable the person to meet particular life situations and to become better able to accept responsibilities. It must be remembered, however, that elements of the physical environment are closely related to the psychosocial environment and the social positions and roles of individuals. In assisting individuals in their development, it is not enough to supply resources. It may also be necessary to show them how to use these resources and in some instances to share them.

Providing a developmental environment is valid in many areas of living. It should be used in families, in child care institutions, in nursing homes, in schools, in hospitals, and in other organizations where human beings live or work together. The effectiveness of this method of assisting depends in large part on the helper's creativity and his or her appreciation, knowledge of, and respect for people. An environment conducive to development is also conducive to learning and participating and is, therefore, of value if used in conjunction with teaching and other helping methods.

Teaching Another

Teaching another is a valid method of helping a person who needs instruction to develop knowledge or particular skills. Learning may not take place if the person to be taught is not in a state of readiness to learn, is unaware that he or she does not know, or is not interested in learning.

To use teaching as a method of assisting requires that the helper know thoroughly what the person to be helped needs to know. For example, a nurse cannot help a patient learn how to select foods according to a prescribed diet until the nurse knows whether the patient knows the nutritional components and caloric values of various foods. The ability to make adaptations in light of a patient's food preferences is also required. The nurse must consider the patient's background and experience, lifestyle and habits of daily living, and modes of perceiving and thinking and must have knowledge of self-care requisites to be able to impart knowledge to the patient.

In teaching another, appropriate educational experiences must be provided. Teaching is not restricted to classroom activity. A nurse who is near a patient at mealtime is providing the patient with an opportunity to ask questions pertaining to diet. The nurse who explains to a patient how to perform a measure that will eventually be a self-care component (the care of a colostomy, for example) may stimulate the patient's interest in listening, observing, and asking pertinent questions about the activity. Learning to change one's behavior as it relates to self-care may require considerable time and a prolonged relationship with nurses who are able to fill a tutorial role effectively. Under some circumstances, group teaching may be an effective way of helping individual patients become efficient in self-care activities.

The interested patient may learn much from observations of competent nurses who provide care. Learning in such situations almost seems to be a matter of absorption. In other instances, a patient must engage in specific and planned learning experiences, such as reading and discussion. The learning experiences may also be related to solving problems, such as how much bread, potatoes, or rice will supply a specific amount of carbohydrate in a diet. In a self-care situation, a patient may need to recognize certain effects of a prescribed medication, how to adjust the dosage, or when to call the nurse or physician. Frequently, patients in self-care situations must learn to limit their physical activities. Not infrequently, patients must acquire psychomotor skills in applying supportive bandages to an extremity, skill in changing dressings, or skill in measuring and administering medication by injection.

When teaching is the helping method being used, persons being taught ideally see themselves as learners and realize that study, learning exercises, observation of others, and practice are needed. Helpers see themselves as teachers who direct and guide learning activities. Because children and adults approach learning differently, assisting through teaching must be adapted to age as well as to past education and experience.

Methods: Individuals and Groups

In nursing a single individual in contrast to a group, all the methods of helping may be necessary for effective nursing. What self-care the patient can or cannot manage and the reasons he or she cannot manage it guide the nurse in the selection of appropriate methods of helping. For example, a nurse may decide that the judicious use of *acting for another* and *supporting another* are most appropriate for a patient who is convalescing from a debilitating illness but whose activity must be limited. The nurse would no doubt also use *guidance* and *teaching* and provide appropriate *environmental conditions.* In each specific nursing situation, one or two helping methods will probably be used more frequently than others. A change in what patients can do for themselves would require that the nurse reexamine and adjust the methods.

Specialized adaptations of the helping methods, with the development of appropriate techniques, are essential in multiperson nursing situations. The most commonly used helping methods in these situations are guiding, providing psychological support, providing an environment for personal development, and teaching. In this type of nursing situation, nurses may help family or group members develop proficiency in the use of some or all of the methods of helping. Some adaptations can be identified in the literature on health care for families and groups. Nurses must be aware of the common methods of assisting and select the methods most appropriate under the circumstances.

Understanding Nursing as a Helping Service Summary

Nursing is a specialized helping service. Nurses help others because of action limitations that are within the domain of nursing. Nurses' understanding of nursing's proper object and their dynamic conceptualization of nursing as a health service are basic guides in ensuring fulfillment of their nursing responsibility. In the course of providing nursing, nurses also provide the ordinary kinds of help that members of families and communities give to one another within the context of day-to-day living, for example, securing reading material and sending messages. However, nurses do not cross boundaries of other helping services and attempt to help with matters for which they are not qualified. Nurses enter into personal situations as nurses to provide help in the form of nursing, not to meet all existent and emerging needs of persons under nursing care. Nurses have knowledge of needs that can be met only by other specialized helpers. Nurses help individuals under nursing care to secure needed help from others by referral, by representing needs for a specialized service, or by helping individuals represent their own needs for such services.

DELIBERATE ACTION

Nursing, self-care, and dependent-care are forms of practical endeavor, each concerned with bringing about new or changed conditions in others (nursing and dependent-care), in self (self-care), or in the environment. Persons who effectively engage in these or other forms of practical endeavor have knowledge of existent conditions (present state of affairs), as well as insights about desired future states of affairs and how to bring about the change from the current state to the desired state of affairs.

Practical endeavor requires the presence and efforts of persons with practical insight into what can or should be brought about under current and foreseen changing conditions and circumstances. Learning is required for engagement in practical endeavor, sometimes at the professional level of education and training or, at the other extreme, learning through trial and error by doing or observing others. Basic to all practical endeavor is what is known as *human action* or **deliberate action** performed by persons to achieve or to move toward achievement of some foreseen end or result. Nurses should have understanding of the nature of deliberate action in order to develop, in concrete nursing practice situations, insights about the action demands that engagement in self-care places on patients and the forms of deliberate action nurses must effectively perform in their own work of nursing others.

Examples

Deliberate action includes simple acts like the actions performed in turning an electrical appliance, such as a lamp, on or off. It includes complex or compound acts for which sets of organized and consecutive actions, individually and together, are coordinated to achieve a common end.[6] Compound actions can be performed by one individual, as when a person accomplishes the purpose of being in Boston on a particular day by driving there in an automobile, or they can be performed by a number of individuals, as when two individuals coordinate their actions to move a heavy object from one location to another. Self-care is a complex of compound actions.

Sets and series of organized, coordinated actions to achieve specified goals are connected in the sense that one action is made possible or facilitated by another action, or an action may interfere with the performance of a contemplated action.[5] The terms *organized* and *coordinated* thus refer to *relations between and among actions* performed by one or more individuals.

Organized and coordinated actions, for example, of a nurse and the person under the nurse's care, demand that the performer(s) or agent(s) have prior knowledge of the nature, timing, and duration of each action within the coordinated set or series and have the performance skills required.

Knowing what actions to perform and *having the skills to perform the actions* are combined with knowledge of the events and results that should accrue from their performance. For example, in a specific instance the deliberate turning of the ignition key of an automobile to the *on* position brings about a series of events resulting in the desired and anticipated starting of the motor. This result may be one of a series of results sought, as when the *purpose* of the person who turned the ignition key is to arrive at work by automobile within some time interval. However, if a person's purpose is to determine whether the car battery is dead, then the purpose is achieved when the motor starts or does not start.

In the foregoing examples, the person who turns the ignition key to achieve either purpose would have relevant information about the situation of action. The person knows whether the key is inserted, recognizes when insertion has occurred, and, when relevant, considers whether the car is cold, and so on. The *agent,* the person performing the actions, has incoming *sensory knowledge and awareness* of the reality of the situation of action. The agent *reflects* on the meaning of existent conditions and circumstances for the set or series of actions in process and for attainment of results toward purpose achievement. Reflection terminates in a particular situation with the agent's *decision* about the action that will be taken.

Nature of Deliberate Action

As illustrated in the examples, *deliberate action* refers to actions performed by *individual* human beings who have intentions and are conscious of their intentions to bring about, through their actions, conditions or states of affairs that do not at present exist. Deliberate action has *intentional aspects or phases,* as well as a *productive* phase. Each of these phases has distinct action components.

Deliberate action has been investigated by philosophers since antiquity. Human action has been and continues to be investigated by psychologists, sociologists, anthropologists, logicians, and others with a variety of foci. Foci of these investigations range from attention to the psychology of human actions, to philosophical bases for studying human action, to the nature of the learning required for it, and to activity theory constructed from a sociological perspective.

As previously mentioned, Parsons[4,5] development of the structure of a *unit of action* (unit act) within the context of a larger system of action has been helpful in aspects of development of the self-care deficit theory of nursing. The components of a completed *human act,* presented by Wallace[7] and by Gilby[8] and extracted from the writings of Aristotle and further elaborated by other philosophers, have been helpful in the work of conceptual development of the *agency variables* of self-care deficit nursing theory, *self-care agency,* and *nursing agency.* Wallace and Gilby identify three types of component actions within a "complete human act," namely, those (1) concerning the end, (2) concerning the means, and (3) concerning execution, that is, the practical or productive actions.

The schema for a "complete human act" that is presented by both Wallace[7] (p. 179) and Gilby[8] (pp. 211-217) identifies action components within the three named types. Components related to the *end* and to the *means* are the *intentional phases* of action, and components concerning *actions to produce the end* constitute the *productive phase.*

The following expressions of the component actions of a "complete human act" are modification of the originals.

1. Components related to the end
   a. Apprehension of some perceived good (an end) as achievable and desirable
   b. Wanting to achieve the perceived good
   c. Judgment that it is possible to achieve the end
   d. Formation of the intention to achieve the end
2. Components related to the means
   a. Deliberation and reflection about the situation of action and the means available
   b. Study of opposing courses of action to reach the desired end
   c. Judgment about and selection of the course of action to be taken, the means to be used
   d. Decision about the course of action to be taken, the means to be used
3. Concerning execution, productive practical action to attain the end
   a. Command to self that action should begin
   b. Operationalization of powers and capabilities to execute the actions through which the end can be attained
   c. Judgment that the end is or is not attained
   d. Satisfaction that the end is attained or regret that it is not: in either instance, there is a *stillness* as action comes to an end

The value of the foregoing schema rests in the identification of forms of action required when persons act deliberately to attain an end, for example, perceiving and apprehending, deliberating and reflecting, making judgments, making decisions, and engaging in productive practical action. In concrete situations of nursing or daily living, the primary focus is on persons who take action. Persons as unitary beings act deliberately to achieve the ends or the states of affairs sought. Nurses in concrete practice situations must have information about the powers and capabilities of persons under care to perform the forms of actions required if they are to effectively engage in self-care or dependent-care. They also require information about persons' willingness to initiate action and to persevere in it.

It is necessary to understand that the named components of deliberate action are forms of action. They in no way suggest the content of the actions; content arises from the concrete conditions and circumstances with which the agent or actor is dealing and with the changes in them that he or she is seeking to bring about. In concrete life situations in which persons seek desired ends, their actions can be understood in terms of both form and content. Performed actions will have a structure, the structure arising from the relations between and among the deliberately produced action components. Specific essential structural arrangements of actions are referred to as *action systems.*

The named action components in the listing are performed in some time sequence. Their performance may be narrowly or widely separated in *time* and may be separated in *place* of performance. This separation in *time* is readily understood from everyday experiences. For example, an individual forms the intention of fulfilling his or her desire to own an automobile of a particular make and vintage. A place of purchase must be located, money or credit must be available, negotiations must be entered into and completed, and the car possessed. The time span between these different sets of actions may be days or weeks or years. Separation in *space* is exemplified by a person's decision to seek health care and the need to move self to the place where it can be secured.

Nurses require the ability to see the wholeness of action systems in which they and their patients are participant actors. A good example, because of its concreteness, is surgical removal or surgical repair of bodily structures. Here the action moves from patients' decisions to undergo surgical therapy, to presentation of self for the surgery, to the complex practical endeavor of preparation for it, to the performance of the surgical procedure itself, to patients' recovery and rehabilitation. Each of these aspects of undergoing surgical therapy involves the necessity of not one but a series of "completed human acts," each of which bears specific relations to the other "human acts" and to the final end or result being sought. The required amount and kind of organization and coordination of actions between and among participant agents of action are extensive. Each participant in this complex, coordinated surgical act has requirements for specific and different enabling powers and capabilities.

In concluding this account of deliberate action, a set of assumptions about human beings relevant to their engagement in deliberate action such as self-care is offered. This is followed by a set of conditions that may encourage persons' action tendencies to pursue needed and desirable ends, such as the regulations achievable through self-care.

Some Conditions of Action

Accepting the generalization that deliberate action involves reflection as well as judgment and decision making requires the acceptance of human beings as having intrinsic activity rather than passivity or strict reactivity to stimuli. A minimum set of assumptions about human beings would include the following (Arnold, pp. 193-204).[9]

- Human beings know and appraise objects, conditions, and situations in terms of their effects on ends being sought.
- Human beings know directly by sensing, but they also reflect, reason, and understand.
- Human beings are capable of self-determined actions, even when they feel an emotional pull in the opposite direction.
- Human beings can prolong reflection indefinitely in deliberations about what action to take by raising questions about and directing attention toward different aspects of a situation and different possibilities for action.
- To act, human beings must concentrate on a suitable course of action and exclude other courses of action.
- Purposive action requires not only that human beings be aware of objects, conditions, and situations but also that they have the ability to contend with them and treat them in some way.
- Persons, as unitary beings, are the agents who act deliberately to attain ends or goals.

If the foregoing assumptions are accepted, it is possible to identify human and environmental conditions and factors that must be developed and operational if individuals are to appraise, select, and proceed with courses of action. Arnold's position about deliberate action and motivation led in 1987 to the expression of six conditions that may encourage action tendencies for self-care. Because the conditions are general and not specific to self-care, they are relevant to all deliberate actions.

- Persons must have available the knowledge necessary to distinguish something as good or desirable from bad and undesirable and to reflect on its desirability or undesirability. The goal and ways to achieve it must be conceptualized or imagined.
- Reasons for selecting certain actions to attain what has been appraised as good or desirable and afforded the tentative status of a goal should be known.
- Time as well as knowledge are required for persons to form ideas about particular actions or to form images of how each action relates to the goal.
- Reflection should be directed to these questions: Is this way of acting good or desirable? Is it more desirable or less desirable than other ways of acting to achieve the goal?

- Reflection about choosing a way of action could go on indefinitely; therefore, reflection should be brought to a close with a decision when the ways of action have been conceived as clear ideas or clear images are formed.
- A person owns his or her appraisal of possible ways of action to attain a goal and his or her decision to act according to one or a combination of these ways, when this way of acting is formalized and incorporated into the person's self-image or self-concept.[10]

Given acceptance of these conditions, for example by nurses, rules and standards of nursing practice can be developed for situations when patients are confronted with choices and decisions with respect to self-care or dependent-care or about choices to engage in the exercise or development of self-care agency or dependent-care agency. Nurses should view the six conditions as applicable to their own choices, as well as to patient choices.

Deliberate action has been examined in terms of essential human qualities and capabilities that are operational when individuals pursue the achievement of desired ends or goals. More detailed insights about these qualities and capabilities can be gained from study of them within the framework of specific sciences. Such insights are necessary for understanding the power (or the agency) of individuals to engage in self-care, dependent-care, nursing, or any other field of endeavor.

SUMMARY

Nursing requirements of individuals are directly linked to the human need for the continuing production of care regulatory of human functioning and development to maintain each within norms compatible with life, health, and human well-being. This care is conceptualized as self-care. The history of the formalization and validation of the concept by members of the Nursing Development Conference Group is recounted. Self-care is described broadly as human action, deliberate or voluntary action. More specifically, it is identified as a human regulatory function.

The concept of self-care requisite is introduced and described. Three types of self-care requisites are identified, and the assumptions basic to their formulation are expressed. Adequate modes of expression of self-care requisites are represented as including both the nature of the action to be taken and the required regulation sought. The need to particularize generalized expressions of self-care requisites for individuals and the selection of means or technologies for meeting each requisite are developed in some detail.

The concepts of therapeutic self-care demand and self-care deficit are introduced and explained. This leads to the description and explanation of nursing as a helping service with identification and descriptions of the five ways in which one person can help another person do what that person needs to do. Nurses' selection and use of some combination of ways of helping defines in part the roles of patients and nurses in practice situations. The chapter is concluded with a detailed exposition of deliberate or voluntary action, understanding of which is a foundation for developing insights about the human action features of self-care, dependent care, and nursing.

References

1. Neufeldt V, Guralnik D, editors: *Webster's new world dictionary,* ed 3, New York, 1988, Prentice Hall, p 127.
2. Nursing Development Conference Group, Orem DE, editor: *Concept formalization in nursing: process and product,* ed 2, Boston, 1979, Little, Brown, pp 129-180.
3. Guyton AC: *Textbook of medical physiology,* ed 8, Philadelphia, 1991, WB Saunders, p 777.
4. Parsons T: *The social system,* New York, 1951, Free Press, pp 8-9n.
5. Parsons T: *The structure of social action,* New York, 1937, McGraw-Hill, pp 44-45.
6. Kotarbinski T: *Praxiology: an introduction to the sciences of efficient action* (Translated by Wojtasiewicz O), New York, 1965, Pergamon Press, pp 47-54.
7. Wallace WA: *The modeling of nature,* Washington, DC, 1996, Catholic University of America Press.
8. Gilby T: Appendix I, structure of a human act. In St. Thomas Aquinas: *Summa theologiae: psychology of human acts,* vol 17, 1970, Blackfriars, Cambridge. In conjunction with McGraw-Hill.
9. Arnold MB: *Neurological and physiological aspects, Vol. II: Emotion and personality:* New York, 1960, Columbia University Press, p 198.
10. Orem DE: Motivating self-care—the reality, persons as self-care agents. Conference papers. Hospitals in the community—a vision, The Wesley Hospital, Auchenflower, 4066, Queensland, Australia, 1988, pp 12-13.

CHAPTER 4

Nursing and Society

Once a society introduces and establishes nursing as a human health service, persons who seek to provide nursing for others or who seek to prepare themselves to do so must earn and be afforded the status of nurse within the society. The recognition of individual women and men as nurses affords them the right to represent themselves as able and willing to provide nursing and the obligation to provide nursing in situations they enter into as nurses. Nursing students and nurses must come to understand, accept, and manage themselves within their public status. Understanding nursing as an available service in communities and societies emphasizes the societal facets of the relationships of nurses to persons they nurse and to the society that recognizes them as nurses.

The differentiation, development, and maintenance of nursing as a human service in societies and culture groups and the provision of nursing to individuals

68

and groups proceed within processes of group life and societal relationships. Differentiation and institutionalization of nursing as a health service are usually brought about by concerned persons in locations where people are who need nursing. Movement toward this end occurs at the international and national levels when the need for, the value of, and the means for providing nursing are understood and communicated by innovators and developers.

This chapter introduces some societal features of nursing. These features have origins in societies (see Prologue) in contrast to purely personal or interpersonal origins (as expressed, for example, in self-care deficit nursing theory).

REFERENCE TERMS

In groups where nursing is provided, reference terms are used to signify individuals who are accepted as providers of the service of nursing, and those who are being provided with the service. In English-speaking countries, the word *nurse* signifies persons qualified through education, training, and experience to provide nursing to persons in need of this special service. Because nursing education in the United States remained outside the national system of education for so many years, the title *nurse,* as previously stated, signified persons with a wide range of nursing knowledge and capabilities. Reference terms within nursing have changed and will continue to change as nurses continue the development of their science and art.

The term **nursing practitioner** is used in this book to signify persons professionally qualified to practice nursing and who are engaged in its regular provision. At times, the terms *nurse* and *nursing practitioner* are used interchangeably. In this book, the term **nurse** is used to refer to women and men prepared either through high-level technical education or professional-level education. However, *nursing practitioner* is used to refer specifically to professionally educated nurses working at the entry or advanced level of professional nursing practice. Nurses prepared through high-level technical education work with nursing practitioners or work under established nursing protocols.

The use of the term *nursing practitioner* presumes that within the broad domain of human service and health professions there is a field identified as nursing. The professionally educated nurse knows the field of nursing and may specialize in one or more areas of its practice. Knowing nursing as a field of practice and knowing the relation of areas of specialization to the whole field is one characteristic of persons who function as nursing practitioners.

The term *nursing practitioner* as used in this text is not equated with the term *nurse practitioner.* The latter term came into use to designate nurses with a technical to technological level of preparation for performing selected tasks or managing certain subsystems of operations traditionally within the domain of medical practice. Some nurse practitioners function as primary care agents who do initial physical examinations and prescribe for common ailments, while they also function as nursing practitioners. Other nurse practitioners function within medical protocols with a medical orientation to care sometimes as physician assistants. *Nurse practitioner* is viewed as an *ambiguous term* because it does not indicate what is being practiced by the nurse who carries the title. The settings in which nurse practitioners function may provide clues to how they function.

Persons under the care of nurses, physicians, or other direct health care providers, as well as persons under care in hospitals, have been and are identified by the term **patient.** The same person could be a nurse's patient, a physician's patient, and a hospital patient. The word *patient* means a receiver of care, someone who is under the care of a health care professional at this time, in some place or places.

Some nurses use the term **client** in place of the term *patient.* This effort seems to be directed toward recognition of the contractual nature of the relationships of nurses to persons under their care and to avoid the philosophical use of the word *patient* to mean *that which is acted upon.* It is customary to use the term *client* in the practice of law, in business, and trade. In the legal profession, clients are persons who *employ* or *retain* an attorney or counselor for advice and assistance. Clients place their affairs in the hands of an attorney who acts for them in legal matters. *Client* also means a customer who *regularly* buys from another or receives services from another.

In the health care professions, it would seem that the terms *patient* and *client* are not interchangeable. Persons who are regular seekers of the services of—that is, who are clients of—this or that nurse may not be under nursing care at particular times and, therefore, would not have patient status. In child nursing situations or in situations in which adults have legally appointed guardians, parents or guardians are the nurse's clients, but it is the child or dependent adult who is the nurse's patient. The terms *patient* or *nurse's patient* will be used to refer to persons under the care of nurses.

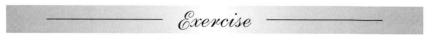

Exercise

Exercise on Nurses' Use of Reference Terms for Persons Under Nursing Care

1. In your contacts with at least five nurses who are engaged in nursing practice determine whether they are willing to respond to a number of questions about their use of general terms in referring to persons under nursing care.
2. If they are willing, ask them already formulated questions to determine:
   a. Whether they use the term *patient* and why.
   b. Whether they use the term *client* and why.
   c. Whether they use other ways of referring to individuals under their care.
3. Express your findings about general terms used by nurses.
4. What conclusion did you reach?

ESTABLISHING AND MAINTAINING NURSING

Nursing as a service is the provision of professional aid that combines features of helping with features of taking care of others when the reasons for the need for help and for being taken care of are within the boundaries of nursing as these boundaries are understood at particular periods in the life of a society. The initiation and development of a system(s) and method(s) of providing people in communities with nursing include (1) offering education and opportunities for training that are enabling for men and women to prepare themselves to provide nursing and (2) the development of means for persons with nursing require-ments to come into relationships with nurses who are able and willing to nurse them. The history of the institution of nursing as a health service in various societies reveals commonalities and differences. Once nursing is instituted, maintaining nursing as an available service within social groups is a continuing problem.

Establishing Nursing

The initial establishment of nursing as an organized health service is brought about in societies because insightful persons recognize the need for it. These enterprising persons provide ways and means to secure and prepare interested women and men to provide nursing. Dock and Stewart[1,2] note that the founda-tions for nursing were laid in the seventeenth century by Vincent de Paul and Louise de Marillac and the French women who worked with them to bring nursing first to the people of Paris and later to those in outlying French villages. Men as well as women were active in the initial establishment of nursing in countries throughout the world. In the United States, it was recognized that medical care without concomitant nursing care was not productive of results sought. The value of nursing was recognized in the Shattock Report of 1850.[3]

The process of distinguishing nursing begins with the recognition that human beings under some range of conditions (1) cannot provide continuing care for themselves or their dependents because of existent situations of personal health and (2) cannot control internal and environmental factors in such a way as to prevent pathology and maintain, promote, or restore human integrity and well-being. Being physically ill or injured and not having the necessary knowledge and skills were some of the conditions identified by the early developers of nursing. The process of developing nursing continues with the formal preparation of persons to provide a kind of care known as nursing. This is followed, in the sociologic sense, by the institutionalization of forms of nursing education and practice.

The process of distinguishing and establishing nursing begun in several countries at different times during the eighteenth and nineteenth centuries continues. Regardless of the time and place of its initiation, the process is a continuing one and includes at least seven sets of actions:

- Recognizing that some persons in their time-place localizations are unable to completely care for themselves or their dependents in whole or in part because of their own or their dependents' states of health and the factors that are conditioning it, or because day-to-day requisites for self-care or dependent-care are novel or complex.

- Naming the help or care that is required nursing.
- Studying human and environmental conditions under which requirements for nursing arise, including the duration of requirements.
- Identifying and adapting effective and socially acceptable ways for selecting and preparing men and women to provide nursing.
- Identifying and adapting ways to bring about associations between nurses who are prepared, able, and willing to provide nursing, and persons in need of it.
- Extending the work of persons prepared as nurses to more and more individuals who need nursing.
- Establishing just means for the financing of nursing.

Each of these seven sets of actions should be continuously performed because the process of distinguishing and establishing nursing to make it continuously available in a society is never ended. The complex process of distinguishing and establishing nursing involves nurses, as well as others who understand the human conditions associated with needs of individuals and groups for nursing. Community-based and governmental agencies are also involved.

Maintaining Nursing

Initial and continuing efforts to make nursing available depends on societal interest and support and on the willingness of women and men to prepare themselves initially and subsequently through continuing education to function in society as nurses. The strength of nursing in a society does not rest in the number of persons who support nursing, but rather in the ability of practicing nurses to continue to advance their nursing knowledge and capabilities and at the same time to manage and reduce stress associated with day-to-day demands to be with and in communication with others as they provide nursing for an ever changing

Exercise

Exercise to Compare What a Nursing Journal Publishes by Time Periods

1. Select a single issue from a specific year of a national nursing journal for the 10-year periods of the 1960s, 1970s, 1980s, and 1990s.
2. For each issue identify the subject matter, the expressed problem, or the issues that were the focuses of editorials.
3. For each issue read the table of contents and the articles as necessary to make a judgment about the subject matter of each article. Make notations about the number of articles by subject matter for each issue selected.
4. Compare and contrast your findings about the subject matter of editorials and articles.
5. Express conclusions about similarities and differences in editorials and articles.

population of men, women, and children in time-place localizations singly or in groups. Nursing's strength also is associated with (1) recognition afforded nurses; (2) satisfaction nurses receive from the effectiveness of their nursing; from their relationships with persons they nurse and with colleagues, and from their own advancement in the profession; and (3) support nurses receive from colleagues and administrators of health care agencies and from their own families. Management of stress involves nurses' development of realistic expectations of themselves in all aspects of their living, including their nursing endeavors.

Maintaining nursing in societies requires deliberate effort by nurses, nursing organizations, community groups, government agencies, educational agencies, and the public. Keeping nursing available and viable is a complex undertaking. The parts or elements of the undertaking must be identified, their meaning and relevance understood, and ways and means instituted to ensure nursing's continued presence and effectiveness. A number of such elements are identified:

- Clear identification of nursing practitioners within social groups, along with prerequisites for their practice in types of nursing practice situations.
- Clear distinctions between nurses prepared through technical education and persons vocationally trained as aides or attendants.
- A public image of nursing practitioners and nurses that is in accord with their contributions to the health and well-being of members of social groups and the responsibilities they bear in a range of health care situations.
- Clear distinctions between the contributions of nurses to health care of individuals, families, and communities and the contribution of members of other health professions and occupations, with recognition of contributions that are common to all.
- Public and private support of university- and college-level educational programs for preparing nursing practitioners and nurses, including requisite access to liberal arts courses directed toward personal development and to science courses that are foundational for understanding nursing.
- Assurance that nursing practitioners and nurses are able to effectively represent themselves and their work verbally and in writing to persons they nurse, to other nurses, to other health professionals, to executives of health service agencies, and to the public.
- Assurance that nursing practitioners have the freedom to practice nursing for the populations they serve, and that contributions of nursing practitioners and nurses that further the effectiveness of the work of physicians are recognized.
- Maintenance of work environments, conditions of work, and remuneration for nursing practitioners and nurses that is protective of their lives, health, and well-being and conducive to personal and professional development.
- Knowledge of existent and emerging or predicted conditions and circumstances of members of communities that are indicators of needed changes in nursing practice and in the number and preparation of nursing practitioners and of technically prepared nurses who work with them.

• Development and redevelopment of ways to ensure provision of nursing to men, women, and children that is effective and economical of time, money, and materials, including new ways of offering nursing, as in nursing clinics, and the development of new nursing positions and titles.

The foregoing elements of the continuing process for maintaining nursing in societies focus on nurses and their education and on ensuring safe and effective nursing. However, additional elements are oriented to the formulation, expression, and validation of nursing knowledge. Developing and validating nursing knowledge is a continuing task that includes the articulation of nursing facts and theories with other established sciences and fields of knowledge. For the task to be done in and over time, there must be university-educated persons with requisite interests, knowledge, skills, and motivation to function in theory development in nursing, nursing research, the design and testing of technologies and techniques of nursing practice (nursing development), and the scholarly endeavor of searching out and organizing existent nursing knowledge.

Needs for these knowledge-related endeavors must be recognized and attended to by the nursing profession, by universities with graduate programs in nursing, by organizations offering nursing as a health service, and by persons who are nurses. Positions for nurses (or other qualified persons) to engage in these nursing knowledge-focused endeavors must be institutionalized and financed.

The four knowledge-focused positions as well as the positions of nursing practitioner and teacher of nursing are represented in Figure 4-1. Interrelations among the positions are shown in the figure. Interrelations of positions indicate either the possibility for combining two or more endeavors, as when teachers are also practitioners, or when there are needs for collaboration, as when developers of technologies and techniques work with practitioners and researchers. All positions show relationships to "structured nursing knowledge" because the work nurses do in each position demands the use of already available knowledge and ideally contributes to knowledge development.

In addition, the positions of teacher, practitioner, theorist, researcher, and developer are related to the position of scholar. The filling of these five positions demands that persons in them are able to and do function as nursing scholars.

Nurses, organizations of nurses, and organizations for the promotion of nursing and nursing education are or should be in the forefront in expenditure of efforts to maintain nursing in social groups. National and state or provincial governments, as well as local governments, community groups, and individual citizens, contribute to ensure nursing's continued availability. Public and private groups under some circumstances and through policy decisions at state and national levels may fail to contribute to the maintenance of nursing, so that nursing becomes less and less available in communities to persons for whom it is an essential service.

The process of distinguishing nursing from other forms of care and establishing and maintaining its availability in social groups requires both

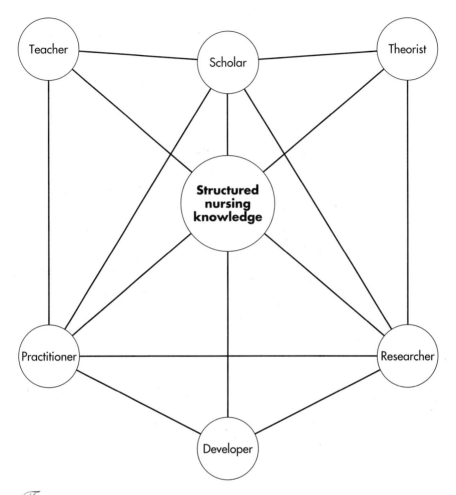

Figure 4-1 Professional roles and role relationships with structured nursing knowledge as common element.

attention and effort. Although this process is distinct from the process of providing nursing to those in need, both are necessary to maintain effective nursing in social groups. Nurses and other concerned persons are involved in ensuring that nursing is available. But it is only the actions of adequately prepared and responsible nurses that result in the kind of care that is named nursing. Because of this, nurses must be aware of the frequency of lack of knowledge or the erroneous knowledge about nursing on the part of political and social activists engaged in policy making about health care and the education of health care providers. Nurses must be effective representatives of requirements of citizens for nursing and requirements for its provision in the society.

THE SERVICE FEATURES OF NURSING

Nursing is a human service in societies in that it meets certain requirements of men, women, and children that arise during day-to-day living. Nursing is but one of an array of human services available to the public in many geographic areas. Like all services, it must be distributed, produced, and financed. The proliferation of services of all types is attested to by the Yellow Pages of telephone books. Nursing meets personal requirements of individual human beings, families, and communities. It is a direct service for persons singly or in groups.

Nursing's helping and taking care of features described in prior chapters express general characteristics of the person-to-person relationships of nurses and nurses' patients. Service features of nursing relate persons who are nurses or aspiring nurses to the larger community and to governmental jurisdictions. These features must be made operative in every situation of nursing practice. Service features of nursing thus provide a societal frame of reference within which nurses function in each situation of nursing practice.

Service connotes action and implies that the results of action or work are beneficial to individuals or groups or whole communities. Services are understood in terms of the functional society where interrelationships come about because of and are dominated by the work performed. One person or group seeks another so that together an objective goal can be attained that could not be attained alone. Plattel[4] states that "in the functional society" relationships between or among persons have "an external character" so that it is possible to talk about "having" or "possessing" a relationship. Individual nurses, their patients, and patients' significant others thus constitute collaborating units within a society.

Service Enterprises

The continuous offering of a service (e.g., nursing) to members of a society requires laborious effort, perseverance, persistent exertion, resourcefulness, and the human and material resources necessary to provide the service. Because services offered should be available in accord with the time at which and the ways in which needs for them are revealed, the availability of services must be timed and the nature and quality of services made known to potential users. Specific services may be offered by individuals or collaborating groups, as in the private or the group practice of nursing or medicine. Specific and sometimes related services may be made available to the public through controlling bodies, such as hospitals that are incorporated as nonprofit or profit-making entities within a governmental jurisdiction. Also national, state or provincial, or local governments may make specific services available to persons who need and qualify to receive them.

Legally constituted bodies, such as hospitals, sponsor the offering of human services by ensuring, for example, that physicians, nurses, and other essential health professionals are available and ready to practice in situations where their specialized work is required. Such institutions make it possible for health professionals to practice within an enabling environment and for members of the public to seek and receive services within this environment. It is important for nurses and nursing students to understand the functional systems needed for the private, group, or large-scale institutional offering of nursing and other health services.

Functions and functional systems are the same in kind but vary in magnitude of performance for private or group practice or large-scale institutional offering. Before offering service, organizations must obtain the legal authority to exist as an enterprise that provides services to the public toward fulfillment of defined purposes. The conditions for receiving this authority must be met initially and conditions for retaining it fulfilled.

For human service enterprises to survive and fulfill their reasons for existence in communities, they must have persons engaged in performing three sets of functions: **governing functions**, **executive functions**, and **essential operational functions**.[5] The main subfunctions of each are identified in the following outline.

GOVERNING FUNCTIONS

1. Acting for the enterprise as a whole
2. Leading the enterprise to achieve its end in the society
3. Providing what is needed and correcting what is out of order

EXECUTIVE FUNCTIONS

1. Defining and limiting the purpose of the enterprise in accord with its purpose for existence and the nature of the current and changing requirements of people for services
2. Securing and maintaining essential effort
3. Providing and maintaining a system of communication

ESSENTIAL OPERATIONAL FUNCTIONS

1. Initial and subsequent distribution of opportunities to individuals or multiperson units to partake of available services
2. Production of services in association with continuing acts of distribution over the time period when services are provided to specific individuals or multiperson units
3. Financing of the services distributed to and produced for individuals and multiperson units

These are dimensions of the mainstreams of functioning of human service enterprises.

Figure 4-2 shows sets of managerial and contributory functions that feed into and out of the three central functional systems. The contributory functions are concerned with the securing, availability, and care of essential resources. The managerial functions are directed to each of the three central functions and focus on the development of designs and plans for execution of each subfunction and on performance evaluation and control.[5] Failure to comprehend the nature of, to provide for performance of, and to perform the identified functions will result in the failure of service enterprises to fulfill their purpose for existence.

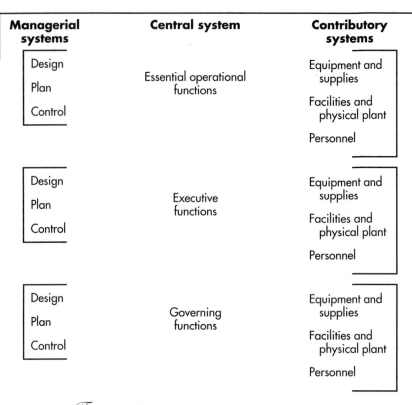

Managerial systems	Central system	Contributory systems
Design Plan Control	Essential operational functions	Equipment and supplies Facilities and physical plant Personnel
Design Plan Control	Executive functions	Equipment and supplies Facilities and physical plant Personnel
Design Plan Control	Governing functions	Equipment and supplies Facilities and physical plant Personnel

Figure 4-2   Functions of human service enterprises.

Nursing's health service features lend specificity of purpose to the types of enterprises that offer nursing in societies.

HEALTH SERVICE FEATURES

Nurses speak and write about nursing as a health service. Insightful nurses have a better understanding of nursing's position in the family of health services than do members of other health professions or the public. From a public perspective, nursing occupies an obscure to invisible position as a specialized health service. The absence of nursing is afforded greater recognition than its presence or its effectiveness as a health service.

Public Recognition of Health Features

Nursing continues to be viewed by health policymakers and others as an adjunct to medical care provided by physicians. Nursing also is viewed by some persons as a service of health care organizations and not as the specialized work of nursing practitioners and nurses, many of whom practice nursing under the jurisdiction of legitimately incorporated health care institutions. Nursing's lack of visibility is due in part to these traditional ways of viewing nursing. It is due also to nursing's lack of visibility because the provision of nursing is a private affair, visible to nurses and to those nursed and at times to physicians.

Nurses are able to articulate the health service features of nursing when they know why people need nursing and how they are or can be helped through nursing. *Self-care* or *dependent-care* is necessary for individuals for life, health, and human well-being. When the health states of men, women, and children or the characteristics of required health-related self-care measures result in action limitations for engagement in self-care or dependent-care, their lives, health, and well-being may be in jeopardy if nursing is not provided. By compensating for or overcoming health-associated human limitations for engagement in self-care or dependent-care, nurses contribute to maintaining health, preventing disease and disability, and restoring or maintaining life processes.

Nurses in their practice of nursing know the human and environmental factors that condition (1) persons' self-care requisites and (2) their self-care capabilities. *Condition** is used in the sense of to affect, to modify, or influence; for example, children's developmental states influence how they express their experiencing of an existent self-care requisite, such as the requisite for food intake, or a requisite to be relieved of discomfort or pain.

The term *self-care requisite* is used in this text as required actions through which individuals regulate factors that affect their human functioning and human development. Care requisites may be met through self-care, dependent-care, or nursing. Self-care requisites, when formulated, express desired results, the goals of self-care.

Persons in Environments

Nurses in concrete nursing practice situations seek nursing-relevant information about both persons who seek or need nursing and their environmental situations. Human beings are never isolated from their environments. They exist in them. For purposes of understanding, **environmental features** can be isolated, identified, and described, and some environmental features are subject to regulation or control. Human environments are analyzed and understood in terms of physical, chemical, biologic, and social features. These features may be interactive. Certain environmental features are continuously or periodically interactive with men, women, and children in their time-place localizations. As is well known, environmental conditions can positively or negatively affect the lives, health, and well-being of individuals, families, communities; under conditions of war or natural disaster, whole societies are subject to disruption or destruction.

---

*Condition as used here refers to the modifying effect of one thing upon another. In other places in the book, *condition* is used to refer to a "manner or state of being," such as the condition of being healthy or ill.

Environmental Features

Some environmental features relevant to the values or presence of self-care requisites are listed in two categories:

Physical, Chemical, and Biologic Features

PHYSICOCHEMICAL FEATURES:

Atmosphere of the earth
Gaseous composition of air
Pollutants—solid, gaseous
Smoke
Weather conditions
Geologic stability of earth's crust
BIOLOGIC FEATURES:
Pets
Animals in the wild
Infectious organisms or agents—viruses, rickettsiae, bacteria, fungii, protozoa, helminths
Persons or animals, including birds and arthropods, under natural conditions affording subsistence or lodgement to infectious agents
Persons or animals harboring infectious agents with manifest disease or inapparent infection

Socioeconomic-Cultural Features

FAMILY:

Composition by roles and ages of members
Cultural prescriptions of authority, responsibilities and rights for family as a unit, dominant family member, other members
Positions of members within families and culturally prescribed relationships
Time-place localizations of members
Family dynamics
Nature of relationships—familial, contractual, coercive
System of family living
Resources of family as a unit
Resources of individual members
Culture prescriptions for securing, managing, and using resources
Culture elements specifying specific patterns of self-care and dependent-care and selection and use of care measures

COMMUNITY:

Population
Composition by family units; by other functional, collaborating social units; and by governmental organs
Availability of resources for daily living of community members and for special needs of the community as a whole

Health services
  Kind, localization, availability
  Openness to individuals, to families
  Accessibility
  Culture practices and prescriptions about use
  Cost, methods of financing

Human Features

In all situations of human living, the health states of involved persons affect what persons do. Health service situations come into being when individuals become concerned about their health states or when they or others perceive changed features or recognize that their health may be in jeopardy. If at the same time they judge that seeking health care and service is a good thing to do and if health services are available, entry to the service is initiated. Existent or projected or potential features of *persons' states of health* are central concerns of health service professionals, including nurses. Nurses view health states of the persons they nurse as a *basic conditioning factor* influencing what persons need to do and what they can do with respect to self-care. Physicians view the health states of persons under their care as a central concern because the focus of medicine is the human potential of persons for health and their subjectivity to ill health, injury, and disability.

The health states of persons in relation to their ages and their developmental states determine in nursing practice situations (1) the amount and kind of help required, (2) the extent of need to be taken care of as persons, and (3) patient and nurse roles in the process of nursing. Nurses must have accurate and reliable information about the health states of their patients throughout the duration of a nursing situation. Nurses, through observation and measurement, obtain information about aspects of patients' health states and also use information obtained by physicians and others.

SOCIETAL ASPECTS OF NURSING PRACTICE

In modern society, adults are expected to be self-reliant and responsible for themselves and for the well-being of their dependents. Most societies accept that persons who are helpless, sick, aged, handicapped, or otherwise deprived should be helped in their immediate distress and helped to attain or regain responsibility within their existing capacities. Thus both self-help and help to others are valued by society as desirable activities. Nursing as a specific type of human service is based on both values. In most communities people see nursing as a desirable and necessary service.

Historical works and the investigations of anthropologists provide evidence that, in the past, societies recognized the social position of nurse and provided ways and means to have nurses. In some situations, persons became nurses because of their position in the family or in the larger society. In other situations, individuals were recruited to become nurses, as is now done in many countries. Preparation for nursing was both formal (through prescribed systems of training) and informal. Modern society introduced science-based education preparatory to nursing practice. The continued presence of active nurses in a society indicates that nursing is a desired and utilized service.

What is nursing? What are the nurse's contributions to the health and well-being of individuals, families, and communities? Is it to give care? Is it to bring about psychological adjustment so that a person will be able to accept and to live with illness or disability and develop personally, using his or her human potential? Is it to implement physicians' prescribed measures of care for the patient? Although the answers to each of these questions is yes, the answers do not adequately describe how and why nursing is specifically different from other human services.

Requirements for Nursing

When do nurses enter into the life situations of individuals or groups? Societies specify the conditions that make it legitimate for its members to seek the various kinds of human services that are provided. These conditions become the criteria that members of the society use in determining whether a particular human service can or should be used. As stated in Chapter 2, the condition that validates the existence of a **requirement for nursing** in an adult is *the health-associated absence of the ability to maintain continuously that amount and quality of self-care that is therapeutic in sustaining life and health, in recovering from disease or injury, or in coping with their effects.* With children, the condition is the *inability of the parent (or guardian) associated with the child's health state to maintain continuously for the child the amount and quality of care that is therapeutic.* The word *therapeutic* is used to mean supportive of life processes, remedial or curative, when related to malfunction resulting from disease processes, and contributing to personal development and maturing.

Requirements for nursing cannot be met unless they are recognized. Physicians identify the need for and seek nursing for their patients. Friends and family members also may recognize when a person needs nursing, and adults may recognize their own needs for nursing. The family is often the first line of assistance when its members are in need. When family, friends, or neighbors are unable or unwilling to help, assistance with management or maintenance of self-care may be sought from organized nursing services. Nursing may be provided in the home or in health care institutions, on an inpatient or outpatient basis. There may or may not be a sufficient number of nurses to provide the needed service. Organization for the delivery of nursing is a need of every community.

Physicians traditionally have had as the focus of their service the health and disease states of individuals. Their concern is with life processes, body structure, and interferences with life and developmental processes. Physicians evaluate health states, determine evidence of the presence or absence of disease, and prescribe and give therapy to maintain health and to cure or control disease or the effects of injury and disease. When able, persons under medical care are expected to manage their own health affairs and maintain the type of self-care they require.

When they are unable, assistance from persons other than the physician is required. Nursing is required whenever the maintenance of continuous self-care requires the use of special techniques and the application of scientific knowledge in providing care or in designing it.

It is an accepted practice for the physician to see patients periodically. The time a physician spends with a patient varies with the patient's health state and the medical care techniques used. Some patients see their physicians once a year, once a month, or more frequently. Physicians do not remain continuously with chronically ill or disabled patients. In the event of serious injury or when life processes or rational processes have been seriously interfered with, the physician may remain with patients for prolonged periods, sometimes working closely with nurses and other health care workers. Patients, nurses, and other specialized workers carry out measures of care prescribed by the physician, and nurses and others assist patients in preparing themselves for measures of care to be performed by physicians. In such instances, a person's self-care becomes linked not only to the medical care given by the physician but also to care or services given by other health personnel, sometimes working as a team. Nurses must often synthesize or unify a variety of care elements into a process of self-care action for the patient.

Nursing as a human service has its foundations, on the one hand, in persons with needs for self-care of a positive, therapeutic quality and limitations for its management or maintenance and, on the other, in the specialized knowledge, skills, and attitudes of persons prepared as nurses. Societies provide ways and means to bring individuals in need of nursing into relationships with qualified nurses. These relationships should be sustained as long as specialized techniques of care are required or until the person or a family member becomes able to manage and maintain the required self-care.

Effecting Nursing Contacts

Nurses who practice nursing engage themselves in the regular provision of nursing to persons who require it. Nurses function as members of the occupation and profession of nursing in particular geographic areas and governmental jurisdictions. Nurses must be educationally qualified, not exceed their practice capabilities, and be personally willing to provide nursing. Furthermore, nurses must meet standards and conform to regulations that make their practice legitimate in particular jurisdictions.

Although nursing is a valued service in many groups, it is frequently in short supply for those who need it. A critical factor is the availability ratio: the number of persons in diverse places who require nursing at the same time and the deployment of nurses in relation to those persons. Nurses, as designers and providers of nursing for populations, should be aware of indexes of the objective need for, the demand for, and the supply of nursing. It is a continual struggle to bring together those who can benefit from short- or long-term nursing and those able and willing to produce and manage systems of nursing. This problem should be a concern of organizations that offer nursing as a community service.

A related problem is financing the provision of nursing in social groups. How much does it cost to produce effective nursing for those who need it? How should these costs be distributed within social groups? These questions have not been answered adequately in the United States, where for decades available nursing was produced in large part by nurses-in-training. This practice has changed, but the problem of financing nursing remains partly unaddressed.

Contact and communication among persons who can benefit from nursing and persons able and willing to provide it define the first prerequisite for the provision of nursing. Social groups have provided and continue to provide ways and means to effect this contact.

People generally come into contact with nurses in one of two ways: Either they find nurses who publicly represent themselves as being engaged in the private or joint practice of nursing, or they come in contact with nurses through a health care institution that employs nurses. These two methods differ in terms of the way agreements are established and the number and nature of agreements among individuals and institutions. In the early and middle years of the twentieth century, hospitals, state and district nurses' associations, and training schools for nurses maintained registers of nurses in private practice. These registers were the primary means of effecting nurse-patient contacts. Nurses would make their availability known by placing their names on a register, and individuals, families, or physicians whose patients needed nursing would contact nurses directly or

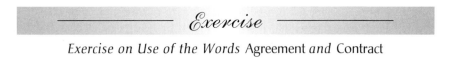

Exercise

Exercise on Use of the Words Agreement *and* Contract

1. Read about the meanings attached to the words *agreement* and *contract* in:
   a. An unabridged dictionary.
   b. A law dictionary, for example, *Black's Law Dictionary.*
2. Identify and record the meaning expressed for each word.
3. Reflect upon these meanings and think and make judgments about the following:
   a. *Expressions*
      "I contracted with my teacher to do B level work this semester with respect to assignments X, Y, and Z." Express what the verb *contract* means in this context.
      "I contracted with my patient Mr. Jones to reach X goals in 2 weeks." Express what the verb *contract* means in this context.
   b. *Situation*
      Miss Burns, RN, was designated as nurse for five individuals hospitalized on Unit A. She agreed with the head nurse of Unit A about the designated assignment. Miss Burns, RN, contacted each of the designated individuals, introduced herself as their nurse, and elicited their questions or expressions of their interests or concerns about the relationship. If each of the five patients accepted Miss Burns as his or her nurse, how would you designate the mutual acceptance of the nurse and the five persons on Unit A?

through such a register. More recently, nurses have been maintaining their own offices, sometimes in group practice with other nurses or physicians, which has made the office visit another method of effecting nurse-patient contacts.

In the second and more prevalent arrangement, persons who need nursing associate themselves with health care institutions, such as hospitals and visiting nurse associations, where nurses as well as other health workers are available. Under this arrangement, nurses are usually employees of the institution as well as practitioners of nursing. Some of them, however, may be attached to registers.

Where nursing is provided in private or group practice, there is a contract or agreement between the nurse and the patient (or the patient's legitimate representative). Where nursing is available through a health care institution, there is a contract or agreement between the patient and the institution. In this case, patients have contact with nurses who have been assigned to them by a manager or supervisor, who is usually also a nurse. Individuals who accept care from assigned nurses indicate explicitly or implicitly that they agree to this relationship.

Nurses have not always been aware of the complexity of the relationships in the second arrangement. Nurses who are institutional employees should understand clearly that they occupy two social statuses: that of employee of a health care institution and that of nurse. This situation sometimes creates boundary maintenance problems and role conflict. The legal perspective in such situations is that the person who is the nurse in the status of *employee* is the *agent* (in the legal sense) of the employing institution. Figure 4-3 illustrates facets of this type of arrangement for nursing.

In both methods of bringing together nurses and persons who can benefit from their care, nurses may go where patients reside, or patients may go to the location of the nurse. From this perspective, nursing as a service can be classified into four categories:

- Home nursing—nurse goes to home of patient.
- Ambulatory nursing for adults—patient comes to location of the nurse (clinic or office) and returns home after the visit.*
- Infant and child nursing in clinics or offices—patient is brought by parents or guardians to where the nurse is and returns home after the visit.
- Nursing for persons in any age-group who are short- or long-term residents of health care institutions, such as hospitals or extended care facilities—nurses come to the institution where patients are in residence.

Health care organizations, such as medical centers with hospitals and health maintenance organizations, may offer services in all of these forms and locations.

From an occupational perspective, nurses should accept nursing cases in accord with the fit between their individual nursing capabilities and the nursing requirements of those seeking nursing care. Determining whether individuals or groups evidence needs that nurses can legitimately meet is an essential nursing

---

*Nonambulatory adults at times come to clinics by ambulance.

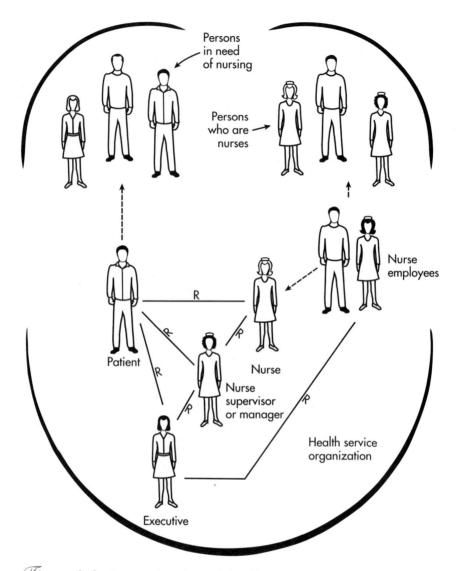

Figure 4-3 Nurse and patient relationships in health service organizations. *R*, relationship.

action. After this determination has been made, nurses should make a more detailed investigation of the nursing requirements of the individual or group. Finally, in light of a precise knowledge of their own nursing capabilities, nurses, as persons responsible for their own nursing acts, must make the judgment that they do or do not have the nursing capabilities required. If the nurse judges that he or she has the requisite capabilities, the nurse can enter into an agreement with the person seeking care (or those acting for the person) about the required form of the nursing that will be provided. At this point the nurse in private or group practice or the nurse who is an employee of a health care institution is in a position to negotiate with patients (or those acting for them) about the provision of nursing.

Nurses and persons who are their patients must be aware of the reasons for their relationships. Hospitalized individuals may be unaware that they have agreed to receive nursing when they contract for hospital care. Such individuals are surprised and at times unaccepting when nurses seek information to determine their nursing requirements. Persons who expect to receive nursing may be concerned and frightened when they are attended by aides, technicians, or orderlies and have no contacts with nurses. Ideally, nurses foster the development of mutual respect and trust in their relationships with patients. They maintain the frequency of contact and the kind and amount of communication with patients and their families essential in determining and meeting patients' requirements for nursing.

As previously indicated, why individuals require nursing is a critical question to be answered by nursing practitioners. The answer provides nurses with knowledge necessary to identify persons with whom they can have legitimate nursing relationships.

Nurses' previously developed (antecedent) knowledge about the domain of nursing practice, about the elements and relationships of nursing practice situations, and about nursing science is used in making observations, as well as in judging and making decisions about the legitimacy of nurse-patient relationships.

NURSE AND PATIENT ROLES

Individuals who receive help and care from persons qualified as nurses are referred to as *nurses' patients.* The term symbolizes the social status and roles of persons under the care of nurses. From a sociologic perspective, the terms *nurse* and *nurse's patient* signify related statuses or positions in social groups. Each status carries with it a *role,* that is, a set of prescriptions for organized action through which the status is filled. Nurses must be aware of the professional-occupational prescriptions for their roles as nurses and the role prescriptions for nurses and patients that are part of the general culture of social groups. General cultural prescriptions about the nurse and nurse's patient roles may vary from one social group to another. The specific understandings individual nurses and those under their care have about their roles operate as underlying assumptions about the expectations and actions of the nurse and the nurse's patient in each nursing situation.

In nursing situations, nurses' **patient roles** are specified by the reasons why the nursing is required and by what can and should be done under prevailing conditions. Nurses can help their patients to know and fulfill their roles only when nurses themselves know why and how their patients can be helped through nursing. **Nurses' roles** become specific in actual nursing situations by their knowledge of why and how an individual, singly or as a member of a family or group, can and should be helped through nursing.

Status and Role

The sociological concept of *status-role,* when combined with an understanding of when, why, and how people can be helped through nursing, can aid nurses in their efforts to develop insights about the *fit* or the *relatedness* of their actions to those of patients. A nurse's domain of action within a nursing situation may extend to some or to all or nearly all matters related to the existence and functioning of those under nursing care. How many aspects of the patient's daily life are encompassed in the nurse-patient relationship indicates the *extensity* of the relationship. The extensity of nurse-patient relationships varies with the patient's capabilities for self-care. For example, the extensity of a nurse-patient relationship is great when persons under nursing care have little or no capability for self-care because of their health state and the health-related nature of their continuing self-care requirements. This is so because nurses' roles extend to and encompass matters related to the moment-to-moment existence of such individuals.

The *intensity* of a nurse-patient relationship reflects the meaning that nurse and patient attach to their role relations. A nurse, for example, may know that nursing care can facilitate a patient's movement toward relative self-sufficiency in self-care. The patient, however, may view some types of help proffered by the nurse as intrusions into his or her life, or a patient may fear to be alone and may desire a nurse's presence continually, or a patient may dread being in the physical presence of a nurse who is rough or verbally abusive. Ideally, in adult nursing situations the extensity as well as the intensity of a nurse-patient relationship has an objective basis in (1) the patient's self-care abilities, limitations, and potential for self-care and self-management and (2) the meaning that nursing care has in relation to the patient's current and future well-being and to the nurse's effectiveness in filling the status of nurse.

Nurses at times have misconceptions about the rights and responsibilities of those who are seeking or are under nursing care. The nurse-patient relationship is contractual in nature. This means that the functions and responsibilities of nurses are necessarily limited to matters within the domain of nursing, that the help sought is for a limited time, and that nurses are remunerated (directly or indirectly) for the help provided. There should be an initial agreement between the nurse and the nurse's patient or between the nurse and those responsible for the patient's affairs about the general characteristics of the nursing required and the nursing to be provided. The responsible person may be the parents of a child, the legal guardian of an adult, a person with the power to act for an adult, or the next of kin. At times executives of health care institutions employing nurses may need to be informed about these agreements. As previously indicated, each nursing situation requires that nurses must establish that persons or groups who have been represented to them as being in need of nursing are indeed in need of it and that they, as nurses, are able and willing to provide nursing. When nurses are employees of health care institutions, such as public health organizations, hospitals, or nursing homes with which patients have contracted for care directly or through their insurance company, there should be a second, preferably explicit, verbal agreement between the nurse and each patient or individuals acting for the patient about the nurse's willingness to provide nursing and the patient's willingness to receive nursing from assigned nurses. Patients and their families should be informed about the goals to be sought through nursing.

Ideally, in health care institutions, explicit verbal agreements about the nursing to be provided should be made by the nurse who has determined the particular patient's nursing requirements, who has designed a system of nursing care, and who bears continuing responsibility for nursing the patient. A number of nurses may contribute to the provision of nursing according to the original or adjusted design; this contributory care includes continuous observation of the patient. These nurses as well as the patient should know their own roles in addition to the role of the nurse who bears nursing responsibility for the patient. Nurses should understand that nursing requirements cannot be met unless they are known. Such knowledge comes only through directed and controlled observation, which necessitates contact and communication with the patient or with persons who know the patient.

Agreements to provide nursing to individuals, families, or groups bind nurses to the provision of nursing in accord with objective nursing requirements. Nurses may be aware that they are not capable of providing the amount and kind of nursing required. At other times they are capable but know that external conditions, including the number of persons requiring nursing, their locations, and the amount and complexity of their care, will sometimes preclude the provision of sufficient nursing. When such conditions predominate, nurses, as responsible persons, must be able to represent the existing situation prudently to the patient, to the employing executives, or to their own supervisors by indicating how all involved can best contribute to ensuring the safety and well-being of a patient. Nurses too often remain silent about situations where nursing is inadequate in quality or quantity or where patients have no contacts with nurses but are charged for it. One problem related to nursing charges within health care institutions results from the failure of those institutions to compute the costs of nursing for persons with differing nursing requirements. For example, the cost of nursing in some hospitals has been and continues to be included in a blanket charge for room accommodations. In some instances such charges are made when no nursing has been provided. Health care administrators sometimes seek to keep costs down by employing vocationally trained workers rather than nurses. This is attendant service, not nursing.

The relation of nurse to patient is *complementary*. This means that nurses act to help patients act responsibly for their health-related self-care by making up for existent health-related deficiencies in the patients' capabilities for self-care, and by maintaining or increasing capabilities for self-care. The complementary nature of nurse-patient relations is a core concept in a nurse's development of insights about nursing and its practice. It is also the reason why nurses and patients or those who act for patients should seek to develop cooperative working relationships. Individuals, families, or groups under nursing care may be receiving other forms of health care, for example, medical care from one or more physicians, sometimes accompanied by a vast array of paramedical services. A nurse's patient, more likely than not, will be in contact and communication with relatives, friends, and work colleagues. The complementary nature of nurse and patient roles is also manifested by nurses' contacts with others to represent patients' desires and needs and health state features.

Nurses require insights about conditions that militate against cooperative working relationships. For example, nurses should seek to understand the cultural elements involved in the prejudicial attitudes or discriminatory practices in groups. These elements may affect both nurses and patients in their role fulfillment. Such elements include the prevailing attitudes of members of a culture group about skin color, national origin, religion, degree of affluence and influence, social status, social deviance, or even being male or female. Such cultural elements can influence how nurses help patients in the development or exercise of self-care abilities.

Patients, too, are influenced by such factors and may be reluctant or initially refuse nursing care or care from particular nurses. If nurses are to become safe and successful practitioners, they must learn to deal with their own prejudices and discriminatory practices. They can learn to recognize such attitudes in their patients, help patients express their difficulties, and at times move to an early resolution of problem situations. Persons as well as societal and interactional features of nursing are summarized in Figure 4-4.

Role-Set

The sociological concept *role-set* can add an essential dimension to nurses' understanding of the complexity of the nurse role in some nursing situations. The term *role-set* stands for the idea that each status—for example, that of nurse or nurse's patient—involves the status-holder not in a single role but in a set of roles that may include contact with persons in other social statuses. The totality of roles is known as the set of roles associated with a specific status.

In situations of nursing practice, the role of nurses encompasses functions performed for and with patients in the provision of nursing. It also includes contacts and coordinating functions with patients' family members, their physicians, other professional or technical providers of health care, social workers, and others. Other role functions may be associated with the place where nursing is provided, with prevailing environmental conditions, or with the procuring of resources needed for nursing purposes.

The concept of role-set, which is associated with a specific status and role, must be distinguished from that of *multiple roles*. For example, a person qualified in a society as a nurse may act to provide nursing care to patients. In addition, this person may also assist physicians in their performance of medical care measures for patients or may function as a medical care technician, a clerk, or a manager

Persons | Nurses, nurses' patients, and their significant others in time place localizations

Societal aspects

Service features

Professional, occupational features

Legal features

Legitimate nursing goals

Actors — Status and role

   Nurses — Qualifications and capabilities

   Nurses' patients — Reasons why nursing is required

   Significant others — Relationship to patient, authority and responsibility for patient

Actors' dynamic sense of duty — active, operative in each

Interactional aspects

Role relationships

   Agreement about general characteristics of nursing required and provided

   Interdependence in role performance

   Coordination of actions

Contact and interactional features

   Communication

   Cooperation of persons

Collaborating units of nurses, nurses' patients, and their significant others

   Association, interaction, integration

   Interpersonal unity

Figure 4-4   Persons and societal and interactional aspects of nursing practice.

of a total system of health service. That nurses in health care institutions have historically had multiple roles has tended to obscure their central role of providing nursing to those in need of it. The fact that nurses have performed, and in some settings continue to perform, in the roles of physicians' assistants, medical care technicians, clerks, housekeepers, or managers does not make these roles nursing practice roles because they involve activities outside the domain of nursing practice. In organizations, however, combining a number of roles into one organizational position is common.

A related consideration in nursing is that the majority of nurses in health care institutions are employees as well as nurses. The role-set associated with the status of employee differs from the role-set associated with the status of nurse. Nurses' and their employers' failure to recognize the differences in these roles and to effect a legitimate alignment of them have hindered the progress of health care institutions and those nurses who are employed in them.

Nurses' patients as well as nurses may be operating concurrently within a number of other statuses and roles. Nurses and their patients may experience role conflicts in trying to fulfill the responsibilities of two or more roles. For example, a nurse's patient who is also a mother may find that fulfilling her responsibilities to herself for health-related self-care conflicts with her homemaking role and the role expectations she holds for her husband and children with respect to contributing to the conduct of the household. Persons under nursing and medical care who are confronted with a need to change life-style in order to care for themselves may not be able to do so until they have attended to the pressing duties of another role, for example, occupational role. Nurses should become able to help patients who have the necessary capacities to work out methods to become free enough, and therefore responsible enough, to provide or to manage their own self-care. Nurses and patients must learn to recognize and resolve role conflicts in order for them to achieve nursing goals.

THE PROBLEM OF VARIETY AND NUMBERS

In 1893 Florence Nightingale's descriptions of the "art of nursing the sick" and "health nursing or general nursing" were published and made available to nurses.[6] Nurses historically have served the sick and the well in a variety of settings. Nurses have worked in the homes of persons in need of nursing, in clinics, and in hospitals. They have worked with community groups and in industry in the interests of the prevention of injury and illness and toward the maintenance and promotion of desirable health states for individuals and communities. They have worked to improve sanitary conditions in hospitals. They were in the forefront of recognizing the importance of understanding the social and behavioral dimensions of health care and in caring for individuals based on a recognition of their uniqueness as persons.

It is questionable, however, whether nurses have adequately explored the problems of providing nursing in terms of (1) the variety of nursing requirements and (2) the numbers of individuals with a range of types of nursing requirements who need nursing at the same time in different locations. The problem of supplying the numbers of people who need or want a service is a perennial problem in all human services. But the combined problem of numbers of people and varieties of requirements is the perennial problem of the health care services.

The ability of nurses to creatively design adequate means for identifying and describing nursing requirements and to design, put into operation, and manage systems of nursing assistance for individuals, families, and groups is one characteristic of the *professional nurse*. Throughout nursing history there has been an inadequate number of nurses who could function to achieve these goals. Traditionally, nurses were trained to relate to individuals or groups under nursing care in order to (1) perform standardized nursing care measures for them and (2) socialize patients to institutional regimens to which nurses and patients were expected to conform. For many years the prevailing forms of education for nursing militated against the availability of nurses who were prepared and willing to accept professional responsibilities. For too long, nurses were unable (and some continue to be unable) to make the focus of nursing explicit and to speak knowingly about nursing to patients, co-workers, and health care administrators. How to look at people from a nursing perspective continues to be a problem in nursing circles. This problem will not be solved until nurses are able and willing to ask and answer the question: When and why can people be helped through nursing as distinguished from other forms of health care?

The problem of the variety and numbers of persons requiring nursing in many places at the same time requires the thoughtful and concerted work of both nursing administrators and nursing practitioners. Nursing administrators (for example, nurses who fill positions of supervisor, coordinator, or director of nursing divisions or units) bear an enabling responsibility that, when fulfilled, makes it possible for nursing practitioners in particular settings to proceed with nursing persons who have requirements for this service. Persons nursed may be members of relatively stable or rapidly changing nursing populations.

Over the years, organized nursing services, especially in hospitals and other resident care institutions, have tended to emphasize a hierarchy of administrative positions and deemphasize the positions of nursing practitioners. The enabling function of nurses in administrative positions in nursing services centers on the population to be provided with nursing, on the settings in which nursing is to be provided, and on ensuring that nursing practitioners and nurses are continuously present, qualified, and willing to nurse, and nurse effectively in a manner satisfying to their patients and to themselves.

The enabling function of nursing administrators has been thoughtfully examined and is effectively carried out by some nursing administrators. Some administrators have made and continue to make contributions to developing knowledge about providing nursing for populations.

A dimension of the problem of the variety of requirements for nursing and the numbers of persons in need of it is the need for continued study of the nursing requirements of populations and their subgroups. On an institution or agency basis, this is viewed as a responsibility of nursing administrators. On a local community basis, it should be a function of professionally qualified practitioners of public health nursing working in collaboration with nursing administrations. On a state and national basis, special projects and programs sponsored by nursing and other health care organizations, including federal agencies, are required. Because the nursing requirements of individual members of populations vary with conditioning effects of factors such as age, developmental state, and health state, studies of nursing requirements of populations must be continuous. Such studies could be articulated with a foundational structure for a developing science of nursing economics.

ROLE COMBINATIONS

The primary work of nurses is to provide nursing in accord with the needs people have in assuming responsibility for, in producing, and in managing their health–related self-care. The practitioner of nursing, the nurse, is the designer and provider of nursing. Nurses cannot become and remain competent practitioners, however, unless they know and are able to apply nursing and nursing-related knowledge in their practice. This knowledge should be continuously formulated and validated through the work of nursing theorists, researchers, and the developers of nursing technologies, techniques, and rules of practice. The status and role of nurse, therefore, should be linked always to that of *scholar or student of nursing* and *of nursing-related disciplines.* Too many nurses remain intellectually impoverished in their chosen field in an age characterized by explosions of knowledge in the health care disciplines and the disciplines related to them. Anyone entering nursing should understand the essentiality of combining the status and role of nursing practitioner with that of nursing student or scholar. The dual role is necessary for the adequate provision of nursing.

Individuals cannot develop themselves as practitioners of nursing and as students of nursing without teachers. Some members of the nursing profession elect to teach nursing students. Ideally, teachers of nursing are prepared and are advancing in proficiency as nursing practitioners while becoming advanced scholars in one or more areas of nursing and in one or more nursing-related disciplines. Some teachers of nursing have not advanced themselves as nursing scholars. It is difficult, if not impossible, for nurses and nursing students to develop as scholars in fields as new as nursing science when they are without adequate guidance from advanced nursing scholars.

Because of the type of education they elect and the roles in which they choose to become proficient, nurses contribute to the maintenance of nursing in social groups in different ways. Nurses who function in the roles of nursing theorists, researchers, developers of nursing technologies, and teachers should be contributing to the advancement and further development of present and future nursing practitioners (see Figure 4-1). The role of *developer* should be afforded greater recognition in nursing. It is the nurse developer who moves the findings of nursing science into a nursing practice frame of reference by inventing processes, technologies, techniques, artifacts, and rules for their use and by determining their effectiveness and reliability in practice settings. At times, developers invent valid and reliable ways of doing things, and only later are the scientific foundations of these new practices identified.

SUMMARY

Endeavors associated with provisions for nursing's availability and its production have societal features. **Societies** as enduring unities of interdependent persons function to maintain themselves and relate individuals to the total unity, the whole that is the society. This relating of individuals to the whole is accomplished, for example, by definition of roles, establishment of organized human groups, and exercise of constraint through regulations and laws to guide individual and group behavior. A society also can be viewed from the perspective of the ordered patterns of relationships and action patterns of its members. This social system view is relevant to understanding the societal features of nursing.

Nursing and nurses in societies where nursing is provided become parts of a number of organized human groups and related action systems. Systems include systems of education (for the occupations and professions), systems for the provision of health care, and systems of rules and laws that regulate the practice of various professions, the establishment and operation of businesses, and the establishment and operation of corporations. These systems have considerable public recognition. Other societal features of nursing, however, are more obscure. These include the demand to maintain nursing as an effective, available health service, the need to effectively formalize the structure of nursing in service enterprises and to provide for the proper functioning of nurses in them, the need for continuous study of and making provision for meeting existent and projected requirements of populations for nursing, and the need to foster understanding of and preparation for the essential roles of nurses in order to keep nursing viable in societies. These are heavy demands.

In summary, several general statements about nursing practice can be made. The statements may stimulate thought or discussion of nursing as a human service:

1. Nursing relationships in society are based on a state of imbalance between the *abilities of nurses to prescribe, design, manage, and maintain systems* of therapeutic self-care for individuals and the *abilities of these individuals or their families to do so.* In other words, the nurses' abilities exceed those of other individuals. When the imbalance is in the opposite direction or when there is no imbalance, there is no valid basis for a nursing relationship.

2. Nursing practice has not only technologic aspects but also moral aspects, because nursing decisions affect the lives, health, and welfare of human beings. Nurses must ask if it is right for the patient as well as if it will work.

3. Solutions proposed to problems of the management and maintenance of therapeutic self-care for patients and families with limited ability to maintain their own care may give rise to other problems, solutions to which may be difficult if not impossible.

References

1. Dock LL, Stewart IM: *A short history of nursing,* ed 3, New York, 1931, GP Putnam's Sons, pp 99-103.
2. Stewart IM, Austin AL: *A history of nursing,* ed 5, New York, 1962, GP Putnam's Sons, pp 84-87.
3. Roberts MM: *American nursing,* New York, 1959, Macmillan, pp 7-17, esp. p 8.
4. Plattel MG: *Social philosophy,* Pittsburgh, 1965, Duquesne University Press, p 53.
5. Developed in the 1950s, the Division of Hospital and Institutional Services, Indiana State Board of Health, revised by D Orem, 1975 and 1989.
6. Nightingale F: Sick nursing and health nursing. In Hampton IA et al, editors: *Nursing of the sick 1893,* New York, 1949, McGraw-Hill, pp 24-25.

CHAPTER 5

Interpersonal Features of Nursing

Nursing has been described as a human service concerned with the health and well-being of individuals and groups. More specifically, nursing has been described as a helping service concerned with aiding individuals to accomplish goals for themselves that they are unable to accomplish without help from others. Knowledge about human health services and helping services provides broad frames of reference for developing insights about nursing. Nursing itself has been explained as a service provided by persons who are legitimately qualified as nurses to produce systems of care for individuals (patients or clients) with health-associated limitations for regulating their own functioning or that of their dependents by meeting their own or their dependents' therapeutic self-care demands. Nursing care directed to knowing and meeting patients' therapeutic self-care demands and to patients' regulating the exercise or development of their capabilities for engaging in self-care or dependent-care is a form of health care.

All human services demand **social encounter** if one person is to serve and another person is to be served. Social encounter in all human service has societal, interpersonal, and technological features. Societal features that link nurses to persons who become their patients or clients include the legitimacy of the nurse-patient relationship, the contractual nature of the relationship, features of contractual relationships, rights and responsibilities of contracting parties before the law, legal and professional limits on the conduct of nurses, and the legality of refusals and demands of patients. Some of these societal features of nursing were addressed in Chapter 4.

This chapter addresses the person-to-person relationships and interactions of nurses and patients through which the technological features of nursing are made operational. The object or subject matter considered is nurses and patients as *persons* who relate to one another within a societal frame of reference for nursing purposes. Purposes of such relationships can be defined broadly in terms of the continued life, health, development, and well-being of the person who is patient and more narrowly in terms of nursing. Person-to-person relationships and interactions produce enabling conditions for nurses' design and production of nursing care; this includes patients' participation in care in accord with their developed deliberate action capabilities, their health-associated action limitations, and their potentials for overcoming existent or projected self-care limitations.

Some of the societal and interactional aspects of nursing were named in Fig. 4-4. The societal aspects named are of a static nature; they place individuals by their orientations to health care, their roles, and their dynamic sense of duty into a structure of positions and roles. The interactional aspects of nursing named in the figure are dynamic; they include the working or instrumental features of nursing, such as contact, interaction, and collaboration in decision making and production of care. The interpersonal features of nursing can be viewed as instrumental means for the design and production of nursing care.

It must be understood by nurses and nursing students that action demands for and existence of interpersonal relationships of nurses and patients do not explain the reasons for such relationships. The self-care deficit theory of nursing expressed in Chapter 2 is offered as an explanation of the reasons for the interrelated societal, interpersonal, and technological features of nursing in concrete nursing practice situations.

The development of the interpersonal features of nursing begins with consideration of the nature and limits of nurse-patient relationships. Variations in nurse-patient interactions are identified. This is followed by examination of factors affecting persons in relationships in nursing practice situations. The chapter is concluded with a consideration of types of interpersonal systems generated in nursing practice situations and relevant nurse characteristics.

NATURE AND LIMITS OF NURSE-PATIENT RELATIONSHIPS

The interpersonal features of nursing are based on existent contractual relationships of nurses and patients. As described in Chapter 4, how these relationships are brought about varies from direct agreements between nurses in private practice and their patients to institutional and agency arrangements for patients to receive nursing and for nurses who are institutional or agency employees to produce nursing. The nurse-patient relationship from a contractual perspective is for the purpose of patients receiving and participating in nursing and nurses producing it. If institutions and agencies do not provide nursing but provide types of task-oriented services, persons seeking nursing should be so informed and not be led to expect nursing and be charged for nursing.

The nurse-patient relationship is a *complementary relationship.* Complementary is used in the sense that the production of nursing care by nurses and patients' participation in care produces a *whole system of action* to achieve the human regulatory purposes expressed by patients' calculated therapeutic self-care demands. The emphasis here is on the interpersonal cooperative action of nurses and patients to produce organized systems of action in time and over time to know and meet the self-care requisites of patients, including selection of ways and means for meeting them. When nurses' patients are unable to cooperate or participate because of their physical or psychic conditions, nurses must produce whole systems of required care, making up for patients' total to near total incapacities for voluntary action. In some situations of this type, dependent-care agents contribute to care production.

Existent and concrete nurse-patient relationships are interpersonal relationships. Adults, adolescents, and older children will have reached some state of personality development. The personalities of persons who come together in a social encounter for nursing or other purposes affect what can and what will occur. This area of knowledge is of importance to nursing students and nurses. Gordon W. Allport's volume of essays titled *Personality and Social Encounter* is an important authoritative historical source about this area of knowledge.[1]

Nurses are young or older adults; patients are of all ages, infants to aged adults. Patients of nurses can be at any one of the known stages of growth and development and in various stages of personality formation. According to their ages, nurses and patients may vary in life experiences and in understanding demands of living under a range of sociocultural-economic conditions. In their interpersonal encounters, nurses and patients reveal themselves to one another, including their beliefs, how they value things, and the meanings they attach to the environmental features of situations in which they find themselves.

There are experienced nurses, and there are persons experienced in being patients of nurses. But there are also neophyte nurses and neophytes at being patients of nurses. Nurses as well as patients may have limited to highly developed social skills for being with and working with others. Abilities of each to initiate contacts and communicate will vary. The ability to be one's self, to be natural yet properly reserved with strangers in accord with conditions and circumstances, is a mark of personal maturity in the initiation of contacts and in interpersonal deliberations.

Nursing students often express desires to take care of people, to help people. To fulfill such desires nursing students must (1) continuously engage in forming themselves as nurses and (2) form or re-form themselves as persons with a "basic affectional relationship in the world around them that gives a sense of kinship and belonging" (p. 215).[2] According to Arnold, variations of the positive emotion of human love that reflect union with others include "fellow feeling," "empathy and sympathy." These variations of human love are indispensable for nurses in fulfillment of their desires to help people. Other variations of the positive emotion of love that may affect the interpersonal relations of nurse and patient include love of beauty, the joy of making and doing, mirth and laughter, religious emotions, and happiness that is the fulfillment of the whole personality in what is good and beautiful.[3]

These variations of the positive emotions of mature human love may be operational in both persons who are nurses and persons who are patients in nursing practice situations. They may be absent in one or both. When present, they are beneficial to each.

The foregoing types of expression of *human love* in interpersonal situations are expressions of the *essential humanness* of individuals. This essential humanness also is understood in terms of *personal freedom* or *liberty.* As expressed by Rahner, individuals use their innermost resources to form themselves, to determine the shapes of their lives as a whole and their ultimate realization of their own natures. Freedom here is understood not in the sense of power to constantly change one's course of action, but the power to decide what is to define one's life.[4] Both the giving that is the active element of mature love (Chapter 2) and the personal freedom of individuals as defined by Rahner foster effective interpersonal relationships. The essential humanness of persons also is expressed in the *unrestricted desire* to know.[5] This desire, when deliberately directed, fosters voluntary attention and can lead to systematic investigation.

These ideas about aspects of the essential humanness of men, women, and children can be keys to nurses' understanding of their own development as persons and their needs for self-development. Nurses should understand that the existence of men, women, and children lies in their development. They are beings in process.[6] Perfection from the viewpoint of development belongs not to the present but to the future (p. 495).[6] Actuality is just what happens to be. Nurses seek to know and work with themselves and their patients as they are but with some vision of what can be.

Nursing students are sometimes instructed that the *role of nurse* is to care for the "whole person" or the "whole patient." This advice may confuse or mislead students who are not helped to understand that the persons who are nurses' patients have requirements for nursing and at the same time have requirements for other kinds of care and help, for example, support from family and friends, spiritual support, medical care, and instruction. Nurses associate and communicate with the *persons* who are their patients and provide the specialized kind of care that is named nursing. They also cooperate with patients and their families to ensure that other kinds of care needed or desired are provided. Nurses sometimes elect to help persons who are their patients, as people commonly help one another as needs arise. When this occurs, both nurse and patient should know that what is done is outside the nurse role. Nurses must exercise prudence in not taking on professional role responsibilities from other fields of human service.

Contact and interpersonal exchanges between nurses and patients in practice situations vary in frequency, duration, and initiator of contact. Nurses need to manage the interpersonal components of practice toward the production of required nursing and at the same time to protect and foster the well-being of patients. Interpersonal contact and communication require effort and energy expenditure by both patient and nurse. This is illustrated by a seriously ill patient who said to his nurse, "Don't tell me one more thing; just take care of me." Patients vary in their tolerance for contact and associations in accord with their temperament, their degree and kind of illness, and their available energy.

Ideally, the interpersonal relationship between a nurse and a patient contributes to the alleviation of the patient's stress and that of the family, enabling the patient and the family to act responsibly in matters of health and health care. A relationship that permits a patient to develop and maintain confidence in the nurse and in himself or herself is the foundation for a deliberate process of nursing that contributes positively to the patient's achievement of present and future health goals.*

NURSE-PATIENT RELATIONSHIPS AND INTERACTIONS

If nurses are to come to know how their patients or clients can and should be helped through nursing and proceed to help them, they must be in person-to-person relationships with them. In social encounter and through interaction with patients and their significant others, nurses, in accord with existent conditions and circumstances, take nursing histories (Appendix A) and engage in nursing diagnosis, including gathering information about what patients are experiencing, how they perceive their own needs for care, and their health states, as well as physical appraisals, developmental appraisals, and mental health appraisals of patients. Nurses prescribe and collaborate with patients and their significant others about components of patients' therapeutic self-care demands and work out designs and plans for meeting them.

The Relationship

The message here is that the interpersonal relation of nurse and patient is not an end in itself. Such relationships in society are deliberately brought about and

---

*Ida Jean Orlando, *The dynamic nurse-patient relationship,* Putnam, New York, 1961, and Ernestine Wiedenbach, *Clinical nursing: a helping art,* Springer, New York, 1964, focus on behavior of nurse and patient during the nursing process. Dorothy Johnson, The nature of a science of nursing, *Nurs Outlook* 59:291-294, 1959, and Dorothy Johnson, A philosophy of nursing, *Nurs Outlook* 59:198-200, 1959, indicate the nurse's role in alleviation of the patient's stress.

continue for brief or prolonged periods of time so that nursing-related health care needs of members of society can be determined and met by persons qualified to do so. In the 1960s, a psychiatric mental health nursing specialist remarked, "I sometimes get the impression that nurses understand nursing as being nothing but an interpersonal relationship."* One wonders if the same belief is not having a resurgence among nurses.

A **relation** implies a connection, an order between a class of entities having at least two members. Interpersonal relations imply connections, order between and among persons. The connections, the order between persons who are nurses and persons who need and can be helped through nursing, must be deliberately brought about. As previously described, a contract or agreement to provide and to receive nursing legitimates the relationship of a nurse and a patient. Given such an agreement, it is necessary for the persons involved to relate themselves to one another as persons unified in action for the benefit of the person who is the nurse's client or patient. When patients because of their states of health, for example, comatose states, cannot relate themselves, nurses must relate themselves not only to the patients through contact, observation, and care but also to the person(s) socially responsible for each patient.

Nurse-Patient Interactions

Interaction means reciprocal action or influence. Within the context of a nursing practice situation, the consideration is what each one (nurse and patient) says and does and their influences upon one another. In concrete situations of nursing practice, nurse and patient are present to one another. Each (when patients are capable) knows the other as *you* and self as *I;* each, if willing, can speak intelligently about himself or herself, about what has been or is being experienced, or about what can or should be done within the situational context. The tangible **interdependence** of nurse and patient with respect to their functioning and their actions and reactions is the essential feature for their generation of systems of interaction or reciprocal influence during the duration of a nursing practice situation. If there is no *nurse,* there is no relationship, no interaction, and no nursing.

Nurses function in a professionally responsible position with respect to the life, health, and well-being of persons who are their patients. Nurses must manage themselves as persons who are nurses. The interpersonal dimensions of a nursing practice situation can interfere with or enhance (1) nurses' endeavors to provide patients with safe and effective nursing according to their needs or (2) patients' search for nursing care. The fear or anger of a patient will influence what a nurse experiences and what he or she does. Nurses who are not at ease with patients affect patients' responses to them. The degree of socialization of nurses to people within a broad range of sociocultural-economic orientations is a major influence on nurses' interpersonal effectiveness with patients.

---

*A personal conversation of J. Backscheider and the author.

Nurse-patient interactions in concrete nursing practice situations, all things being equal, vary with the personalities of the parties involved. Granted personality differences, the question arises whether there are other factors that condition what is offered, given, or manifested in nurse-patient interactions. Related to this is the question, How can the modalities or forms or characteristics of systems of nurse-patient interactions be described? The second question is addressed first because the form or characteristics of systems of social interaction provide categories within which to locate answers to the question about factors that can condition, that is, affect the characteristics of nurse-patient relationships and interactions.

FORMS OR MODALITIES OF INTERDEPENDENCE AND INTERACTION

In his study of relationships among members of groups, *Social and Cultural Dynamics,* Sorokin identifies and names characteristics of human **interaction systems.** These include the overall conditioning effect of each person on the other person; the extensity, intensity, duration, and continuity of interactions; the differences in the aspirations of interacting persons; and the organization or lack of organization of the positions and roles of interacting parties.[7]

Overall conditioning effects are identified as *two-sided or mutual conditioning* and *one-sided conditioning* or *one-sided dependency* (p. 438).[7] Sorokin identified one-sided conditioning with the power that one person can exercise over another person, placing the person in a psychologically as well as socially dependent relationship to the person exercising power, as with prisoners and their guards. In nursing and in health care situations, *mutual conditioning* should prevail even when patients are not aware or rationally conscious. Nurses and health professionals observe and respond to patients as they are, and their actions are performed in the interests of the life, health, and well-being of patients. *One-sided conditioning* as described by Sorokin is approximated when nurses respond to patients as objects, distance themselves from patients, or refuse to listen and take into consideration patient requests or what patients say about existent conditions. It may exist in an outright form when so-called health workers victimize persons under their "care," abuse them physically or psychologically, or prevent persons from doing what they can and should do with rationality and reason under existent conditions and circumstances.

Extensity of interaction in interpersonal situations refers to the proportions of each individual's activities and experiences out of their whole system of living that are conditioned by their interactions (pp. 438-439).[7] Extensity of interactions can range from encompassing all or nearly all aspects of daily living to a narrow segment of it.

Mothers and fathers caring for their infants over the 24 hours of the day and closely knit families have highly encompassing systems of interaction. In health care settings, for example, patients under intensive care from nurses and physicians may have all or nearly all aspects of living conditioned by their dependence on health care professionals. Nurses and other professionals who are with patients during segments of each day because of on- and off-duty hours have periods of freedom from interaction with patients. All-encompassing demands on nurses or family members for interaction with persons who are suffering physical or psychic illnesses or disabling conditions are both physically and psychologically exhausting for them as care providers.

Nursing situations, in terms of extensity of systems of interaction, vary from the foregoing types of situations mentioned, to the moderate extensity of nurses' systems of interactions with their patients who suffer chronic illness and who do engage in self-care, to the narrow extensity of a system of interaction with a patient having a routine health assessment or for whom a nurse performs a care measure that a patient cannot perform for self.

Intensity of interaction has reference to the influence within a system of interaction of what one person experiences or does on the feelings, thoughts, and actions of the other (p. 440).[7] One individual's actions and experiences may be profoundly influenced by everything that the other individual does or by what happens to him or her, as in a highly integrated family. In other interpersonal relationships only major events in the life of one person influence the other. Intensity, including depth of influence of one person on the other, varies with the meaning that they attach to actions and experiences. Some patients respond with a depth of insight and feeling to nursing care that brings relief and comfort and freedom from fear that they will not be cared for. Nurses and other health professionals may be deeply influenced by their interactions with patients who show courage and fortitude under disabling and life-threatening conditions. What is happening to family members of patients may deeply affect nurses and other care givers.

Duration and continuity of interaction refers to the time span of a concrete system of interaction. It also takes into consideration the influence of prior interactions on subsequent actions and experiences of individuals (p. 440).[7] Interactions may take place and endure for only a brief time, as when a customer purchases groceries from a specific store; such episodic interactions may occur only once or may continue for years. Interaction within families, by contrast, may continue throughout the lifetimes of family members, and the influence of some family members on others can continue even after their deaths. Duration and continuity of nurse-patient interactions vary over a range that is positively definable in terms of the nature of patients' requirements for nursing.

The *direction of interaction* and the *organization of interactions* are modalities described by Sorokin (pp. 441-444).[7] *Direction* refers to the concurrence or lack of concurrence of the aspirations and efforts of one person with the aspirations and efforts of the other person. When there is lack of concurrence as well as resistance and antagonism, the direction is *contrary* and the interaction is "mutually antagonistic." Persons may concur only in part of what they aspire to do and in the efforts they expend. They may be antagonistic in other parts. Such interactions are *mixed*. All of these directions of interaction can be found in nursing practice situations. Resolution for the well-being of patients is demanded. Discussion and negotiation are required.

Organized and unorganized interactions refer to the existence of or lack of defined positions, role responsibilities, rights, and functions of interacting persons. Defined positions and roles and so forth would be based upon goals and values of services institutionalized within the group or the society. A functional family is an example of a system of organized relationships and interactions. In unorganized groups with undefined positions and role responsibilities, relationships and interaction are confused and vague. In concrete situations in society there may be gradual movement from the unorganized to well-organized groups of interacting persons.

In nursing practice situations the basis for organization of positions and roles is defined in terms of the nurse as provider of nursing and the patient as being in need of nursing. The role responsibilities of each are partially defined by the status of each. Within this organizational frame the number of nurses assigned to patients, their duties and their modes of relating must be worked out and understood. The methods of helping selected and used in nursing practice situations further define role responsibilities of nurses and patients.

Sorokin's modalities of systems of interaction is a general descriptive means for examining nurse-patient interdependence and systems of nurse-patient interaction. Reciprocal influence and action must always be understood by nurses within the frame of reference provided by the reason for the existence of nursing practice situations and the contractual nature of nurse-patient relationships. Nurses, however, cannot function therapeutically for their patients unless they seek to know and believe in the humanness of themselves and the persons for whom they provide care.

AN EXAMPLE OF THE ABSENCE OF NURSE-PATIENT INTERACTION AND THE ABSENCE OF NURSING

Excerpts from a document titled *Some Comments of a Patient (Mrs. K) about Her Experiences at X Hospital** are presented to illustrate what patients experience in the absence of systems of nurse-patient interaction directed to the well-being of patients. The *Comments* are illustrative of the absence of nursing care directed to helping patients know and meet their existent and emerging therapeutic self-care demands and in the safe use or development of their powers of self-care agency. The person, Mrs. K, who is the patient, is ignored and appears to be considered simply as an environmental feature to whom some work operations are directed.

The *Comments* are those of a mature woman, a nurse, written after a prolonged hospitalization. Mrs. K, at the age of 70, was admitted to the hospital by her physician, an internist, so that she could receive nursing while undergoing

---

*Unpublished, handwritten manuscript presented by Mrs. K to the author.

medical diagnostic procedures, some of which were intrusive. During the hospitalization, Mrs. K experienced a severe drug reaction and a series of pulmonary emboli. The experiences mentioned in the *Comments* are interspersed with generalizations and principles.

Mrs. K wrote, "I am interested as a professional person to help improve the situation." The *Comments,* written some years ago, express what persons continue to experience when nursing is not provided to persons in need of it.

The absence of effective nurse-patient relationships and an ongoing system of nurse-patient interactions was stressful to Mrs. K. With reference to interactions she made this statement: "It should be recognized that every conscious patient has a role in the design of the plan of care and in the execution of care measures."

Admission to the Nursing Unit

On my admission I was taken to my room by a candy striper [a young volunteer worker] and introduced to no one. It was approximately an hour and a half before anyone entered the room. Finally, a nurse came into the room and said: "How did you get in here?" I told her I had been brought to the room some time ago by a candy striper.

Some time later she came dancing into the room. She had, apparently, heard I was a nurse. She gave me a urine specimen bottle, cotton and other material and said: "Now be a good girl and let me have a mid-stream specimen." She gave no further instruction. When she returned for the specimen some time later she picked up the specimen joyfully and said: "That's a peach." I did not know whether she was referring to me or to the specimen.

The head nurse was on the unit that afternoon but she did not visit me, nor was I given any further information about tests that had been ordered, times of serving meals, how to use gadgets in the room and on the bed or anything else. Believe me, I felt ill-at-ease and rather lonely until the doctor arrived who did tell me what to expect about some things.

Off to a Bad Start

I did not see the head nurse the next morning until after the Patient Visitor* came into the room. She asked if I was comfortable and had what I needed. I told her the technicians had been having trouble in collecting blood and I said I would like to see the head nurse to see how we could proceed. (I had asked to see the head nurse twice before this.) The Patient Visitor immediately went to get the head nurse and things began to happen—including visits by a couple of technicians, the head nurse, and the supervisor.

By this time I felt that I had created a scene and had probably placed myself in the category of a difficult patient. It immediately made me reluctant to make even slight requests at times that might seem trivial or unnecessary. This set the stage so that I took care of myself for the most part during my entire hospital stay, even when I was very ill and was really unable to do much for myself.

No Nurse, No System of Interaction

I never really was conscious of having a specific person assigned to me in the role of nurse. All who came into my room, except the head nurse, seemed to be concerned with getting specific tasks done without evidence of awareness of how these tasks or jobs related to my personal well-being or for the achievement of my health-care goals. Most of the tasks performed were concerned with bed making and removing soiled linen from the room.

As far as I could determine, no one was assigned as "my nurse"—someone for me to talk

---

*Patient Visitors were assigned to hospital units as official representatives of the hospital.

with, confide in and ask questions of. After I was in the hospital for several weeks I finally realized that I was not expected to ask questions of anyone but the head nurse. And, of course, she was not on the unit at all times, and I had the feeling she was really too busy for me to take her time.

In my situation it appeared that the only person on the unit who really knew anything or very much about me was the head nurse—but as I pointed out I did not see her until the second day I was in the hospital.

Those members of the nursing personnel who came into my room to do anything, except for the administration of medicines, were practical nurses and aides, most of them being aides.

In this connection it is difficult for me to reconcile myself to the practice that a nursing aide be assigned to the full care of a patient. It would seem that her job is to assist the nurse and to be under her immediate direction and supervision at all times even though she may be performing many of the nursing care procedures.

An Emergency, No Nursing

When I had the first pain with the pulmonary embolus (early afternoon) I asked to see the nurse in charge (a relief nurse). I told her when she came in some time later that I thought my doctor was still in the building and perhaps she could reach him before he would leave. Without going into the details of all that happened that afternoon, I had no relief until my doctor's associate happened to come into my room about 6:30 P.M. He immediately ordered appropriate treatment. One order was to use a hot water bottle which arrived a couple of hours later. I was tense for several days after that experience. My own doctor advised me to call him direct in his office if I ever had a similar experience.

Exercising Power Over Patients

Most of the nursing personnel who came into my room were concerned with getting isolated tasks done, as I have said elsewhere. There was little or no observation of me or my surroundings by those assigned to take care of my room (I cannot say they were assigned to take care of me) except by the head nurse who was extremely observant. Those who took note of me and my surroundings were the head nurse and the Patient Visitor.

One communication barrier between me and the nursing personnel was the impression given that the nursing personnel were overworked and that they had no time to listen to patients, to observe symptoms and patients' environment, and to make the patients feel at home and comfortable in their surroundings.

One thing that bothered me was what seemed to be a general concept of what was considered to be the "good" or "ideal patient." This was evidenced by such remarks as: "Mrs. _____ is such a wonderful patient. She never asks for anything." "Mr. _____ just lies there without a word of complaint about anything that is done for him. He knows when we are too busy to do things for him." This sort of talk makes the usual patient conform to what the nursing personnel seem to describe as "good or appropriate patient behavior."

Meaning of the *Comments* for Nursing

The foregoing excerpts from a patient's *Comments* illustrate the absence of nurse-patient relationships and the absence of an effective system of nurse-patient interaction during the period of hospitalization. These excerpts as well as other material in the *Comments* also illustrate the absence in nurses or the inability of nurses to engage in nursing diagnosis, to prescribe the patient's therapeutic self-care demand, to identify her abilities as well as limitations for knowing and meeting the components of her therapeutic self-care demand, or to regulate her engagement in self-care in accord with health state factors. There was no evidence of a design for nursing care and planning for execution of the design to give direction to nurses, practical nurses, and aides.

The fact that Mrs. K initially was mobile and rationally conscious seemed to blot out any consideration that she could be unknowing about her condition and about how to care for herself in terms of her symptoms and the reason for hospital admission. There is no evidence that nursing personnel understood or maintained a nursing focus (see Figure 9-1). Nor is there evidence that there was understanding of the health focus(es) specific to Mrs. K and its meaning for health care and nursing. At the time of admission to the hospital, Mrs. K's health focus was oriented to "illness or disorder of undetermined origin with concern for the degree of illness, specific effects of the disorder, and the effects of specific diagnostic or therapeutic measures used." (Group 3, Classification of Nursing Situations By Health Focus, Chapter 9).

During the period of hospitalization with the occurrence of Mrs. K's experiencing the effects of pulmonary emboli and the illness associated with the severe drug reaction, the health focus became a Group 5 type. The health focus in this type is "oriented to regulation through active treatment of a disease or disorder or injury of determined origin, with concern for the degree of illness; the specific effects of the disease, disorder or injury; and the specific effects of the therapeutic measures used."

The offering of these excerpts descriptive of one individual's experiences and thoughts during a period of hospitalization serves two purposes. They illustrate the meaning of continuing nurse-patient relationships and interactions, and requirements for the presence of nurses who are interacting with patients and who know what nursing is and are able and willing to produce nursing for patients.

FACTORS CONDITIONING THE FEATURES OF NURSE-PATIENT RELATIONSHIPS AND INTERACTIONS

The legitimacy of occupancy of positions of nurse and nurse's patient derives from societal standards, laws regulating the practice of nursing, and qualifying conditions possessed by persons with the statuses of nurse and patient. Nurses and nurses' patients who are related under some type of agreement for the provision of nursing seek a relationship of instrumental effectiveness between the nursing capabilities of nurses and the nursing requirements of patients as defined by the nature of and the reasons for the existence of patients' self-care deficits. It is nurses' initial and continuing judgments about the presence of and reasons for patients' self-care deficits that establish and maintain the linkages between the social and technologic components of nursing practice.

The *interpersonal components* of nursing practice are enabling for both the social-contractual components and the technologic components of practice. Contact, association, and communication are essential interpersonal components required for bringing particular nurses into a nursing relationship with particular patients and for effecting arrangements for the provision of nursing. One result sought from interpersonal relations of nurses and patients and their families is a level of coordination that is enabling for the performance of the technologic work of nursing practice (see Table 12-1).

The level of cooperation attained among nurses, their associates, their patients, and persons with significant relations to patients is a function of the quality of the interpersonal relations among them and the effective designing of nursing systems. Mutual cooperation and effectively managed division of labor within nursing practice situations is *high-level* coordination. A high level of coordination allows considerable independence of cooperating individuals. Such a level of coordination requires role differentiation, acceptance of role responsibilities, knowledge of role articulations, and developed social, interpersonal, and communication skills of involved individuals. The world of the nurse is not the world of the patient. Nurses and their patients ideally search for some common ground from which they can move to relate and communicate so that what patients need is revealed and how nurses can help is communicated.

Conditioning factors that can affect the characteristics of nurse-patient relationships and interactions must be known to nursing students and nurses. They must have the knowledge and skills to understand and recognize the relevance of specific factors to their relationships with patients. Some of the same factors considered here as affecting nurse-patient relationships are treated in different ways in later chapters that focus on the technological aspects of nursing. In the later chapters the focus is on how factors named *basic conditioning factors* affect the values of the two patient variables *therapeutic self-care demand* and *self-care agency*. Here the focus is on the interpersonal rather than the technological features of nursing.

The question of interest here is, Given factor X, for example, a debilitating illness of a patient, how can and should nurses relate to patients and manage their interactions with them, and what relational and interactive behaviors can be expected from patients? Some factors that affect the interpersonal features of nursing are clear-cut and overtly evident to observant nurses in their initial and subsequent periods of contact with patients. Other factors reveal themselves throughout the course of the nursing practice situation to observant nurses. Factors affecting interpersonal relations and interactions are considered in three groups.

- Factors that condition the possibilities for and the quality of adaptive interchanges between nurses and patients, and nurses and others.
- Factors that affect the extensity, duration, and continuity of nurse-patient interactions.
- Factors that affect the quality of patient participation in the design and production of nursing.

The factors now considered relate to individuals who are patients. Relevant factors descriptive of nurses are considered under nurse characteristics. Some factors identified in these groups can remain relatively stable throughout the duration of nursing situations; other factors may change. Stability can be associated with the factor, such as gender or adulthood, or with how the factor is operative in an individual, such as a sensory deficit resulting from loss of vision. Change in factors is associated with both the nature of the factor and how the factor is operative in individuals. *Factor*[8] is used in the sense of a constituent element or component that is an effective force in a complex thing enabling the whole thing to do a particular kind of work or helping it in the production of a definite result.

Factors that remain stable or relatively stable throughout the duration of nursing situations should be understood and accepted by nurses as *conditions of action* that must be taken into account whenever nurses select ways and means to facilitate effective interactions with patients who, for example, have various forms of sensory deficits or language comprehension problems.

Factors Affecting Patients' Abilities to Relate to and Interact with Nurses

These are factors that are operative in enabling persons to be aware of themselves and their surroundings, to know what is going on, to respond to what they experience, and to know how they and others fit into situations in which they find themselves. Each factor can vary over a range of values and therefore have a range of effects on the performance or behavior of individuals. For example, attentiveness can range from the narrowly focused attention of an angry person, to the alert attentiveness of the interested, involved person, to absence of awareness as in sleep or comatose states.

Examples of factors that in some way affect patients' rational and interactive behaviors include:

- Arousal level and attentiveness as when:
  Awake and alertly attentive
  Awake and aware of surroundings but not attending to them
  Drowsy
  Asleep
  Anesthetized
  Confused
  Stuporous, comatose, delirious
  Alert with narrowly focused attention as in states of fear or anger
- Ability to maintain attention and exercise vigilance with respect to self and to environmental features so that perceptions and judgments have validity
- Ability to initiate and pursue contacts with others as ability is affected by age and developmental state, language skills, and developed social skills associated with personal, family, or group culture
- Ability to represent to others with adequate forcefulness existent conditions and circumstances, differentiating them from what is imagined
- Ability to converse and engage in dialogue about specific matters relevant to what is ongoing in a situation
- Needs of persons for solitude and their minimization or avoidance of social encounter, as in some forms of psychic illness
- Outright rejection of being under health care and nursing

- Rejection of individuals in the position of nurse by patients because of attitudes and values that may be related to age, gender, and other factors specific to persons in the position of nurse

The foregoing factors affect what patients can and cannot do or are willing to do in interpersonal situations with nurses to generate effective systems of interaction toward the production of nursing for patients. Recognition of the presence of factors such as the ones represented and their operation in individual patients places demands on nurses for regulation of the number and frequency of contacts with patients, the selection and use of valid interpersonal techniques including communication techniques, development of the art of conversation, overcoming reluctances to initiate contacts with persons or enter their personal space under conditions that are foreign to the cultural practices of the person who is nurse, development of the art of representation of facts and conditions, and circumstances and possibilities for effective action and consequences if action is not taken.

The presented listing of patient factors affecting patients' interactions with nurses is not exhaustive and not even adequately formulated. Nurses, in situations in which patients experience difficulties with relating to and interacting with them, should record and describe what is ongoing. If this is done, there would be movement toward more adequate identifications and description of factors. This would be a necessary, beginning movement toward the formulation and testing of interpersonal technologies of nursing practice.

Factors Affecting the Extensity, Duration, and Continuity of Interaction

The approach taken here is oriented to health care in the form of nursing or dependent-care. The question is, What factor(s) recognized by nursing practitioners (and dependent-care agents) should affect the extensity, duration, and continuity of their directed contacts and interactions with individuals for whom they bear care responsibilities? The critical human encompassing factor affecting the named modalities of interaction is the *self-management capabilities* of individuals being cared for. Self-management includes ability to manage self in stable or changing environments and the ability to manage one's personal affairs. In nursing or other types of care situations, *extensity and continuity* of contacts and interaction should *increase* with decreases in or absence of self-management capabilities of persons under care.

Some specific factors that negatively condition self-management capabilities of individuals are clear-cut, including states of dependency associated, for example, with:

- Infancy, early childhood, and extreme old age
- Developmental and functional states of infants born prematurely, of low birth weight, or with genetic or developmental defects
- Acute illness or serious injury at any age
- Uncompensated disabilities, physical or psychic
- Instability of vital human functioning, at any age, that endangers the continuance of life or future normalcy

- Debility with or without confusion
- Delirium
- Depression
- Chronic fear, chronic worry
- Panic

The foregoing examples specific to self-management capabilities of individuals and resultant needs for nurse contact and specialized communication requirements represent one extreme of dependency of individuals on nurses or dependent-care agents in their daily living. The other extreme is represented by persons who are able to manage themselves and their affairs but lack at a particular time the required knowledge and the skill adaptations needed to proceed effectively with an aspect(s) of self-care or dependent-care. Such individuals may have extensive knowledge of their own modes of functioning and about care of self or dependents. Interacting with these individuals may be difficult for nurses who lack confidence in their abilities, in what they know and what they can do. There is, of course, a middle range where persons have periodic needs for nurse contact and interaction about some aspects of self-care or dependent-care on a daily, weekly, or monthly basis.

The requirements for extensity and continuity of interaction with patients provide *one basis* for judging time requirements for nursing. Specific factors affecting extensity of interaction also may be indicators of the importance of nursing for the life, health, and well-being of patients and the meaning that the provision of nursing has for patients and persons related to them.

The duration of nurse-patient interactions varies with the nature of factors that gave rise to the need for interactions. Factors may necessitate interactions of extreme extensity, continuity, and long duration, as with seriously ill, incapacitated persons. Factors, such as experiencing pain or being uncomfortable, apprehensive, or fearful, that can be brought under control by appropriate use of care technologies may require interactions of relatively short duration over some time period. This also holds for patients' needs for guidance and direction as they perform care measures or engage in skill development or when nurses routinely perform care measures for patients.

Factors Affecting the Quality of Patient Participation

Patients' participation and cooperation with nurses in the receiving and giving of nursing care is influenced by age, developmental state, degree of maturity or personalization, and arousal levels and abilities to attend to themselves and their environments. Given values of these factors that are enabling for participation, other factors also affect patient participation. These factors include the following:

1. Self-image as responsible person and as self-care or dependent-care agent identified from:
   a. Self-reference expressions, for example, "I have been doing my best to manage my care," or "I have been taking good care of my child."
   b. More specific expressions about role in current health care situation, role expectations of others, role relationships to others

    c. Expressions of patients about how they are affected by what they are or have been experiencing

    d. Explicit statements about what has been done in self-care or dependent-care, what can no longer be done, and the effectiveness or ineffectiveness of care

    e. Explicit statements about present requirements for care

2. What patients attend to voluntarily, what they are preoccupied with.

3. Interests and concerns as revealed by recurring conversational themes or as deliberately communicated by patients or persons related to them:

    a. Expressions of interest in and concern for their health state or specific features of it

    b. Expressions of interest in and knowledge of health and health care

    c. Expressions of interest and concerns about personal matters other than their health care that precludes their attending to self-care matters, for example, family affairs

4. Evidence of developed and operable human powers that indicate how patients do conduct themselves when they must act deliberately to attain sought-after results. Such evidence need not be related to self-care or dependent-care. Evidence would relate to what patients do and do not do with respect to:

    a. Initiating action sequences and carrying them through to completion of the task, including:

        (1) Eliciting aid as needed to complete a task

        (2) Directing and maintaining attention on self, on actions in process, and on relevant environmental conditions

    b. Modes of thinking about reality situations, for example, at the level of the concrete or abstract*

    c. Being reflective about actions performed and expressing judgments about them

    d. Making decisions

    e. Conserving available energy

    f. Controlling positioning, ambulating, and engaging in manipulative movements

Information about these factors that affect the quality of patient participation is important to nurses in all situations in which patients are adult and capable of managing themselves in their environments. Information about named factors reveals action abilities and action limitations of a general nature that are indexes of how patients can participate and the adjustments that nurses need to make in using various methods of helping. For example, when patients think concretely, directions and instructions should be phrased in terms of specific things to be done and the sequences in which they are to be done.

---

*See Nursing Development Conference Group, Orem DE, editor: *Concept formalization in nursing: process and product,* ed 2, Little, Brown, Boston, 1979, pp. 215-229, esp. pp. 219-229, for an account of Joan Backscheider's work in classifying intellectual operations of an adult ambulatory nursing population with indications of meaning for nursing.

SYSTEMS OF INTERACTION

It is understood in concrete situations of nursing practice that the social, interpersonal, and technological features of nursing practice together constitute an action process. The separation out and analysis of some interpersonal modalities of nursing practice are for purposes of understanding interaction demands on nurses that arise in different contexts.

Interactional systems in nursing are divided in two groups according to the age and the sensory and rational consciousness of persons who are patients.

Group One. Patients are adults, environmentally aware, rational, capable of self-management, but not necessarily able to control their position and movement in space.

- Patient and nurse roles (including role content) are clearly defined and accepted; there is an active cooperative relationship between nurse(s) and patient characterized by an effective communication process, current conditions and circumstances are attended to in the design and performance of care operations, and goals sought through self-care and nursing operations articulate with the patient's broader health goals and with care operations performed by other health care professionals.
- Patient and nurse roles continue to be in process of definition; some ideas of nurse and patient about self-care and nursing operations or performance responsibilities are in conflict; resolution of differences or conflicting goals is an ongoing part of the communication process; the nurse(s) proceeds with performance of nursing operations necessary to protect the life, health, and well-being of the patient with patient's acceptance of them, however reluctantly.
- Nurse role is clearly defined, effectively performed, and acceptable to the patient; the patient's role responsibilities, what the patient can and should do now and in the future with respect to self-care and in establishing and maintaining cooperative relationships with health care professionals or with persons taking on dependent-care responsibilities, are under investigation.

Group Two. Patients are adults or infants and children whose powers of self-management are undeveloped, developed but limited, or when developed are not operational; patients have limited or no awareness of the environment and limited or no ability to attach meaning to what is sensed and perceived; patients' powers to contact and deliberately communicate with nurses or other care givers is limited or nonoperational; contact and communication with and responsiveness to patients is dependent upon the presence and the operations of nurses.

- Infants and young children by stage of development who are well or ill
- Older children and adults with limited power to attend to environmental features and to make rational and reasonable judgments and decisions on which to base their actions
- Children and adults with loss of awareness and no ability to attend or to attach meaning to environmental features

These suggestions about features of systems of nurse-patient interdependence and interaction are offered as guides to further understanding of the interpersonal features of nursing practice situations. They may lead to insights about conditions that guide nurses' selection and use of methods of helping (Chapter 3). They also point to the kinds of knowledge and the opportunities for interpersonal skill development that should be provided for in professional-level education for nursing.

The descriptions of features affecting nurse-patient interdependence and systems of interaction set some developmental requirements for nursing students and nurses. Developmental endeavors are to ensure that they are or are becoming capable to be with and work with patients as persons who have requirements for health care in the form of nursing. Capabilities included in the following list (as well as ones previously identified) are offered as examples.

- Establish contacts, negotiate agreements, and maintain contacts with persons who need nursing and those who seek it for them
- Interact and communicate with persons under nursing care and their significant others under ranges of conditions and circumstances that facilitate or hinder interactions and communication
- Direct interactions and communications toward the development of interpersonal, functional unities
- Allow persons under nursing care time to reflect about and appraise what has been represented to them as desirable courses of action
- Provide for the privacy desired and required by persons under nursing care
- Through attitudes and behavior show respect for persons under nursing care
- Know and represent to others the interactional capabilities of persons under nursing care
- Maintain a dynamic sense of duty in all nursing practice situations

Development of the personal capabilities to function in the described ways requires not only developed skills but also experiential and speculative knowledge organized around nursing considered as a human service to persons in a range of states of dependency on nurses and others.

FURTHER CONSIDERATIONS

To be able to view themselves realistically as persons who render nursing care, nurses must have the time and preparation to give the care required by the patient. Education and experience in nursing and the scope of responsibility for nursing patients should influence that view. Many factors affect the willingness of the nurse to render care. Some nurses frequently specify lack of time as a result of the many demands on them. Other nurses refer to patients as "difficult" or "easy," thereby implying the kind and degree of effort involved in rendering care. The patient's age, gender, race, culture, social status, or disease factors also have an effect on the nurse's willingness to render care. In fact, some nurses develop preferences about the types of patients for whom they are willing to render care. In the last analysis, the quality and availability of nursing care in specific nursing situations is based on the unconditional willingness of individual nurses to render care.

Socialization in nursing situations is required because nurses and patients are usually strangers and they must enter into helping relationships. A patient may need preparation in fulfilling the patient role in the nursing situation. Temperament, self-image, and pattern of living may affect the patient's ability to accept the role of patient. Further, the nurse's gender, age, culture, or socioeconomic status may facilitate or hinder the patient's performance in the patient role. Similarly, these same factors, as they relate to the patient, may have an effect on the nurse's performance of the nurse role.

The socializing process may continue throughout the period the patient requires nursing care. It is not merely an initial effort on the part of the nurse and the patient to adjust to their roles in the situation, but a continued effort to carry out their roles and to understand their relationships with other persons who are providing care in the situation. The nurse sometimes must ask, Is the patient able to participate in his or her own health care by giving essential information to the physician or to others? The following excerpts from recorded material about a nursing case present an example of a need for help in this direction. It is evident from these excerpts that the nurse and the patient had established an effective nurse-patient relationship and that the patient trusted the nurse. The progress made by the patient as a result of his own socializing efforts is also evident. The observations were made and recorded by Sister Gretta Monnig.[9]

> The patient was sitting in a chair when the surgeon made rounds. The doctor remarked that this was enema day. The patient said nothing about the enema but told the surgeon he felt fine. After the surgeon had left the room, the nurse remarked that she would get the enema. The patient replied, "I do not need an enema; I had a bowel movement this morning." The nurse asked why he had not told the surgeon.
>
> "I take a look at all those doctors and can't think of a thing to say. Do the other patients feel this way?" he asked.
>
> The nurse replied, "Most patients think of their questions after their doctor has been in to see them. It must be hard to ask questions in front of a large group of people."
>
> "All those people scared me. I was afraid that my questions would sound silly," replied the patient.
>
> The nurse asked, "Is it easier to talk to the doctor when he makes rounds to change your dressings?"
>
> "He always seems to be in a hurry," replied the patient.
>
> "How about the doctor who comes in the evening?" asked the nurse.
>
> "He is a fine doctor," said the patient. "I usually save my questions for him, but I still forget to ask him."
>
> "Would writing the questions on a slip of paper help you to remember what you want to ask the doctor?" asked the nurse.
>
> "I will try that," replied the patient.
>
> In the evening the patient said, "I wrote down my questions today. The doctor answered every one of them. He talked to me quite a while. I never realized how interesting doctors are." After that evening the patient appeared more at ease when the doctors made rounds.

Ideally, then, the socializing efforts of nurses help them to know their patients and how to direct their efforts in encouraging patients to better cope with socializing activities in health situations. When children are involved, their developmental state and physical dependence on adults are of prime importance in the socializing aspects of the nursing situation. The nurse who gives care to children has a dual function in socialization activities. The nurse must continue, along with the parents, to aid the child in normal development. Under the conditions imposed by illness or special health needs, a child is confronted by physicians and other adults who place a variety of demands on both the child and the parents. Fostering the child's movement toward independence during illness through socializing activities is an important nursing task. Supervised contacts with other children may be of great importance in the socialization of children in institutional settings. Some 3-year-old children, for example, can effectively demonstrate to another child how to behave under conditions new to them—where and when to wash the face and hands, where to eat, and the proper use of utensils.

Closely related to socialization is the nurse's and the patient's awareness of overt and covert problems in health care situations. The case material on the socialization of the patient demonstrated that the patient was aware of his inability to communicate with the physicians attending him and recognized his need to change that behavior. It was up to the nurse to assist him in changing. The nurse cannot do this effectively unless he or she understands and accepts the nurse's and the patient's role in the nursing situation.

Personal factors that help to describe the nurse include (1) *age, gender, race, and physical and constitutional characteristics;* (2) *health state, socioeconomic status, culture, and roles in family and community;* and (3) *maturity as a person.* These personal factors are the ones most likely to influence nurses' relations to patients. The age and gender differences between the patient and the nurse are of considerable importance. A male patient, for example, may be either willing or reluctant to accept assistance from a female nurse. Health and the changes that normally occur with aging may limit what nurses can do regardless of what they are willing to do. For these reasons some norms related to personal factors are specified as pertinent considerations in certain types of nursing positions.

A nurse's socioeconomic and cultural background may influence the requirements for socializing efforts in a given situation. Nurses must be cognizant of the similarities and differences between the patient's pattern of living and their own that may have an influence on both the patient and themselves. Some nurses have a tendency to look at certain patterns of living as inferior merely because these practices are different from their own or from their ideal.

The nurse's maturity as a person determines how he or she will perceive himself or herself and the patient within a helping relationship. Mature nurses have a realistic view of themselves. Family and community demands may exert a desirable or an undesirable influence on a nurse. Lack of energy, lack of interest, and preoccupation with matters outside the nursing situation are some of the effects family and community demands may create. There are also positive effects; for example, the demands of family and community may stimulate the nurse's interest in people and in solving problems of living. Enlightened motivation and wisdom in helping and working with people in interpersonal situations are important positive effects that accrue to the mature nurse.

Nurses make judgments and decisions about themselves, their families, and their patients. The quality of the judgments and decisions they make gives expression to their personal commitments and their sense of responsibility in life situations. The state of personal moral development achieved by a nurse affects the characteristics of the decisions the nurse makes in nursing situations as well as in other situations. Nursing students should have learning experiences that will facilitate their moral development. Nurses in practice should examine the decisions they make in nursing situations in order to achieve understanding of themselves, the deliberate choices they made, their understanding of the options open at the times the choices were made, and the relationship between what they know and what they do. A nurse may know what should be done when particular conditions prevail in a nursing situation, but of vital concern to both nurse and patient is the actual decision the nurse makes.

Responsible nurses evaluate their own nursing performance in light of the patient's requirements for care. They seek and accept nursing supervision and strive to develop as nurses. They identify factors in nursing situations that interfere with patient progress and are able and unafraid to act to bring about change or represent these conditions to other responsible persons. Changes in nursing practice come about to the degree that nurses are both knowledgeable and responsible.

The relationships between nurses and patients vary in duration from hours to days to months to years. Nurses must be able to enter into short-term and long-term relationships with patients with a view toward rendering effective help for short periods of time or over a prolonged period of time with either periodic or continuous contact.

Nurses must know why persons are under health care as well as the nature of their requirements for nursing. Nurses' patients at times reject or react unfavorably to an aspect(s) of their systems of nursing care or medical care and at times to the total system of health care. Nurses (and physicians) must be alert to personal responses and reactions of their patients to particular aspects of care and to the patients' levels of tolerance for the totality of the health care system.

An important interpersonal feature of nursing is nurses' awareness of and insights about what patients are experiencing in the health care situation, such as the demands placed upon them, conflicts being experienced, or not knowing what to do or how to represent their beliefs about their needs for care. Nurses should be aware of the stress-producing features of each person's health care situation. Demands on patients for interactions with nurses and other health professionals can produce stress. But nurses' awareness and insight are not sufficient. Nurses must have the creative capabilities to help patients in resolving and in seeking solutions to problem situations, or to identify for patients persons who can help them.

When demands of particular health care situations become sufficiently burdensome, patients may withdraw. Withdrawal may take a number of forms, for example, psychological withdrawal, as in depression or failure to cooperate or making the decision and taking action to remove oneself from the health care situation. Hospitalized patients sign releases or simply walk away without informing anyone of their plans. Patients no longer attend clinics. Withdrawal may be evidence of the ineffectiveness or inefficiency of the operation of a health care institution or agency, including the absence of or inadequacy of nurses or other health care professionals. It may be an expression of hopelessness or fear or anger on the part of a patient, or it may reflect a lack of resources.

SUMMARY

Some interpersonal features of nursing have been separated out from the social and service dimensions of nursing practice to emphasize their importance in nursing practice. The nature of nurse-patient relationships was described as contractual and complementary. The interpersonal features of the relationships were related to nursing as a human service and the necessity for social encounter of nurses and persons who are nursed. The essential humanness of persons who are nurses and persons who are patients was described in terms of the operation of variations of the positive emotion of human love, including fellow-feeling, sympathy, empathy, personal freedom or liberty, and the unrestricted desire to know.

The purpose of a nurse-patient relationship was identified not as an end in itself but as a necessary means for the design and production of nursing care. Characterizing features of nurse-patient interactions were identified. Sorokin's modalities of interdependence and interaction were briefly described with adjustments to the professional responsibility of nurses in interpersonal situations with patients. Sorokin's modalities were related to nursing practice situations.

An example of the absence of a system of nurse-patient interaction and the absence of nursing was presented. The example was taken from a document developed by a mature woman following a hospital experience.

Three types of factors conditioning the nurse-patient relationship and interactions were presented. These were factors that condition the possibilities for and the quality of adaptive interchanges between nurses and patients; factors that affect the extensity, duration, and continuity of nurse-patient interaction; and factors that affect the quality of patient participation in the design and production of nursing. Following this, two variations of interactional systems in nursing situations were identified on the basis of the rationality and self-management capabilities of persons under nursing care. Related nurse capabilities were identified.

The chapter concluded with further considerations of the characteristics of nurses and demands on them arising from the interpersonal features of nursing. The emphasis throughout the chapter was on the person-to-person features of nursing practice and not on persons' requirements for nursing or nurses' capabilities to provide nursing. The approach taken in this chapter is viewed as necessary for the formalization of the knowledge and the interpersonal skills required for the practice of nursing.

References

1. Allport GW: *Personality and social encounter, selected essays,* Boston, 1960, Beacon Press.
2. Arnold MB: *Emotion and personality, psychological aspects,* vol I, New York, 1960, Columbia University Press, pp 212-215.
3. Arnold MB: *Emotion and personality, neurological and physiological aspects,* vol II, New York, 1960, Columbia University Press, pp 312-330.
4. McCool GA, editor: A Rahner reader [Karl Rahner], New York, 1975, Crossroad, pp 352-353.
5. Arnold MB: Emotion and personality, neurological and physiological aspects, vol II, New York, 1960, Columbia University Press, p 311.
6. Lonergan BJF: Insight, a study of human understanding. Crowe FE, and Doran RM, editors: *Collected works of Bernard Lonergan,* Toronto, 1992, University of Toronto Press, pp 494-504.
7. Sorokin P: *Social and cultural dynamics,* revised and abridged by the author, Boston, 1957, Porter Sargent Publisher, pp 436-452.
8. Webster's dictionary of synonyms, ed 1, Springfield, Mass, 1951, G&C Merriam Co, p 288.
9. Monnig Sr. NG: Identification and description of nursing opportunities for health teaching of patients with gastric surgery as a basis for curriculum development in nursing, Master's dissertation, School of Nursing, Catholic University of America, Washington, DC, 1965, pp 89-90.

PART II

Formalization of Nursing Knowledge

CHAPTER 6

Views of Nursing and Views of Humankind

Each nurse has his or her own view of nursing. **View** is used here in the sense of a more or less clearly formulated idea or judgment about something, implying the exercise of mental rather than physical vision. Nurses' *views* may be clearly formulated and expressed as *concepts,* concepts that express nurses' formulated *insights* about what nursing is. Other nurses have and express opinions about nursing that may have some reality focus but are colored by their sentiments and feelings, as well as their biases. There are, however, too many nurses who have insights about the reality that is nursing but are unable to formulate and express their insights in language that communicates their ideas and the meaning that nursing holds for them.

A nurse's view of nursing affects what he or she focuses on and attends to in nursing practice, in scholarly endeavors, in teaching nursing, or in nursing research and theory development. Ideally, nurses in the professional roles shown in Figure 4-1 have available to them structured bodies of nursing knowledge and at the same time contribute to the development of these bodies of knowledge. One of the difficulties that nurses face, and have faced for some time, is that knowledge that nurses have acquired and use is not organized around the enduring realities that confront nurses in their work of nursing.

One knowledge-organizing approach was to extract from medical and other nursing-related fields textbook material that nursing educators judged to be relevant to the work of nursing and then to attach to the extracted content what was often referred to as "nursing implications." What nurses ordinarily *did for* their patients and their approaches to patients were organized in textbooks usually referred to as "fundamentals of nursing." Types of care measures, referred to as nursing procedures, that nurses *performed for patients,* with step-by-step instructions about the processes of performance, were included in textbooks of fundamentals, as well as in what were referred to as "procedure books" available to nurses on hospital units. There was no consideration that at times, ideally, the patient should be the performer, not the nurse. These two approaches to organizing nursing knowledge had their foundations, respectively, in what are commonly referred to as the *medical model of nursing* and the *task orientation to nursing.*

VIEWS OF NURSING: FINDING THE ENDURING REALITIES OF NURSING PRACTICE

Nurses in the latter half of the twentieth century were concerned with **approaches to the question: What is nursing?** with less attention to the critical question: *Why do people require nursing?* The first question is not adequately answered by statements such as nursing is a *human health service, nursing is help,* or *nursing is caring.* The response demanded is a statement about the human focus of nursing and what nurses make or produce for others when they engage in nursing them. The statement would specify how nurses' exercise of their powers and capabilities to produce nursing for others is deliberately related to realities (verified or verifiable) about these others that are indicators of their legitimate need for a specific health service that has the form and the name of nursing.

An Early Approach to the Questions

In 1859 Florence Nightingale's *Notes on Nursing: What It Is, and What It Is Not*[1] was published in London. This educated woman, who with other women volunteers had nursed the sick and the wounded during the Crimean War, wrote in the preface to her book, "Notes . . . are meant simply to give *hints for thought* to women who have personal charge of the health of others." Later in the preface she wrote, "If . . . every woman must at some time or other of her life, become a nurse, i.e., have charge of somebody's health, how immense and how valuable would be the produce of her united experience if every woman would *think* how to nurse" (italics added).

Nightingale in her preface equates sanitary knowledge with nursing knowledge and describes it as knowing "how to put the constitution in such a state as that it will have no disease, or that it can recover from disease . . . " Throughout her *Notes* there is explication of Nightingale's meaning of the term "sanitary knowledge," which includes "proper use of fresh air, light, warmth, cleanliness, quiet and the proper selection and administration of diet. . . ." There is also development within the text of notes about nursing (good and bad) for persons with diseases, those with injuries, and those receiving forms of medical care.

Based on her education and experiences and the cultural features of the period within which she wrote, Nightingale addressed elements of nursing practice. A detailed content analysis of her *Notes on Nursing* would yield her 1859 partial answers to our questions: What is nursing? and Why do people require nursing? Some of her "general principles" are unacceptable; nonetheless, her points of emphasis are revealing and enduring. They include, for example, the focus on women becoming able "to think nursing"; her emphasis on sanitary knowledge in relation to prevention, including the "health" of places such as hospital wards; and a view of the nurse as "having charge of somebody's health." Prevention of disordered health and restoration of health appear to be the broad goals of nursing. The more specific result sought through nursing "is to put the patient in the best condition for nature to act upon him" (pp. 74-75).

Some Later Approaches to Answering the Questions, 1950s and 1960s

During the latter half of the twentieth century, there was evidence of developing interest on the part of nurses to answering the question: What is nursing? This interest seemed at least in part to be associated (from my experience) with demands on nursing students and nurses "to make plans for nursing care that patients should have" and the demand that nurses should teach patients how to provide some elements of their own care. Nurses' interest was no doubt associated with their awareness of the inadequacies of a "medical model of nursing" (seeing nursing as an adjunct to medicine) and the impersonal nature of "the task approach to nursing" (focusing on the tasks and not on the patient). The need to bring both the nurse and the person nursed into explicit focus and the need to reveal nursing as a field of practice in its own right were bases for nurses' growing interest in the question: What is nursing? and in efforts to answer it.

Another factor operating during this period was the rapid (after World War II) development of rehabilitation medicine and its various technical support fields, with its emphasis on restoration of persons' natural functioning or substituting for it when it was impaired or lost. The demand on patients to participate fully in their own rehabilitation—to learn self-management, self-care, and active engagement in activities of daily living—was the outstanding feature of this emerging system of health care. Rehabilitation revealed to me and to others the inadequacies of nursing's seemingly single emphasis on doing for patients, the inadequacies of nurses' approaches to teaching patients, and the importance of patient participation in their own health care. Virginia Henderson's 1955 definition of nursing[2] and my own 1956[3] (p. 21) definition of nursing were products of this period.

A 1967 survey by Horgan[4] revealed information about how nurses were viewing nursing during the 1950s and 1960s. Horgan identified that the question: What is nursing? is found repeatedly in the nursing literature of that period. She reviewed issues of the *American Journal of Nursing* and *Nursing Outlook* for the years 1950 to 1965. Thirty articles, reports of interviews, or reviews were identified and abstracted. Following are some of the conclusions Horgan reached about the content of the expressed ideas about nursing (p. 32).

1. Nursing as a health service in society is not emphasized.
2. The expressed focus and ultimate end of nursing seem to be the meeting of the needs of the patient.
3. The reason for nurses being in nurse-patient situations is not stated other than in terms of meeting patient needs.
4. The technologies of assessment and validation of needs are emphasized; the technologies of fulfillment of needs are not a central focus.

The emphasis on assessing and meeting patient needs presented nurses with the problem of having organized knowledge of patient needs and the problem of identifying patients' needs. Both problems are addressed by Black[5] in a paper titled "Assessing Patients' Needs." She discusses the general classification of needs—physical, psychologic, social, and spiritual—and states that "we in nursing keep before us the objective that *all* the needs of our patients will be met." Black goes on to state that "in so far as possible, we attempt to obtain need satisfaction for each patient on a specifically individual basis."

Black notes that although "this mode of grouping needs does serve to remind us that there is breadth to our concern for patients, it fails to point to particulars that are specific enough to guide us in a detailed assessment of needs." Her paper continues with various approaches to aid nurses in understanding need satisfaction and fulfillment, with a focus on the then current psychologic theories, including motivational theories.

Black's paper is referenced because it is a scholarly, insightful exposition of what is demanded of nurses and nursing students when the question: What is nursing? is answered with "meeting patient needs."

Approaches to Answering the Question, the 1970s and 1980s

The Nursing Development Conference Group in the first and second editions of their book, *Concept Formalization in Nursing: Process and Product,*[6] expressed the object of their work as "the need for and the problems associated with the organization and continuing development of authoritative knowledge about (1) the realities that nurses observe and regulate as nurses and (2) how nurses can effectively observe and regulate these realities." They define authoritative knowledge as "knowledge that has been formulated and tested by mature nursing scholars functioning in collaboration as members of the discipline of nursing" (p. 3).

During the period of the 1970s, professional nursing organizations in the United States and Canada advocated the selection and use of a concept of nursing or its related developed conceptual framework to guide nursing education and nursing practice. The Nursing Development Conference Group in the early 1970s studied nurses' expressed concepts of nursing, found not in published articles but in books on nursing that were published during the period 1859 to 1971 (pp. 59-100).[6] (See listing of authors in Table 6-1.) Statements of the concepts were extracted and examined to reveal points of emphasis and developments that indicated increases in expressed understandings of the reality foci of nursing. The expressed concepts studied were analyzed to reveal their similarities

 Table 6-1   Names of Fourteen Nurses Who Published Their Generalizations About Nursing (Concepts) in Nonspecialized Nursing Books Between 1859 and 1977

Name	Dates of Published Works
Florence Nightingale	1859, 1893
Clara Weeks-Shaw	1885, 1902
Bertha Harmer	1922 and three subsequent editions
Hester Frederick and Ethel Northam	1938
Virginia Henderson	1955 in her revision of Harmer; 1959, 1971
Dorothea E. Orem	1959, 1971, 1973
Faye Abdellaha, Irene Beland, Almeda Martin, Ruth Matheny	1960, 1973
Ida Jean Orlando	1961, 1972
Martha Rogers	1961, 1970
Ernestine Wiedenbock	1964, 1970
Myra E. Levine	1969, 1973
Imogene King	1971
Pamela H. Mitchell	1973, 1977
Sister Callista Roy	1974, 1976

Addendum: Nurses recognized for their contributions to nursing theory development who published their concepts of nursing in specialized nursing books or in journal articles

Hildegard Peplau	1952
Joyce Travelbee	1966, 1972
Dorothy Johnson	1961

This listing is taken from the work of The Nursing Development conference Group's study of "selected concepts of nursing in the public domain"[6] (pp. 59-102). The works were identified in collections in four libraries, two university libraries, the Johns Hopkins Medical Institutions, and the National Library of Medicine. Sarah E. Allison conducted the search and secured permissions of authors for the extraction of their concepts and their publication.

and differences. Commonalities among the analyzed concepts included the following ideas:

(1) nursing is result producing activity that involves nurses in helping relationships with recipients of nursing; (2) nursing is a unique service, an entity because of its own proper activities and, therefore, distinct from medicine; and (3) nursing is related to the state of health or well-being, or the absence thereof, in recipients of nursing.[6] (pp. 85-86)

The differences in the analyzed statements of general concepts of nursing clustered around ways of symbolizing recipients of nursing, the focus of nursing actions, and the results of nursing (p. 86).[6]

In the 1970s these expressed general conceptualizations of nursing, as well as others, were available for consideration by teachers of nursing, nursing practitioners, and administrators of nursing education and nursing service as organizing frameworks for constructing designs for nursing education and nursing practice. The Nursing Development Conference Group viewed "concepts of nursing in the public domain" as representing "incipient nursing theory open to change and validation" (p. 59).[6] It is an open question whether the advocates of the use of general concepts of nursing and conceptual frameworks as guides for nursing practice and nursing education understood the effort and the nature of the work involved in putting concepts to work. This included mastery of the selected general concepts of nursing, the uncovering of the substantive structure of each conceptual element in it, the formalization of theories, and the *structuring or organization of nursing knowledge* around *theoretic elements* or *hypothesized relations between elements*. It seems that there was an assumption that nursing already had the form of an organized, structured discipline of knowledge available to all.

During this period and subsequently in the 1980s and continuing into the 1990s, the adoption of specific conceptual frameworks to guide nursing education and nursing practice in some situations resulted in continuing development of specific conceptualizations of nursing and determination of their usefulness in the endeavors of nurses in nursing education and nursing practice. (See Fawcett[7] for the use of and developmental work related to specific nursing conceptualizations and theories).

Perhaps the most important outcome of this period was the increased ability of *individual nurses* to *think nursing* and to organize their already acquired knowing of nursing around conceptual elements of the nursing theories they espoused. The period of the 1970s and 1980s was marked by the formation of nurse-managed and nurse-operated clinics (for example, the nursing clinics at the Johns Hopkins Institutions organized by the Center for Experimentation and Development in Nursing, 1968-1974) in the outpatient departments of hospitals or as free-standing nursing clinics and other movements that illustrate nurses' growing acceptance that nursing is a health service unique unto itself with situational requirements for nurse-physician coordination and communication.

During the 1970s and 1980s, **self-care deficit nursing theory**[8] was used to guide curriculum development for nursing educational programs, to guide individual nurses in their nursing practice, and to provide insight about the organization and operation of nursing services in hospitals and community agencies. During this period and into the 1990s, the work of development of the theory continued, and it is used by nurses in the United States and in other countries.

SELF-CARE DEFICIT NURSING THEORY AND VIEWS OF HUMANKIND

The conceptual elements within productive general theories of nursing identify human points of reference, views of humankind that reveal the human entities that nurses focus on in nursing practice situations and investigate in the practice of nursing science. The main conceptual constructs of productive theories are descriptively explanatory of the *what* and *why,* the *who* and the *how* of nursing. A valid, comprehensive theory of nursing has as its reality base persons who need and receive nursing care and those who produce it, as well as the events of its production. It answers the question posed previously. The specific views of humankind expressed in theories of nursing fit within one or more broader views of human beings. These views were proposed by the Nursing Development Conference Group in the 1970s.

Broad Views

Five broad views are identified as necessary for developing understanding of the main conceptual elements of self-care deficit nursing theory and for understanding the societal and interpersonal aspects of nursing. These views are (1) person, (2) agent, (3) user of symbols, (4) unitary human being or embodied person, and (5) as individuals (objects) subject to physical forces. These broad views subsume more specific nursing views. They also point to the sciences and the fields of knowledge that nurses must master to be effective nursing practitioners and scholars. These five **broad views of humankind** are as relevant for nurses viewing themselves as they are for nurses viewing persons in need of nursing. At times nurses must help persons under their care to view themselves in one or more of these ways.

The *person view* of individuals in society is basic to understanding the other views. As expressed by Weiss, a mature human being "is at once a self and a person, with a distinctive I and me; he [or she] has private, publicly viable rights and is able to possess changes and pluralities without endangering his [or her] constancy or unity"[9] (p. 128).

The *person view* is the enduring, stable view that individuals have or should have of themselves and others. As individuals develop as persons, ideally they grow in self-knowledge, with convictions about themselves as responsible for their own lives and well-being and as contributing to the functioning and stability of their families and communities. The *person view* encompasses individuals' self-understanding, their spiritual functioning, and their religious orientations, as well as their orientation to their world and to persons in it.

The view of *person* is central to and an integrating force for understanding other views. It is the person who takes on the role of agent or actor, who uses symbols to communicate and to express feelings and concerns, who is alive and aware of bodily functions, and who must contend with physical forces in the environment.

The *person view* is the view that nurses should use in all interpersonal contacts with men, women, and children under their care and with their families and friends. The *person view* is central to nurses' use of other views of men, women, and children.

The *person-as-agent view* is central to understanding self-care deficit nursing theory. It is an operational view of both nurses and those nursed that incorporates the view of agent with the view of person. The concepts self-care, nursing, nurse, self-care agent, self-care agency, and nursing agency require the person-as-agent view. The structure of the processes of self-care and the processes of nursing also require the person-as-agent view. This dual view is emphasized because individuals, when they act deliberately to bring about conditions in themselves or their environment that are sought but do not presently exist, do so as persons who think and are knowing and willing to act as agents.

The person-as-agent view is critical as persons seek to organize their environments, cooperate with others, and communicate with them.

The *user of symbols view* is a critical view in nursing practice situations and in all human contact situations. Persons use symbols to stand for things and attach meaning to them; they use them to formulate ideas and to communicate. Communication requires the use of language or other means of conveying information to others. In nursing practice situations, the use of symbols includes the language of the cultures of nurses and the cultures of those for whom they provide nursing. Nurses must master the language of nursing and the language of the health care disciplines that articulate with nursing. Language differences among individuals in these situations constitute obstacles to be overcome.

The ability to use symbols to communicate with others requires not only learning but also specific skills. Ideally the use of symbols in communication develops in individuals as an art form. Nurses' failure to formalize the lanuage of nursing has hindered their ability to communicate about nursing to the public, to their patients, to colleagues in other health services, and to health service administrators.

The *unitary being or embodied person view* encompasses the views that human beings are living, functioning beings who grow and who develop as persons throughout their life span; who exhibit features of physiologic, psychologic, and spiritual functioning; and who may exhibit a religious habit of mind as they live within families and larger social units. Viewing men, women, and children as unitary embodied beings brings into focus the internal structure, the constitution, and the human functions that are the objects of study of the life sciences. The life span of humankind and the stages of growth and physical, emotional, and cognitional development are parts of this view. Aberrations of human structure and human functioning and their effects on individuals and what they can and cannot do and what they need to do are important insights in reaching an understanding of this view.

The *view of individuals as objects subject to physical forces* is a necessary nursing view whenever a man, woman, or child is unable to act to protect self from environmental forces. The view carries with it the understanding that persons, to protect themselves from physical force, must be able to control their position and movement in space, have awareness of impending danger, know what to do under existent or predictable conditions, and have the requisite power, capabilities, and resources to act. This is a necessary view whenever nurses provide care for infants, young children, or older children and adults who are unable to control their position and movement in space or contend with physical forces that threaten their safety.

Nurses who take the *object view* of persons in concrete nursing practice situations understand these persons' requirements for protective care. The nature of the required protective care is understood in terms of the incapacities of individuals to manage themselves and defend themselves against physical forces, including physical force exerted against them by other human beings. This view of humankind articulates with the universal self-care requisite of *protection from hazards*. Meeting this requisite is a critical component of both self-care and dependent-care systems.

VIEWS OF HUMANKIND WITHIN SELF-CARE DEFICIT NURSING THEORY

Self-care deficit nursing theory (described in Chapter 2) answers the questions: What is nursing? and Why do persons in specific time-place situations require nursing? The theory adequately models nursing as a *specific human health service,* naming the nature of and the reasons for the time-place requirements of individuals for nursing and the nature, structure, and results sought through nurses' production of the service of nursing. This general theory of nursing is focused on the concrete world of men, women, and children and on the concrete conditions and circumstances of human living in families and societies.

The theory is reality focused with respect to its origins, the reason that people require nursing, and the conceptual elements of its structure that name the characterizing features of both the providers and the recipients of nursing. The theory also specifies the features and the structure of the nursing systems of care that are produced by nurses for and with persons with health-associated limitations for maintaining systems of self-care of a therapeutic quality for themselves or their dependents. Views of humankind that are explicit or implicit in the theory are addressed first in terms of persons who have requirements for nursing and then in terms of persons who produce nursing.

Persons Who Have Requirements for Nursing

Persons in need of nursing are embodied beings, living, functioning, and developing in relatively stable or changing environments. Their functioning is subject to internal neuroendocrine regulatory processes. As all of humankind, they must be supplied with the materials (air, water, food) and the environmental conditions that regulate and support life processes and functioning within human norms. These materials and conditions must be supplied through the deliberate exercise of human effort and the performance of deliberate actions (self-care or dependent-care) to meet human regulatory requirements that are named **self-care requisites.**

Self-care as performed by or for individuals is assumed to be a **human regulatory function** that is essential for continued life and functioning, as well as growth and development within human norms. As a regulatory function, self-care demands continuous production. Failure to produce self-care systems of a therapeutic quality for self or dependents is a hazard to their lives and to the normalcy of their functioning.

Persons who as agents of action produce self-care or dependent-care have the requisite powers and capabilities to do so. Such powers and capabilities are named, respectively, **self-care agency** and **dependent-care agency.** These terms stand for *theoretic concepts* that encompass the whole complex of powers and capabilities that persons must possess and exercise to produce self-care systems and dependent-care systems. Such systems are formed from performance of the deliberate actions through which specific methods or technologies are used to meet the existent or projected particularized self-care requisites of individuals. The totality of actions that should be performed at specific times and over some time duration is conceptualized as the **therapeutic self-care demand.** When the powers and capabilities of persons to meet their own or their dependents' therapeutic self-care demands are not adequate because of health-associated reasons, there arises **self-care deficits** or **dependent-care deficits.** These deficits give rise to requirements for nursing.

Persons Who Produce Nursing Systems of Care

Nurses are *persons* who become active as *agents* when they exercise their powers and capabilities in determining if and why individuals require nursing and proceed to design and produce sequences of deliberately performed actions *to meet these persons' personalized self-care requisites* and to regulate the exercise or development of these persons' self-care agency by using methods of helping adequate to overcome their action limitations, their *deficits for meeting* their *prescribed therapeutic self-care demands.*

Nurses as persons *use symbols* to communicate with persons for whom they provide nursing. They attend to these persons' use of language or other forms of expression and elicit information from them. Communication demands on nurses also arise from families of persons under care and from these persons' physicians or other health care professionals. The demands on nurses for communication using language and other symbolic forms appropriate to situations are at times extensive and heavy. Nurses also must be concerned about the communication demands placed on persons under their care, for such demands can be stressful and energy depleting.

The powers and capabilities of nurses to determine requirements of persons for nursing and to design and produce systems of nursing care for them must be equal to these demands in each time-place nursing situation where nurses elect to provide service. But above all, nurses must be willing to exercise—that is, operationalize—these powers and capabilities for the benefit of persons under their care at the time and for the duration of time that specific kinds and amounts of nursing actions are required. Nurses develop their powers and capabilities to nurse (their *nursing agency*) through education and experience in concrete situations where individuals need and nurses provide and produce nursing systems of care.

Nursing agency is a *theoretic concept,* the *substantive structure* of which is an artificial construct of required operations, enabling powers, and foundational human capabilities and dispositions. Its hypothesized structure is analogous to that of self-care agency. The quality of *nursing agency,* the power that is *enabling (when exercised)* for the production of nursing, varies from nurse to nurse. It is the quality of nursing agency of nurses that determines their legitimacy or lack of legitimacy to become the nursing agent in specific concrete situations of practice.

COMPLEXITY OF HUMAN POWERS

Self-care deficit nursing theory as previously described offers solutions to a number of problems for which the nursing profession must provide answers. Why do persons require nursing at specific times and over some duration of time? What is the nature of the health service nursing? What powers and capabilities enable nurses to produce nursing? The answers to these problems that are provided by the theory require continued development. Such development is aided through the making or imagining of **models** to fill in gaps of our knowledge of the structure and constitution of things specified by the theory.[10] Hartnett's models of *deliberate action* and the Nursing Development Conference Group's model of *self-care agency* are examples that begin to fill in our knowledge of the theoretic concept of self-care agency. The model of self-care agency, as presented in Chapter 11, is a hypothetical construct of human powers, human capabilities, and foundational capabilities and dispositions. Other developed models are described in subsequent chapters.

Regardless of the nursing theory to which nurses ascribe, each nurse must become able to accept men, women, and children as substantial unities who function as unitary beings. But it is also essential for nurses and nursing students to grasp (1) the complexity of the powers that characterize human nature and (2) the uniqueness of each individual person. W.A. Wallace, in his *The Modeling of Nature,* presents "an overlay model of human nature" (p. 419),[11] using computer graphics to show "models or schemata" as overlapping layers to specify details of what is being modeled. Wallace's model, developed in eight overlays, shows the **powers and habits** of humankind as they are identified through the sciences and philosophy. The *first* layer is foundational, showing *proto matter* (first matter; the mass-energy of science, p. 9) as identified by philosophers and *natural form* (an energizing field). Subsequent layers are identified as inorganic powers; nutritive powers; sensitive powers; rational powers; intellectual habits; the concepts and sciences that perfect the intellect; operational habits, associated with the will; and, in the eighth layer, supernatural habits. Wallace superimposes intellect and will on the layers.

The utility of the overlay model of the powers and habits of humankind for nurses and nursing students is that its schemata present the types of *human powers* and the *developed habits* of themselves and of persons under their care that are in some way enabling for what they experience, think, and do in nursing practice situations. The powers and habits of humankind identified in the model are the foci of specific sciences. As Wallace says in his models of nature, "All sciences stand on equal, and complementary, footing." The *complexity* of the *powers of humankind* is an indication not only of the kinds of knowledge needed by nurses but also of the awe and respect that nurses should have for humankind as unitary beings. Wallace's overlay model should be understood for what it is—a modeling of the powers and habits of humankind. It is not a model of a human being.

SUMMARY

The production of self-care and nursing involves an expenditure of effort and energy. Engagement in self-care or in nursing is work that demands that each person become an active agent in his or her own care or in the care of another. Self-care demands that persons be or become able to accept their own status as embodied beings with numerous powers and capabilities, yet also with demands for self-maintenance and self-regulation. Nursing demands that the persons who function as nurses not only see the other, the *person* nursed, as having all the features and demands of *embodied beings* but also see and attend to themselves from this perspective.

The foregoing views of nursing and humankind constitute guides for nurses and nursing students to look at themselves and the *persons* they nurse in terms of their personal and their "private, publicly viable rights"[9] and their responsibilities in the world where they live and function.

Some of the ideas presented in this chapter were developed in an article titled "Views of Human Beings Specific to Nursing," published in *Nursing Science Quarterly* (10:1, Spring 1997). The article develops the idea that the nursing-specific conceptualizations in valid general theories of nursing "are the human points of reference that reveal the human powers and qualities, that are the entities investigated in nursing science" (p. 26). The critical point is the necessity for nurses and nursing students to use valid general theories of nursing if they are to develop and conceptualize their insights about persons and about humankind that are nursing relevant.

Nurses come to know many things about themselves and others. They, however, must have some basis for determining what is nursing relevant. Nurses come to know, for example, where persons live; their customs and way of life; their values, prejudices, fears, and orientations; and their beliefs about their place in the world and their ancestors and how they come to exist. Insights about the broad views of humankind expressed in this chapter are starting points that lead to fields of science or segments thereof that nurses must master. Developing and using models are necessary in the formalization of the subject matter of nursing. For example, Hartnett's development of physiologic and psychologic models of voluntary, deliberate human action preceeded the Nursing Development Conference Group's development of a three-layered model of *self-care agency* (pp. 135-143).[6]

References

1. Nightingale F: *Notes on nursing: what it is, and what it is not,* London, 1859, Harrison.
2. Harmer B, revised by Henderson V: *Textbook of the principles and practice of nursing,* ed 5, New York, 1955, Macmillan, p 4.
3. Orem DE: *Hospital nursing service, an analysis,* Indianapolis, 1956, Division of Hospital and Institutional Services, Indiana State Board of Health, p 21.
4. Horgan MV: *Concepts about nursing in selected nursing literature from 1950-1965,* Washington, DC, 1967, Catholic University of America (master's dissertation), p 32.
5. Black MK: Assessing patients' needs. In Yura H and Walsh MB, editors: *The nursing process,* Washington, DC, 1967, Catholic University of America Press.
6. Nursing Development Conference Group, Orem DE, editor: *Concept formalization in nursing: process and product,* ed 2, Boston, 1979, Little, Brown.
7. Fawcett J: *Analysis and evaluation of contemporary nursing knowledge; nursing models and theories,* Philadelphia, 2000, FA Davis Company.
8. Orem DE: *Nursing: concepts of practice,* ed 1, New York, 1971, McGraw-Hill.
9. Weiss P: *You, I, and the others,* Carbondale and Edwardsville, 1980, Southern Illinois University Press, p 128.
10. Harré R: *The principles of scientific thinking,* Chicago, 1970, University of Chicago Press, pp 34-35.
11. Wallace WA: *The modeling of nature, philosophy of science and philosophy of nature in synthesis,* Washington, DC, 1996, Catholic University of America Press, p 419.

CHAPTER 7

Self-Care Deficit Nursing Theory

Self-care deficit nursing is identified as a general theory of what nursing is and what nursing should be as it is produced in concrete nursing practice situations. As a general theory, it is not an explanation of a particular nursing practice situation or even of a type of situation. The theory is an expression of a singular combination of conceptualized features and relations among them that are common to all instances of nursing. Valid general theories in practice fields such as nursing should not be considered as static entities but ones that can and should undergo continuing development as they guide the intellectual and practical activities of nursing practitioners, scholars, theorists, and researchers. Nurses' mastery of the conceptual structure of self-care deficit nursing theory and their use of the conceptual constructs of the theory in nursing endeavors were instrumental in the identification of the characteristic ways that the theory serves nurses, expressed as its functions.

FUNCTIONS OF THE THEORY

Eight **functions** of self-care deficit nursing theory have been identified by nurses. The functions are:

- To set forth the views of human beings proper to nursing
- To express the specific focus or proper object of nursing in human society
- To set forth the key concepts of nursing considered as a field of knowledge and practice and to establish a system of symbols or language
- To set limits on and orient thinking and practical endeavor in nursing practice, research, development, and education for nursing
- To reduce cognitive load by providing subsumers for incoming information and enable persons who understand the theory to categorize and form concepts from related insights about features of concrete nursing situations
- To allow inferences to be made about the articulations of nursing with other fields of human service and with patterns of daily living of individuals and families in communities
- To generate in nurses and nursing students a style of thinking and communicating nursing
- To bring nurses together as communities of scholars engaged in the continuing development, the structuring, and the validation of nursing knowledge

Nurses' mastery of the self-care deficit theory of nursing and the results of their use of its principles to guide their nursing endeavors attest to its usefulness.

The eight expressed functions of this general theory of nursing are based on nurses' perceived and expressed values of the theory in guiding their observations, their intellectual activities, their style of thinking, and their use of a developing language in their communications about nursing. The eighth, the last listed function, references the value of the theory in bringing nurses together to deliberate about and seek to develop a practical nursing science, the validated theoretic and practical nursing knowledge that is organized as its constituent components. Additionally, there is need for the identification and development of foundational sciences that support the practical science. The endeavor of doing nursing science is one that nurses have not adequately engaged in and one that some nurses are unable to deal with realistically.

In the 1990s some nurses rejected and negated the value of general theories of nursing. There also was a turning to philosophy and a movement away from the concrete enduring elements of nursing practice as revealing the subject matter of nursing. Philosophy, according to Harré,[1] "concerns the way we think and reason about different subject matters. It is concerned with the organization, nature and modes of generation of the products of intellectual activity; that is with thoughts, theories, judgments, assessments," and with the individual consciousness of the persons who think, judge, theorize, and so on (p. 3).

Persons who do nursing science formalize, develop, and validate the subject matter of nursing. A philosophic system may aid us in developing insight and in knowing how we think about the world and things in it, but no philosophic system can tell us what **subject matter** we are to think about and develop as nurses. The subject matter of nursing practice and its science is *persons in society who require nursing, persons who produce nursing, the relations between them, and the structure of the processes of producing nursing.* The self-care deficit theory of nursing as initially formulated and in its development not only identifies the subject matter of nursing but also provides the concepts and conceptual constructs that guide the initial and continuing development of a practical science of nursing.

SOME DEVELOPMENTAL FEATURES OF THE THEORY

Ideally, persons engaged in doing nursing science have formed or are forming a model of what nursing science encompasses. This section addresses two fundamental and preliminary steps to understanding movement toward nursing science from the standpoint of a valid general theory of nursing, namely, aspects of development of general theories of nursing and the **premises** on which self-care deficit nursing theory are based. This section is concluded with an *introduction* to refinement of the **theory.**

Aspects of Theory Development

Valid general descriptive explanations of nursing begin with nurses' conceptualized and expressed insights about dominant features of nursing practice situations known to them through experience and investigation. Insights, when formulated as concepts and expressed verbally or in writing, constitute static representations of situational features and relationships. Dominant features identified in explored nursing practice situations provide the concrete basis for insights leading to the formulation of theoretic positions about nursing.

Nursing has form as well as situational features with which nurses deal as nurses. The form of nursing is expressed in part by its helping and taking care of characteristics, which lay out its interpersonal form. Other aspects of nursing's form arise from the fact that nurses deal with life situations where results are sought, that is, where new, not at present, existent, conditions are to be brought into existence through the goal-oriented deliberate actions of nurses and their patients. Theoretic positions about nursing include both form and situational features.

A general theory in a practice field is descriptively explanatory of the dominant features and relationships that characterize the field's practice situations. General theories structure what is already known and thus provide organized foundations for the continued development, structuring, and validation of knowledge that is of practical value for practitioners in the field. General theories are of particular value in fields such as nursing in which nursing

─────────────── *Exercise* ───────────────

Exercise in Examining Statements Responsive to the Question:
What is Nursing?

Select a number of written statements of nurses that are responsive to the question: What is nursing?
Identify why you selected these particular statements.

1. Read each statement carefully. Examine it for and identify its structure. Reflect about the meaning of the statement. Reflect about the relationships among the parts of the statement that give it structure.
2. Extract the parts of each statement that express elements or features of nursing.
3. After working with each one of the statements you selected, compare the statements for similarities and differences as related to expressed elements.
4. Discuss the results of your investigation with colleagues in a planned meeting.
5. Note and record the questions that arise during the discussion.

knowledge that should be available to nursing students and scholars is relatively unstructured within a nursing frame of reference, as attested by textbooks in various areas of nursing practice. A general theory of nursing is an effective but general answer to the questions: What do nurses attend to and do when they nurse? What do nurses make when they nurse? A general theory of nursing also provides structure for the organization of nursing knowledge.

The formulation and expression of a general theory of nursing occurs over time. It is based as previously indicated on insights about (1) recurring features of nursing practice situations and (2) relationships between and among features. Analysis of situations of nursing practice and analysis of nursing case material (a nursing case is a particular instance of nursing) yield insights about the recurring features of nursing practice and the relationships between and among them. Identified recurring features—for example, the capability of healthy adults to meet self-care requisites for maintaining adequate intake of water and food under some conditions but not under others—are investigated. Insights are formulated as concepts, and expressed concepts are then validated in concrete practice situations or through analysis of nursing case material. Experiences of members of the Nursing Development Conference Group* in these matters are described in "Dynamics of Concept Development" in the 1973 and 1979 editions of *Concept Formalization in Nursing: Process and Product.*[2]

Formulation and expression of a general theory of nursing proceed as a creative synthesis of the conceptualized recurring dominant features of nursing

───────────────

*This voluntary study group had its origins in 1965 as the Committee on the Nursing Model, the School of Nursing, Catholic University of America, Washington, DC. The name *Nursing Development Conference Group* will be used regardless of time period.

practice situations and the relationship among them. There is, as indicated, the question of form or structure of the synthesis of nursing features.

Nursing, as previously stated, has an interpersonal form. But form also is reflective of the practical service nature of nursing, which gives rise to requirements for nurses to perform operations to determine what is and what can and should be and to decide within the interpersonal frame what will be done and then engage in its production and evaluation. Operations involve the selection and deliberate performance of actions and action sequences by nurses and nurses' patients according to their determined roles. A general theory of nursing is thus a synthesis of postulated entities related within an interpersonal form; within the interpersonal structure, there is an operational structure.

See Appendix B for some detailed highlights of development of self-care deficit nursing theory.

Underlying Premises of Self-Care Deficit Nursing Theory

Five premises about self-evident characteristics of human beings served as guiding principles throughout the process of conceptualizing nursing. They have been referred to at times as assumptions. They are more properly referred to as premises because they were and are advanced as true and not merely assumed. The five premises that follow were formalized in 1973[3] (pp. 3-5).

1. Human beings require continuous deliberate inputs to themselves and their environments in order to remain alive and function in accord with natural human endowments.
2. Human agency, the power to act deliberately, is exercised in the form of care of self and others in identifying needs for and in making needed inputs.
3. Mature human beings experience privations in the form of limitations for action in care of self and others involving the making of life-sustaining and function-regulating inputs.
4. Human agency is exercised in discovering, developing, and transmitting to others ways and means to identify needs for and make inputs to self and others.
5. Groups of human beings with structured relationships cluster tasks and allocate responsibilities for providing care to group members who experience privations for making required deliberate input to self and others.

A general theory of nursing is an account of entities and relationships that serve to organize the outlook of nurses. It also lays a framework that expresses essential variables and relationships and a base for predicting relations. The theory is viewed as descriptively explanatory of the lawlike relationships or universal conditionals implicit in premises 1 to 4 and in premise 5 as this pertains to societies where nursing is established as an available human service.

The *self-care deficit theory* of nursing is a synthesis of knowledge about the theoretic entities self-care (and dependent-care), self-care agency (and dependent-care agency), therapeutic self-care demand, the relational entity self-care deficit, and nursing agency. This general theory of nursing is expressed in terms of the named theoretic entities and introduces existential statements about them, such as *mature adults engage in self-care*. Recognitive criteria are required for verification or falsification of such statements within space-time matrices. Recognitive criteria would be developed to establish that the action expressed in existential statements about instances of persons engaged in self-care is self-care and not another form of deliberate action. See Harré[1] pp. 66-67.

Refinement of the Theory

The self-care deficit theory of nursing as it is expressed in Chapter 2 has been refined and further developed. This was accomplished in part through the separate expressions of a theory of self-care, a theory of self-care deficit, and a theory of nursing system. The named theories in their articulations with one another express the whole that is self-care deficit nursing theory. The theory of nursing system subsumes the theory of self-care deficit and through it the theory of self-care. Self-care deficit theory subsumes the theory of self-care (Figure 7-1).

In each of the three theories, four categories of postulated entities establish the ontology, the realities that are the focuses of the theories: (1) persons in space-time localizations, (2) attributes or properties of these persons, (3) motion or change, and (4) products brought into being.

Table 7-1 identifies the reality focuses of the theory and names the entities postulated within each of the three theories within the general theory.

In subsequent sections, each of the three theories is described with a presentation of the central idea of the theory, the **presuppositions** to the theory, and the **propositions** that flow from the expressed **central idea**.

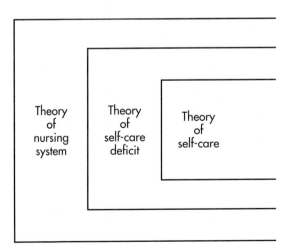

Figure 7-1 Constituent theories, the self-care deficit theory of nursing.

Table 7-1   Postulated Entities for the Theories of Self-Care,
Self-Care Deficit, and Nursing System

Postulated Entities	Theory of Nursing System	Theory of Self-Care Deficit	Theory of Self-Care
Persons in space-time matrices	Nurses, patients with S-CD* Clients with D-CD†	Persons not able to know and meet their own or their dependents' health-associated TS-CD‡	Persons performing operations to know and meet their own or dependents' TS-CD‡
Properties of persons	Nursing agency of nurse Nature of patient's self-care deficit	Health-derived or health-related self-care or dependent-care deficit—partial to complete	Self-management capabilities Self-care agency or dependent-care agency Therapeutic self-care demand
Properties of relationships	Legality of relationship Nursing legitimacy Interpersonal unity		
Motion or change	Change in patients' TS-CD‡ or S-CA§ or D-CA‖ Exercise of nursing agency by nurse Role allocation Role acceptance Role fulfillment by nurse, by patient Role change Change of nurses	Self or another— seeking nursing assistance, agreeing to receive nursing under specified conditions	No performance to complete performance of self-care or dependent-care operations
Product	Nursing system	Agreement to receive nursing Beginning interpersonal relationship with nurse(s)	No care system or a self-care system or a dependent-care system

*Self-care deficit.
†Dependent-care deficit.
‡Therapeutic self-care deficit.
§Self-care agency.
‖Dependent-care agency.

THE THEORY OF SELF-CARE

The idea of self-care has been foundational in the development of the self-care deficit theory of nursing. Conceptualization of self-care and work to understand the substantive structure (parts or elements) of the concept led, in 1990, to the hypothesis that self-care is a human regulatory function. From this base a refined expression of the theory of self-care is presented in the form of presuppositions of the theory, its central idea, and a series of propositions.

Presuppositions

- All things being equal, mature and maturing persons through learning develop and exercise intellectual and practical skills and manage themselves to sustain motivation essential for continuing daily care of themselves and their dependents with some degree of effectiveness.
- Self-care and care of dependents require the availability, procurement, preparation, and use of resources for determining what care is needed and for its provision.
- Available and known means and procedures of self-care and dependent-care are culture elements that vary within families, culture groups, and societies.
- Individuals' action repertoires and their predilections for taking actions under certain conditions affect what persons do and do not do with respect to self-care or dependent-care within the context of stable or changing life situations.
- Experiences of persons in the provision of self-care or dependent-care enables them to accumulate and structure bodies of experiential knowledge about kinds of care, when care is needed, and methods of providing care.
- Scientific knowledge available and communicated to persons in communities is added to their experiential knowledge about self-care and dependent-care.

The Central Idea of the Theory

Self-care is a human regulatory function that individuals must, with deliberation, perform for themselves or have performed for them (dependent-care) to supply and maintain a supply of materials and conditions to maintain life; to keep physical and psychic functioning and development within norms compatible with conditions essential for life; and for integrity of functioning and development.

Self-care as a human regulatory function stands in distinction from other types of regulation of human functioning and development such as neuroendocrine regulation. Self-care must be *learned* and it must be *deliberately performed continuously* in time and in conformity with the regulatory requirements of individuals associated, for example, with their stages of growth and development, states of health, specific features of health or developmental states, environmental factors, and levels of energy expenditure.

Propositions

A number of propositions are presented that are aids in the selection and organization of knowledge relevant to self-care from other fields of knowing.

Propositions may also provide the foundations for formulation and testing of hypotheses about self-care or dependent-care. The propositions presented are not logically related.

Set one
- The materials continuously provided or sustained through self-care or dependent-care are materials essential for life, namely, air, water, and food.
- Conditions that are provided or maintained through self-care or dependent-care are concerned with safe engagement in human excretory functions, sanitary disposal of human excrements, personal hygienic care, maintenance of normal body temperature, protection from environmental and self-imposed hazards, and what is needed for unhampered physical, cognitive, emotional, interpersonal, and social development and functioning of individuals in their life situations.
- The quality and quantity of materials and the conditions provided or sustained through self-care or dependent-care must be within a range that is known to be compatible with what is biologically required for human life, for integrity of human development, and for integrity of human structure and functioning. *Note:* What is known in any time-place localization varies with the state of the arts and sciences and with access of people to what is known.
- Self-care or dependent-care performed by persons with the intention of doing good for self or others may fall short of the focal conditions and goals sought because of their lack of knowledge and skills or other action limitations.

Set two
- Engagement in self-care or dependent-care involves performance of operations to estimate or establish what can and should be done, to decide what will be done, and to produce care. *Note:* These operations conform to the estimative or intentional and the production phases of deliberate action (Figure 7-2).
- Self-care or dependent-care is work or labor that requires time, expenditure of energy, financial resources, and continued willingness of persons to engage in the operations of self-care or dependent-care.
- Self-care or dependent-care performed over time can be understood (intellectualized) as an action system (self-care system, dependent-care system) whenever there is valid and reliable information about care measures performed and the connecting links among them.
- Care measures selected and performed in self-care and dependent-care are specified by the technologies or methods selected for use to meet known or estimated requirements for regulation of functioning or development (self-care requisites). When this is understood and skills are developed, care measures become performance *habits*.

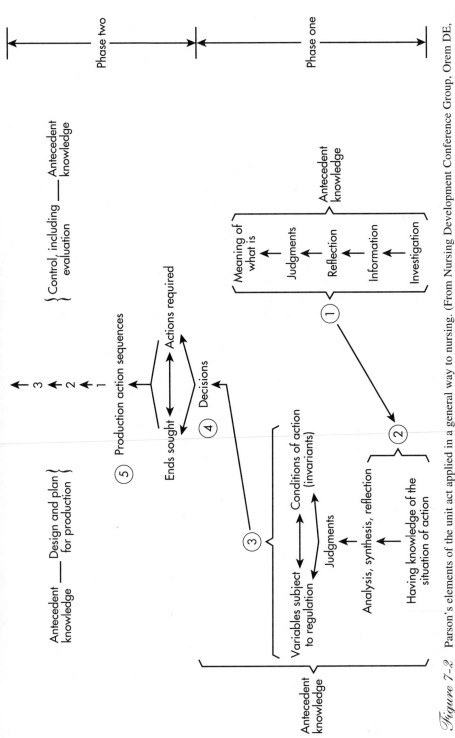

Figure 7-2   Parson's elements of the unit act applied in a general way to nursing. (From Nursing Development Conference Group, Orem DE, editor: *Concept Formalization in nursing: process and product*, ed 2, Boston, 1979, Little, Brown.)

THE THEORY OF SELF-CARE DEFICIT

The theory of self-care deficit is the essential constituent or element of self-care deficit nursing theory. The theory expresses and develops the reason why persons require nursing. The theory is expressed in the form of its presuppositions, its central idea, and propositions that are guides to the further development and refinement of the theory and for determining the validity of its elements and its structure.

Presuppositions

Two sets of presuppositions link the central idea of the theory of self-care deficit to the theory of self-care and to the idea of social dependency.

Set one
- Engagement in self-care requires ability to manage self within a stable or changing environment.
- Engagement in self-care or dependent-care is affected by persons' valuation of care measures with respect to life, development, health, and well-being.
- The quality and completeness of self-care and dependent-care in families and communities rests on the culture, including scientific attainments of groups and the educability of group members.
- Engagement in self-care and dependent-care are affected, as is engagement in all forms of practical endeavor, by persons' limitations in knowing what to do under existent conditions and circumstances or how to do it.

Set two
- Societies provide for the human state of social dependency by instituting ways and means to aid persons according to the nature of and the reasons for their dependency.
- When they are institutionalized, direct helping operations of members of social groups become the means for aiding persons in states of social dependency.
- The direct helping operations of members of groups may be classified into those associated with states of age-related dependency and those not so associated.
- Direct helping services instituted in groups to provide assistance to persons irrespective of age include the health services.
- Nursing is one of the health services of Western and other civilizations.

Central Idea of the Theory

Requirements of persons for nursing are associated with the subjectivity of mature and maturing persons to health-derived or health care–related action limitations associated with their own or their dependents' health states that render them completely or partially unable to know existent and emerging requisites for regulatory care for themselves or their dependents and to engage in the continuing performance of care measures to control or in some way manage factors that are regulatory of their own or their dependents' functioning and development.

Propositions

The following propositions serve as principles and guides for the further development of the theory. The propositions are not logically related.

- Persons who take action to provide their own self-care or care for dependents have specialized capabilities for action.
- Individuals' abilities to engage in self-care or dependent-care are conditioned by age, developmental state, life experience, sociocultural orientation, health, and available resources.
- Relationship of individuals' abilities for self-care or dependent-care to the qualitative and quantitative self-care or dependent-care demand can be determined when the value of each is known.
- The relationship between care abilities and care demand can be defined in terms of *equal to, less than,* and *more than.*
- Nursing is a legitimate service when (1) care abilities are less than those required for meeting a known self-care demand (a deficit relationship) and (2) self-care or dependent-care abilities exceed or are equal to those required for meeting the current self-care demand, but a future deficit relationship can be foreseen because of predictable decreases in care abilities, qualitative or quantitative increases in the care demand, or both.
- Persons with existing or projected care deficits are in, or can expect to be in, states of social dependency that legitimate a nursing relationship.
- A self-care deficit may be relatively permanent, or it may be transitory.
- A self-care or dependent-care deficit may be wholly or partially eliminated or overcome when persons with deficits have the necessary human capabilities, dispositions, and willingness.
- Self-care deficits, when expressed in terms of persons' limitations for engagement in the estimative (intentional) or production operations of self-care, provide guides for selection of methods of helping and understanding patient roles in self-care.

THE THEORY OF NURSING SYSTEM

The theory of nursing system subsumes the theory of self-care deficit, and, with it, the theory of self-care. The theory of nursing system establishes the structure and the content of nursing practice. It is the theory that articulates the nurse property of *nursing agency* with the patient properties of *therapeutic self-care demand* and *self-care agency* (or dependent-care agency).

Presuppositions

These presuppositions are foundational to the theory of nursing system.
- Nursing is practical endeavor, a human health service.
- Nursing can be understood as art, an intellectual quality of nurses designing and producing nursing for others.
- Nursing has result-achieving operations that must be articulated with the interpersonal and societal features of nursing.

• The results sought by nurses through nursing can be expressed as forms of care that ideally and ultimately result in movement to positive health or well-being.

Central Idea of the Theory

All action systems that are nursing systems are formed (designed and produced) by nurses for legitimate recipients of nursing by exercising their powers of nursing agency. These systems compensate for or overcome existent or emerging health-derived or health-associated limitations of the recipients' powers of self-care agency or dependent-care agency* in meeting their own or their dependents' known, existent, or projected therapeutic self-care demands in relatively stable or changing life situations. Nursing systems may be produced for individuals, for persons who constitute a dependent-care unit, for groups whose members have therapeutic self-care demands with similar components or who have similar limitations for engagement in self-care or dependent-care, or for families or for other multiperson units.

Propositions

Some propositions specific to the further development and validation of the theory of nursing system are presented. These propositions are not logically related.

• Legitimate recipients of nursing are persons, as individuals or members of groups, with powers of self-care agency or dependent-care agency that are rendered totally or partially inadequate by their own or their dependents' states of health or by the nature of health care requirements.

• In the design and production of the nursing system, nurses seek and confirm information needed to make judgments about the components (some or all) of therapeutic self-care demands and powers of self-care agency or dependent-care agency of persons under their care.

• The compensatory nature of nursing systems for individuals in their time-place localizations is specified by the immediacy of their need to meet components of their therapeutic self-care demands and by their existent inabilities for taking the required kinds of action.

• The action limitation overcoming the nature of nursing systems is specified by persons' limitations of self-care agency that can be overcome by learning, by skill development and exercise, and by developing, enhancing, or adjusting skills in self-direction and self-management.

• The structure of nursing systems varies with what legitimate recipients of nursing can and cannot do in knowing and meeting their own or their dependents' therapeutic self-care demands and in overcoming existent or projected action limitations.

---

*Limitations of dependent-care agency relevant here are those associated with the state of health care of the dependent person.

- The structure, content, and results of nursing systems in operation in concrete life situations vary with nurses' developed powers of nursing agency, with their willingness to exercise these powers, and with factors internal to nurses or with external circumstances and conditions that facilitate or impede nurses' exercise of their powers of nursing agency.
- The linkages of nursing systems (as here described) to more encompassing interpersonal systems of recipients vary with the powers of legitimate recipients of nursing to interact and communicate with nurses and with nurses' powers of interaction and communication.

SUMMARY STATEMENTS ABOUT THE THEORY

This general theory of nursing is referred to as the *self-care deficit theory of nursing* because it is descriptively explanatory of the *relationship* between the action capabilities of individuals and their demands for self-care or the care demands of children or adults who are their dependents. *Deficit* thus stands for the relationship between the action that individuals should take (the action demanded) and the action capabilities of individuals for self-care or dependent-care. *Deficit* in this context should be interpreted as a *relationship,* not as a human disorder. Self-care deficits may be associated, however, with the presence of human functional or structural disorders.

The self-care deficit theory of nursing assumes that nursing is a response of human groups to one recurring type of incapacity for action to which human beings are subject, namely, the incapacity to care for oneself or one's dependents when action is limited because of one's health state or the health care needs of the care recipient. From a nursing point of view, human beings are viewed as needing continuous self-maintenance and self-regulation through a type of action named *self-care*. The term *self-care* means care that is performed by oneself for oneself when one has reached a state of maturity that is enabling for consistent, controlled, effective, and purposeful action. The unborn, the newborn, infants, children, the severely disabled, and the infirm cannot meet any or some of their own requirements for maintenance and for regulation of their functioning.*

The theory posits two **patient variables**—namely, self-care agency and therapeutic self-care demand—and one **nurse variable,** nursing agency. In conceptualizations of the theory of self-care deficits, the patient variables are viewed as related, and within the theory of nursing system, nursing agency is viewed as related to both patient variables. Persons with health-related self-care deficits are designated as legitimate patients. Nurses view their own legitimacy in terms of their capabilities for providing the kind and amount of nursing required by persons under their care.

---

*The terms *self-care requisites* and *therapeutic self-care demand* are consistently used with respect to all persons of all ages. It is the form of care that is differentiated—namely, self-care and dependent-care.

FOUNDATIONAL CONCEPTS

During the process of development of self-care deficit nursing theory, including the validation of its dominant conceptual elements, the Nursing Development Conference Group[2] identified five concepts of the greatest generality that underlie the theory and its concepts: man (humankind), [deliberate] action, organization, process, and system (pp. 122–125). These concepts were identified because nurses' developed insights about them and their mastery of the meaning of the concepts provide a general organizing foundation in nurses' cognitive structuring of the subject matter of self-care deficit nursing theory and its subsidary theories. In taking this position, the group followed the work of D.P. Ausubel.[4]

The terms that stand for the five concepts have been used repeatedly in this and prior chapters; also used is a sixth term, *good. Deliberate action* was described and explained in Chapter 3, including a word model of the "component actions of a 'complete human act.'" *Views of humankind* were adequately developed in Chapter 6, namely, the person view, the person as agent view, the person as user of symbols view, the embodied person view, and the view of the individual as object, subject to physical forces. The final section of this chapter describes five of these foundational concepts, with additional models of deliberate action, Lonergran's description of the *good,* and descriptive material about *organization, process,* and *system.* Understanding these concepts, and the terms that stand for them, is foundational to dealing cognitively with the subject matter of nursing as set forth in self-care deficit nursing theory and to guiding persons in the practical work of nursing and self-care.

Deliberate Action: Units of Action and Phases of Action

Deliberate actions of individuals at moments in time are directed to bring about conditions or occurrences that are not yet in existence. According to Wallace[5] and Gilby,[6] practical or productive actions involve three different types of component actions: actions related to the end or result sought, actions related to deliberation about the course of action to be taken and the means to be used, and finally productive, practical action to achieve the end. The completion of all three types of actions in achievement of a foreseen and desired end can be viewed as an interrelated system of individual actions and action sequences; a common example would be preparing a meal for four people. The working out of the actions and action sequences to be performed to achieve the end designated in this example is a complex undertaking but one that has been mastered by persons with culinary knowledge and skills. Nurses must engage in such analyses and sequencing of action in nursing practice. Identification of the action components and units of action involved in knowing and meeting a specific self-care requisite is an example.

To adequately identify the components of a complete human act performed to achieve some end in some time-place situation, nurses must be able to envision the whole of the movement from *apprehension of an achievable and desirable end* to *attainment of the end or its nonattainment.* The two models presented in this section may help nurses achieve the ability to envision the whole of a specific action system identified within a situation where action is engaged in by responsible persons.

Units of Action

The first model (a pictorial model) was developed from Parson's expressed conceptualization of a *unit act* (see Chapter 3). Parson's terms *unit act* and **unit of action** refer to the smallest distinct unit of doing something that is meaningful (makes sense) when viewed within the context of a complete human act as represented in the models of Wallace[5] and Gilby.[6] For example, a person engaging in the routine of actions he or she performs to leave his or her home at 8 AM may be considered as a unit act within the whole sequence of actions necessary for the person to be at work at 9 AM. Being at work at 9 AM can be envisioned within the still larger action framework of the person's occupational life.

The model shown in Figure 7-3 is a gross representation of the component actions that identify the end and the means of action within a nursing practice situation or units thereof. The agent of action is represented as nurse. The person within whom there is a requirement for a desirable and attainable future state of affairs is identified as (the nurse's) patient. The model represents action components that are more or less formalized or set when nurses' judgments have been made about: (1) the state of affairs currently existent in the patient and his or her environment, (2) a desirable and attainable future state of affairs for the patient, (3) factors that can be controlled in the patient or the environment, and (4) the means that are nursing appropriate with an adequate degree of reliability and validity for the nurse to use in enabling movement from the "present state of affairs" to the "desirable future state of affairs." The nurse is shown as having ideas of the "desirable future state of affairs" and with the capability to envision movement from the patient's "present state of affairs" to "a future and desirable state" by using the "nursing means" the nurse selects.

The model also shows that associated with the patient's present state of affairs, including the environment, there are "uncontrollable factors" that prevail and influence the nurse's selection of the *means* and become "conditions of action" influencing the judgments and decisions of the nurse as he or she acts to bring about the envisioned "desirable future state of affairs." For example, in meeting the universal self-care requisite *maintain an adequate intake of food,* the amount and kind of food immediately available for consumption are a *condition of action* at the immediate time and place where persons act to meet this requisite. As another example, a nurse makes the judgment and the decision that the position of an unconscious patient should be changed. The nurse's judgments, decision, and actual changing of the person's position form a unit of action within the accomplishment of the larger goal of preventing lung congestion and prolonged pressure on body tissues. The uncontrollable factor at the time of the nurse's decision would be the patient's state of unconsciousness.

The model represented in Figure 7-2 is developed within the frame of reference of nursing as a practice field. Within the boundaries of self-care deficit

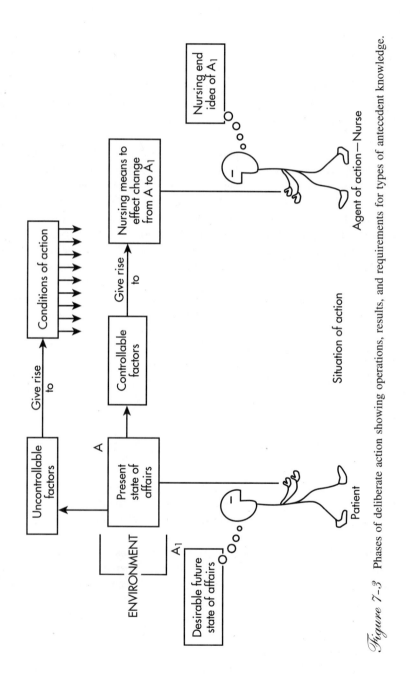

Figure 7-3 Phases of deliberate action showing operations, results, and requirements for types of antecedent knowledge.

nursing theory, the patient's *present state of affairs* would include a patient's powers and capabilities to engage in self-care as well as a patient's self-care action limitations in relation to the therapeutic self-care demand. The model has been helpful to nurses and nursing students in developing for themselves a broad, general frame of reference for viewing nursing practice situations. Parson's concept *unit act* is important for nurses, as well as for other health care workers, because each of their prescriptions for care may need to be broken down into series of unit acts so that patients can understand care prescriptions, choose to follow them, and proceed to follow them.

Phases of Action

The model shown in Figure 7-3 divides the component actions necessary to bring about, within a situation of action, conditions that are sought but do not exist into two **phases of action.** *Phase one* is represented as an *investigative and estimative phase* ending with *judgments* about situational *variables subject to regulation* (the controllable conditions of Figure 7-2) and *conditions of actions* (invariants). *Phase two* is represented as proceeding from *decisions* about *ends* to be sought (the means to be used) and the *actions required* to use the *means* to achieve the end, to *production action sequences* designed to achieve the end sought. *Phase* is used to mean the performance and emergence of different forms of human behavior as persons perform the component actions and action sequences represented in the phases.

The Nursing Development Conference Group separated reflection and judgments about the variables subject to regulation and the invariants from phase one and combined them with *decisions* from phase two to make a *transitional phase.* This phase is so named because it represents action that moves from the investigative, analytical, and synthesizing aspects of phase one to the production aspects of phase two. The three-phase approach identifies investigative, transitional, and production phases of deliberate action. The two-phase approach identifies an investigative and estimative phase and a production phase of deliberate action.

The phase of action model is important for nurses' consideration because it represents nurses' need for **antecedent knowledge** in order to perform observational, perceptual and cognitional, and production actions. The kinds of antecedent knowledge needed by nurses depend on conditions and circumstances that prevail in the situation of action. These conditions and circumstances relate to persons under nursing care, their environments, and time-place factors. Antecedent knowledge also includes experiential and theoretic knowledge of types of nursing cases, models of nursing practice, and valid and reliable nursing means to bring about desired conditions. Because *production action sequences* must be *designed* and *plans* made for their execution, antecedent knowledge must include professional knowledge of *design* and *planning* in the context of nursing practice. This same need for antecedent knowledge holds for *control* of production actions and *evaluation* of results being achieved.

This model shows the complexity of deliberate action from the perspective of the person who is the agent of action. This person in the context of nursing practice may be nurse, patient, or both nurse and patient.

The Good–Desire, Order, Value

Integral to understanding deliberate action, including self-care and nursing, is the foundational idea of **the good.** Because persons have action tendencies toward that which they appraise as good (liked), a consideration of what is good is essential.

Lonergan[7] suggests three levels of the good or desirable. In the first or elementary level, what is good is the object of desire. At this level, the good is particular and is coupled with its opposite bad. For example, "It is good that my dentist will see me today, for my tooth continues to ache." Lonergan suggests that the second level of the good is the good of order, in which recurring desires and aversions of members of social groups through intelligent control and insights into concrete situations result in arrangements for human living, including an "intelligible pattern of human relationships" in the family and in other social institutions. The good of order is dynamic, leading individuals to consider how their own actions are conditioned by existent arrangements, including patterns of relationships, and how their own actions to fulfill desires condition the fulfillment of desires of others. The good of order is viewed as an aspect of human intersubjectivity. The third level of the good is that of value or worth "as the possible object of rational choices." Whatever is desired becomes a value when it is placed within some intelligible hierarchy as a possible object of choice within a situation of action.

The levels or aspects of the good as identified by Lonergan are important in practical endeavors such as self-care and nursing, especially when unfamiliar possible courses of action to change situations are identified and are objects of choice. Persons become concerned with reasons for their action and begin a process of reflection by closely examining what could be done and investigating their motives for choosing courses of action. Desirability and usefulness of a course of action for goal achievement are considered. The fit or lack of fit of a course of action in the accepted order of things—for example, in the family or the health care system—the location of the course of action, and the goal sought within each person's value hierarchy are examined.[7]

Insights about good as the object of desire, the good of order, and good as value or worth add another dimension toward respecting the practical intelligence of men, women, and children and their choices of what to do and what not to do before initiating concrete courses of action to change their life situations.

Organization, Process, System

Organization is commonly conceptualized as a formal organization of persons who interact and coordinate their efforts toward some end. Barnard[8] defines "a formal organization as a system of consciously coordinated activities or forces of two or more persons" (p. 73). However, organization can be conceptualized more generally as that arrangement of elements or parts of real entities, conceptualized constructs, or produced entities so that they function in a unified manner. The cells, tissues, organs, and organ systems of living plants and animals are examples of parts of real entities. The structure of the concept of nursing system (see Box on p. 156) is an example of the second. The coordinated actions of a nurse and a patient in meeting one or more of the patient's self-care requisites is an example of a produced entity, a system of action.

Process refers to the course of something being done or taking place in a definite manner, a continuing movement toward an end, involving many changes. Achievement of a goal or a subgoal sets limits on the time dimension of processes. Process can refer to chemical or biologic processes, to industrial processes, to the reflective thought processes of a person, or to a person's deliberate actions to bring about some change or some new condition. Processes for attaining specific results repeatedly needed in human life situations become formalized as technologies.

System is a term that is used in a variety of ways. Basically the reference is to things or ideas or formalized designs for things to be done or to series and sequences of deliberate actions so arranged that the arranged entities do or will behave together as whole. A concept of system also includes the insight that changes in parts within the system will affect the whole that is the system. In daily living, people refer to the solar system, systems of government, school systems, and so forth. In nursing, for example, there is reference to health care systems, self-care systems, and nursing systems. *System* is a versatile term that is used in conjunction with *process* and *organization.* For example, *process is a system of action,* and Barnard[8] uses the term *system* when he defines a formal organization "as a system of consciously coordinated activities." In fact, when persons understand how a number of entities work together as a whole, they think of it and refer to it as a system.

The Nursing Development Conference Group took the position that W.R. Ashby's concept of *self-organizing system* was "most accurately suited to practical science purposes in nursing." Ashby, as cited by the Nursing Development Conference Group,[2] identifies "self-organizing systems" as those "that exist only when and for the duration that there are self-connecting links between the behavior or state of independent parts or subjects, the connection occurring at some point of conditionality between them" (p. 125) (see Ashby,[9] pp. 108-118). The Nursing Development Conference Group's expressed concept of a nursing system (see Box on p. 156) is illustrative of a self-organizing system. This expressed concept of nursing system can also be thought of as describing "consciously coordinated activities or forces" of nurses and persons under their care.

Commonalities

The three terms just described all subsume concepts of *order* and *relations. Order* refers to the sequence or arrangement of things or events.[10] From a philosophic perspective there are a number of classifications of order. For example, order as the unification of distinct objects by means of intrinsic relations is the ontological

Conceptualization of Nursing System

A *nursing system,* like other systems for the provision of personal services, is the product of a series of relations between persons who belong to different sets (classes), the set A and the set B. From a nursing perspective any member of the set A (legitimate patient) presents evidence descriptive of the complex subsets self-care agency and therapeutic self-care demand and the condition that in A demand exceeds agency as a result of health or health-related causes. Any member of the set B (legitimate nurse) presents evidence descriptive of the complex subset nursing agency, which includes valuation of the legitimate relations between self as *nurse* and instances in which, in A, certain values of the component phenomena of self-care agency and therapeutic self-care demand prevail.

B's perceptions of the conditionality of A's subset objective therapeutic self-care demand on the subset self-care agency establishes the conditionality of changes in the states of A's two subsets on the state of and changes in the state of B's subset nursing agency. The activation of the components of the subset nursing agency (change in state) by B to deliberately control or alter the state of one or both of A's subsets—therapeutic self-care demand and self-care agency—is nursing. The perceived relations among the parts of the three subsets (actual system) constitute the organization. The "mapping" of the behaviors in "mathematical or behavioral terms" provides a record of the system (p. 107).

Entities described and synthesized in the theoretic concept nursing system are summarized.
- Persons in the designated statuses of "legitimate patient" and "legitimate nurse"
- Two properties of "legitimate patient," namely, "therapeutic self-care demand" and "self-care agency"
- An inequality of patient properties, therapeutic self-care demand, and self-care agency within an action frame of reference—the demand for self-care (therapeutic self-care demand) exceeds the existent and operational capabilities of a legitimate patient to meet the demand (self-care agency)
- One property of "legitimate nurse," namely, "nursing agency," which includes capabilities to value legitimate relations between self as nurse and the person(s) in patient status under prevailing values of the component phenomena[*] of self-care agency and therapeutic self-care demand
- Motion or change revealed by events and operations including (1) nurse perceptions of conditionality between patient properties, therapeutic self-care demand, and self-care agency, (2) nurse insights that change in patient properties, dependent on nurses' creative endeavor, is conditioned on the nurse's own state of development of nursing agency and the nurse's exercise of it, and (3) nurse activation of components of nursing agency to deliberately control or alter the state of one or both patient properties.

[*]The reference here is to the substantive components of these two conceptualized properties that point to concrete features of individuals and their environments.

From Nursing Development Conference Group, Orem DE, editor: *Concept formalization in nursing: process and product,* ed 2, Boston, 1979, Little, Brown.

order, the *real order* that persons through use of their reason discover in the concrete world, the world of reality. Persons in life situations also discern relations and establish order in formulating and expressing concepts and discerning relations among concepts. This is the *logical order.* Persons in life situations also discover the order required and produce this order among their deliberately performed actions to move from a current state of affairs to a more desirable state, or to achieve some end that is sought. This is a *produced order,* an *artificial order,* the order required when individuals take actions to know and meet self-care requisites or when nurses take actions to know and meet the nursing requirements of persons under their care[10] (pp. 13-17).

Relation conveys the idea of connection between two or more entities. "It signifies some sort of interdependence, some sort of order between beings"[8] (pp. 249-250). Relation is the binding and unifying element of order. By means of relation, distinct entities are combined into a harmonious and unified whole. Distinct objects, distinct ideas or concepts, or discrete human actions can be related, ordered to one another according to time and place or other ways in which one entity can be said to be prior to the other. What is common to related entities has its basis in qualities existent in each, qualities that bind them together and unify them[11] (pp. 11-14).

SUMMARY

This chapter on self-care deficit nursing theory states what nurses have found and continue to find about the characteristic ways in which this general theory of nursing aids them in their work. Aspects of development of the theory are expressed in terms of what is involved in theory development, underlying premises of the theory and the continued development and refinement of the general theory through expression of theories of self-care, self-care deficit, and nursing system. The three theories express the elements, the relationships, and the propositions that guide model building, hypothesis formation, and continued developmental effort. The chapter concludes with descriptions of concepts foundational to understanding the conceptual constructs of self-care deficit nursing theory. The chapter in its entirety is designed to give nurses and nursing students an overview of the value and complexity of one general theory of nursing and the demands placed on persons who desire to master the theory and gain understanding of its meaning for their work in nursing.

References

1. Harré R: *The principles of scientific thinking,* Chicago, 1970, University of Chicago Press, p 3.
2. Nursing Development Conference Group, Orem DE, editor: *Concepts formalization in nursing: process and product,* ed 2, Boston, 1979, Little, Brown.
3. Orem DE: A general theory of nursing. Presented at the 5th annual post-master's conference, Marquette University School of Nursing, June 1, 1973, pp 3-5.
4. Ausubel DP: Some psychological aspects of the structure of knowledge. In Elam S: *Education and the structure of knowledge,* Chicago, 1964, Rand McNally, pp 221-249.

5. Wallace WA: *The modeling of nature,* Washington, DC, 1996, Catholic University of America Press, p 179.
6. Gilby T: Appendix I, Structure of a human act. In St. Thomas Aquinas: *Summa theologiae: psychology of human acts,* vol 17, 1970, Black Friars, Cambridge. In connection with McGraw-Hill, pp 211-217.
7. Lonergan BJF: Insight: a study of human understanding. In Crowe FE, Doran RM, editors: *Collected works of Bernard Lonergan,* Toronto, 1992, University of Toronto Press, pp 619-621.
8. Barnard CI: *The functions of the executive,* Cambridge, 1938, 1962, Harvard University Press.
9. Ashby WR: Principles of self-organizing systems. In Buckley W, editor: *Modern systems research for the behavioral scientist,* Chicago, 1968, Aldine, pp 108-118.
10. Dougherty GV: *The moral basis of social order according to Saint Thomas,* Washington, DC, 1941, Catholic University of America Press, pp 13-17.
11. Renard H: *The philosophy of being,* ed 2, Milwaukee, 1946, Bruce Publishing, pp 11-14.

CHAPTER 8

The Practical Science
of Nursing

Nurses in practice situations have experiences involving themselves and others. They observe, reflect, reason, and understand as persons who know nursing. Knowing nursing is a dynamic cognitional process and not a static condition of a nurse or nursing student. Developing a cognitional orientation to nursing requires both teaching and learning focused on nursing as a field of practice with its developing fields of knowledge. Teaching communicates insights with empirical meaningfulness that are enabling for nurses' understanding of the complexities of nursing situations. Learning results in the accumulation of related insights by nurses and in nurses' movement to spontaneously seek answers to questions that arise when discussions, actions, or thoughts reveal that understanding is incomplete.

Teaching and learning preparatory for nursing practice should have as their

159

organizing center a core of formulated, expressed, validated, and related concepts that are constituent parts of the *practical science nursing.*

Nurses must be able to think nursing, as well as perform the operations of nursing practice. Nurses who do not develop the ability to think within a nursing frame of reference may tend to be task oriented, viewing persons who require nursing as objects on which work operations are performed. Learning to think as a nurse is facilitated or hindered by the way in which nursing content and experiences are selected and organized in nursing courses in educational programs. The practical science nursing, even in a beginning state of development, provides essential content for courses with a nursing practice focus.

This chapter proposes to explicate the distinguishing features of nursing science and to demonstrate the place of self-care deficit nursing theory in relation to the processes of development of nursing science. What is needed initially by nurses and nursing students is knowing that science primarily is a *search for understanding.* The essential question is: What do nurses seek to understand about nursing practice?

Nursing science is viewed as constituting one of eight fields of knowledge about nurses and nursing (see Box below). Broadly conceived, nursing science seeks to describe and explain nursing practice in terms of its human elements (nurses and patients) and their properties and powers. It is therefore critical content in instructional programs at all levels of nursing education.

Unlike the other seven fields of knowledge, the processes of nursing science do not involve movement from an already developed science or discipline such as sociology or history, with their developed methodologies. Nursing science is a purely creative endeavor of nurses who seek understanding of their field of service in societies and who must find the foundations for doing nursing science.

Nursing science as a process begins with investigations of what, why, or how questions in a search for understanding of nursing practice. The process, when carried to completion, yields conclusions in the form of theories that are hypothesized statements of understandings that are attained. Hypotheses validated through research are added to the compendium of scientific knowledge about nursing practice.

Fields of Knowledge About Nurses and Nursing

1. Nursing sociology
2. Nursing, a profession and occupation
3. Nursing jurisprudence
4. Nursing history
5. Nursing ethics
6. Nursing science
7. Nursing economics
8. Nursing administration

INQUIRY IN PRACTICE FIELDS

The nature of science in practice fields is discussed in its relation to the work of providing nursing.

Nurses work in life situations with others to bring about conditions that are beneficial to persons nursed. Nursing demands the exercise of both the speculative and practical intelligence of nurses. In nursing practice situations, nurses must have accurate information and be knowing about existent conditions and circumstances of patients and about emerging changes in them. This knowledge is the concrete base for nurses' development of creative practical insights about what can be done to bring about beneficial relationships or conditions that do not presently exist.

Asking and answering the questions "what is?" and "what can be?" are nurses' points of departure in nursing practice situations. Answers provide foundations for nurses' judgments and decisions about what should and will be done. Speculative knowing and factual knowing refer to the state of things as they are. Practical refers to that which is useful under some set(s) of circumstances in bringing about needed or desired conditions that are not yet present.

The Factual and the Practical

Nurses, like persons in other human services or persons engaged in result-seeking endeavors, must be conscious of the consistency between what they know and what they do. To achieve this state, nurses must be cognitively active in each nursing practice situation. Nurses search out characterizing features of situations and the patterns and relationships among identified features, including evidence of what should and can be changed. Observation, including the exercise of highly developed perceptual skills, and reflection and judgment are essential in determining nursing-relevant features, both factual and practical, of situations where persons are under nursing care. Nurses reflect on their practical understanding of what can be done to effect more desirable conditions and make critical judgments about what should be done and what should be avoided. Final decisions about what will be done may or may not be in accord with judgments about what should be done.

Engagement in the foregoing types of intellectual activities demands that nurses and nursing students have prior or antecedently acquired authoritative knowledge from a number of organized fields of knowledge, including nursing science and the sciences basic to nursing. In the absence of such *antecedent knowledge,* observations, judgments made, and the courses of action selected will be based wholly on commonsense knowledge of individuals that is uninformed by nursing science and nursing-related science. Nursing is practical endeavor, but it is practical endeavor engaged in by persons who have specialized theoretic nursing knowledge with developed capabilities to put this knowledge to work in concrete situations of nursing practice.

Without knowledge of the practical sciences of nursing, nurses and nursing students are unable to attach *nursing meaning* to what they observe, the factual information they obtain, the complex judgments they make about concrete situations, and the needs for and the possibilities for change that they discern. Situational conditions and relationships among them at times are not known or understood because of nurses' lack of knowledge to guide and attach meaning to observations or because of their inability or failure to observe. At times, persons are moved to and do take action without knowing the appropriateness of what they do and even at times with full knowledge of its inappropriateness.

The complexity of some nursing situations requires that knowing, effective practitioners select courses of action to achieve a sought-after result without full knowledge of the situation. At other times, practitioners know conditions and know what situational changes are desirable, but how to effect change is unclear. Measures to effect desired change may be undiscovered, or, if discovered, they are not validated or have limited reliability. In both of the preceding situations, the nurse's rule is to proceed with caution, use controlled trial approaches, and act to prevent harm as action proceeds. Such situations demand the presence of nursing practitioners with sound theoretical and experiential knowledge of nursing.

Naming Nursing As a Field of Knowledge and Inquiry

A number of terms are used to refer to professional fields such as engineering, medicine, and nursing from the perspective of their accumulated, structured, and validated knowledge and their modes of inquiry. The terms include applied field, applied science, practice discipline, practical science, and science. Nurses have been reluctant not only to take a position about the proper object of nursing but also to take a position about naming nursing as a field of knowledge and inquiry. Nurses have used all of the terms just expressed, but few have expressed rationales for their use or attached meaning to particular terms.

The term *discipline* means a branch or field of knowledge exhibiting a distinctive outlook and style of thinking, as well as distinctive, organized ideas and concepts, methods of inquiry, and modes of understanding data. Disciplines of knowledge with their modes of inquiry are developed and advanced through the work of scholars, theorists, and researchers in the field who communicate their insights and the results of their investigations. The term *practice* in the context of practice discipline means that the ways of knowing and the organized facts, ideas, and concepts associated with the investigations of members of a discipline relate to elements of their practice field and serve to (1) explain and describe elements of the practice field and (2) bring together and organize knowledge in a way that prepares for action.

The term *applied field* is used more frequently in academic circles than the terms *practice discipline* or *practical science* to refer to the knowledge specific to professions and occupations. *Applied field* signifies that persons who engage in, for example, the practice of engineering or medicine or nursing extract from developed disciplines of knowledge, especially the natural sciences, ideas, laws, and theories that are useful to them in the resolution and solution of recurring problems in their practice fields. The term *applied field* minimizes the complexity of practice fields. The term is too narrow to be descriptive of all the constituent kinds of knowledge that constitute well-developed practice fields.

ACCEPTING NURSING SCIENCE AS PRACTICAL SCIENCE

Sciences are reasoned intellectual constructions of men and women that lead to insights about the world of nature and things in it, including humankind. Scientists seek to become knowing in a genuine fashion about the things they investigate, in contrast to having opinions about things[1] (pp. xi-xii). The kinds of knowing recognized as scientific, as well as the beliefs about the truth and certitude of findings attained by scientists, vary by historical periods, from that of Plato and Aristotle to more recent periods. These differences seem to be attributable to how philosophers express in their developed philosophic systems their view of the *real* and how they conceptualize the *nature* of what *persons can know* about the world and the things in it, and how *knowing* is effected.

Sciences have been and are classified in a number of ways. "One of the most basic divisions is that into speculative science, which is concerned primarily with knowing and not with doing, and practical science which is concerned with knowing as ordered to doing"[1] (p. 171). This distinction has been recognized since antiquity; however, the developed literature about the sciences is to a large extent one-sided, with emphasis on **speculative science.** Recognition of the idea of practical science is revealed in the *Ethics* and *Politics* of Aristotle[2] (pp. 180-181). Thomas Aquinas in his *Summa Theologia* expressed the idea and the features of *practical science* and related practical science to the *arts,* through which the thing to be made or the act to be done is constructed[2] (pp. 314-316). The relationship of practical sciences to associated arts, through which results sought are first designed and then brought about, is the basis for the statement that nursing and medicine are arts as well as sciences.

In the twentieth century the philosophers Maritain[2] and Wallace[1,3] wrote about the nature of practical science, including the kinds of knowing and modes of development that characterize them. Simon[4] addressed the sciences of the artificial in his 1969 work, artificial standing in contrast to natural. Natural is that which exists without human influence to bring it into existence. Argyris, in collaboration with colleagues, developed the idea of *action science* as "inquiry into how human beings design and implement action in relation to one another"[5] (p. 4).

In the interest of nurses and nursing in 1967, the philosophers Dickoff and James of Yale University expressed in a symposium on theory development in nursing[6] their "theory about nursing theories." They named, described, and expressed content for four types or levels of nursing theory. A condensed version of the types is as follows: (1) factor-isolating theories, (2) factor-relating theories, (3) situation-relating theories, and (4) situation-producing theories. They indicated that nurses interact with reality for practical purposes and that "situation-producing theories" conceptualize desired situations as well as prescriptions for behavior to bring about the desired situation. Their reference was to nursing as a practice discipline; however, their reference might well have been to "nursing as practical science."

In the 1960s, during the process of developing the self-care deficit theory of nursing and moving from the base of my expressed general concept of nursing, I took the position that nursing as science has the nature of practical science with supporting foundational sciences. This was the period when we, the members of the Nursing Development Conference Group, were engaged in validating conceptual elements and demonstrating causal relations between concepts.[7]

In the academic year 1964-1965, members of the Nursing Development Conference Group and other faculty members of the School of Nursing, the Catholic University of America, through the efforts of Dean Mary E. Redmond, were provided with help in learning about nursing considered as a practical science. W.A. Wallace, of the faculty of the School of Philosophy, conducted a series of conferences on the nature and characteristics of practical sciences, and E.F. O'Doherty, of University College, Dublin, worked with us on the logic of the nursing sciences[7] (p. 105). The practical science models of Maritain and Wallace were and are valuable guides in the development of initial and continuing insights about the form and structure of nursing as practical science.

PRACTICAL SCIENCES

The term **practical science** is used by philosophers and philosophers of science within a philosophic system of moderate realism. Its referent is to modes of inquiry and fields of knowledge associated with the practical order of things, things that are doable. Wallace[3] (pp. 273-293) states that practical sciences are concerned with "principles and causes of things to be done." Practical science is contrasted with "theoretical science" concerned with things that are "knowable" and with "demonstrable knowledge" of the subject of investigation. Wallace[3] and Maritain[2] (pp. 458-459) state that practical science has theoretic or speculative parts, as well as parts that give direction to what to do or what not to do in distinct situations.

Three commonly recognized groups of practical science are identified by Wallace:[3] (1) ethics or moral science concerned with human action in terms of its "being human or moral," (2) the health sciences (e.g., medicine and nursing), and (3) the sciences that deal with forces and objects from a production point of view (e.g., engineering).

The Parts of Practical Sciences

Practical sciences include speculatively practical knowledge and practically practical knowledge.[2] Speculatively practical knowledge brings unity and meaning to the universe of action (action domain) of a practice field and to its elements. The theories and conceptual elements of the self-care deficit theory of nursing are speculative in mode. They describe and explain elements and relations within nursing practice situations, including principles and causes of their existence. The expressed *theory of nursing system,* which subsumes the theory of self-care deficit and the theory of self-care, is an example of how the practical science, nursing, constructs one subject (nursing system) "precisely as capable of being produced" while remaining in the speculative mode.

The second kind of knowledge, practically practical knowledge,[2] is more particularized, dealing with the details of cases, but always within the universal conceptualizations of the practice field, including its domain, elements, and types of results sought. This kind of knowledge is practical in that it is preparatory for action and includes rules and standards of practice; it is compositive in that it brings together knowledge necessary for taking action and organizes it according to actions and results. This form of knowledge is movement closer to concrete practice situations. Experience has a primary role in establishing what is needed for action, and practitioners within the profession have major roles in development of this kind of knowledge.

Practically practical knowledge in nursing science includes, for example, sets of care measures designed to meet a type of self-care requisite particularized for individuals of the same chronologic age, gender, and developmental state living under specified environmental conditions. Another example is rules for selection and use of methods of helping in relation to certain values of self-care agency and the nature and extent of types of self-care limitations.

Theoretic (speculative) nursing science has many of the features of science, unqualified by the adjective *practical.* In its development, methods of inquiry are used to investigate and analyze features of nursing practice situations and nursing cases. Investigators develop insights about perceived features and relations among them. They formulate insights as concepts. Expressed concepts of features and relations among them that are validated in concrete practice situations are the beginnings of descriptions and explanations of nursing's practice domain. Formulated and expressed concepts that are related can be synthesized or unified to form structures of related concepts. Syntheses can be expressed as static unions that express properties of persons—for example, therapeutic self-care demand—or as dynamic processes, as in the theory of nursing system in which nurse and patient properties are conceptualized as necessarily interactive if a synthesis is to occur. (See the conceptualization of nursing system in the Box in Chapter 7, p. 156).

Applied Science

A third kind of knowledge is found within the structure of practice fields. Every practical science includes a number of **applied sciences.** Applied sciences are existent sciences that are put to use or are pursued to achieve some end outside the domain of the science. In practice fields, applied sciences are developed at points of articulation between theoretic or practical problems of a practice field and facts and theoretic formulations of the science that is being applied. The formulations are selected because they are useful in resolving or solving types of problems in the practice fields. Examples of applied sciences include climateo-physiology, medical microbiology, and surgical anatomy. The potential applied nursing sciences can be identified.

Nursing as knowledge essential in achieving nursing results for people would be constituted within this framework from two types of practical nursing sciences and from sets of applied sciences. Nurses, unlike other professionals, rarely use the term *science* with respect to their own discipline. Nurses, however, appear willing to accept the idea of medical sciences and engineering sciences. Science is systematic empirical inquiry. It is concerned with affording meaning to concrete matters of fact. Myriads of facts have been and continue to be amassed within real situations of nursing practice. But facts do not make a science. Neither do the results of research, the fit of which into the structure of nursing science is unspecified. Developing the ideas and concepts, the laws, and the theories that describe and explain the elements of nursing's practice field is essential in making explicit the structure of nursing as a practical science and in opening systematic avenues for research.

SELF-CARE DEFICIT NURSING THEORY IN DEVELOPMENT OF NURSING SCIENCE

Self-care deficit nursing theory, with its conceptual elements and constructs and the defined relations among them, serves in the initial establishment of the subject matter of nursing science. Any effort by members of the nursing profession to develop, validate, and structure knowledge required by nurses in their nursing practice endeavors requires (1) a model of practical science and (2) a valid, comprehensive, general theory of what nursing is and what nursing should be. To be useful, a valid general theory of nursing will have been moved to a stage of development where its concepts have been formally expressed, the substantive structure of concepts uncovered, and relationships demonstrated.

Essential Theory Development

The theories of self-care, self-care deficit, and nursing system described in Chapter 7 and explanations of the nature of conceptualized entities and their structure—for example, self-care requisites—is representative of this stage of development.

Another feature of development began with acceptance that nursing as science encompasses persons performing three types of activities: self-care, dependent-care, and nursing care. These types of activities necessitate a focus on persons as agents. Investigation is required to secure information about the nature and the internal sources of these distinctive types of human activities, for example, the nature of self-care. Such information is grasped at first in a general way that is open to progressive development and refinement on the basis of additional information[1] (pp. 4-5). For example, knowing through observation, perception, and judgment that mature and maturing persons engage in self-care led to the reasoned judgment that persons who engage in self-care would necessarily have the power and capabilities to do so. These yet to be identified powers and capabilities were collectively named *self-care agency.*

Acceptance that self-care is deliberate action to fulfill needs for regulatory inputs to self or environment led to the use of Hartnett-Rauckhorst's models and other models of action to begin to formalize developing insights about how to model the conceptual structure of self-care agency. These insights were enabling for the identification of the powers and capabilities that characterize self-care agency and for understanding and naming the operations through which self-care is performed. These operations were identified as investigative-estimative operations, judgment and decision-making operations, and production operations. (See Chapter 11 for development of the nature and internal sources of the human power named self-care agency.)

These examples illustrate that in a foundational search for knowledge in developing a practical science the mind must reason by analogy. In present-day language, scientists use models and modeling techniques to penetrate the nature of things. Wallace says that in contrast to, for example, models of economic trends, such modeling is "more speculative, theoretical and at ground epistemological"[1] (p. xi). The examples also illustrate Wallace's statement that the work of science involves intellectual movement—reasoning from the "perceived appearance of things to their hidden but underlying causes"[1] (p. xi).

Bringing in the Person Who Is Patient

The continuing development of the conceptual elements of the theories of self-care, self-care deficit, and nursing system contributes to increasing information about the **patient variables** (therapeutic self-care demand and self-care agency) and the nurse variable (nursing agency). (See Chapters 10, 11, and 12.) Recognition and acceptance of the patient and nurse variables must be accompanied by continuing recognition and acceptance that it is persons who are nursed and persons who provide nursing.

In the course of development of self-care deficit nursing theory, members of the Nursing Development Conference Group recognized that certain distinguishing characteristics of persons under nursing care affected or conditioned the values of the patient variables, therapeutic self-care demand and self-care agency, at particular times and under specific circumstances. Such conditioning characteristics of persons were named **basic conditioning factors.***

The Nursing Development Conference Group identified eight basic conditioning factors, with the understanding that factors could be added. In this book Chapter 12 names 10 factors: age, gender, developmental state, health state, pattern of living, health care system factors, family system factors, sociocultural factors, availability of resources, and external environmental factors such as physical or biologic factors of the person's environment.

The nature and nursing practice relevance of these factors are summarized.

1. Basic conditioning factors are not explanatory of patient variables but are **parameters of patient variables** that may actively condition their values at specific times.
2. Basic conditioning factors and the patient variables (therapeutic self-care demand and self-care agency) introduce different but related kinds of subject matter into nursing science.

---

*See Chapter 12 for a development of nurses' use of the factors; also see *Concept Formalization in Nursing: Process and Product*[7] (pp. 169-175) for a description and explanation of basic conditioning factors and their meaning in nursing practice situations.

3. Basic conditioning factors have as their referents human conditions, culture elements, environmental conditions, socioeconomic conditions, and others.
4. Basic conditioning factors can exert a stable influence on the values of patient variables or a rapidly changing conditioning influence, for example, the stable influence of age and developmental state on the patient variables of mature healthy adults in contrast to the effects of a rapidly changing health state on the values of these variables.
5. Basic conditioning factors may affect *not only the value* of persons' therapeutic self-care demands and persons' self-care agency at specific times and over some duration of time *but also the means* that nurses can use to meet persons' therapeutic self-care demands and to regulate persons' exercise or development of their self-care agency. For example, age and developmental states of infants affect the means used to meet the requisites for *intakes* of water and food. Persons' states of cognitional development affect nurses' choice of helping methods.
6. A known relationship between a basic conditioning factor and a patient variable can be expressed as a conditional proposition.

Basic conditioning factors have been described as affecting the values of persons' therapeutic self-care demands and their self-care agency as represented in Figure 8-1. Such factors also can be interactive among themselves. Two such

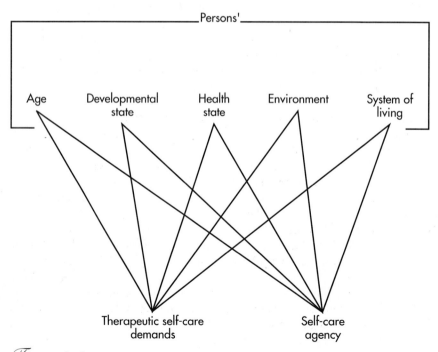

Figure 8-1 A sample of basic conditioning showing relationships to the patient variables.

examples are presented in Figure 8-2. Nurses should understand that such interactiveness is a possibility in every nursing practice situation that requires investigation. Nurses require speculative knowledge about known and validated interactions among factors, existent or projected. This knowledge is a requisite part of educational preparation for nursing.

The factors identified as conditioning persons' therapeutic self-care demands and their self-care agency within the technological dimension of nursing practice can also condition the interpersonal and societal dimensions of nursing practice. These factors are identified in Chapters 4 and 5.

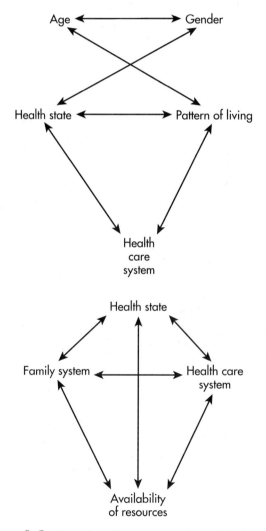

Figure 8-2 Examples of interactive basic conditioning factors.

STAGES OF DEVELOPMENT OF NURSING SCIENCE

Science is activity with respect to entities to be understood not in their individuality in time-place localizations, but in their universality. Doing science is basically intellectual activity. Workers in science function as scholars, theorists, researchers, and, in the practical sciences, also as developers of technologies and techniques for effecting change in concrete situations. Development of technologies and techniques is critical in practice fields because practitioners must move from intellectual conceptions of selected orders or correlations to be brought about to the effecting of those orders or correlations in concrete situations of practice. Technologies and techniques to effect change must be discovered, their validity and reliability under ranges of specified conditions established, and their undesirable effects, if any, set forth.

Workers in a science function with respect to whatever is currently known about their field or areas within their field of knowledge and inquiry that constitute their domain of activity.

Developmental Work

The work of development of nursing science is the result of theorists' and scholars' search for—and their development and expression of—insights about why persons require nursing and the nature of the service, the product, that nurses produce for persons who require it. Development is understood as movement from states of lesser complexity to states of greater complexity. In the development of nursing science, theorists and scholars move *from their perceptions of* persons who require nursing, of persons who nurse, and of the deliberate, coordinated actions that constitute nursing *to a search for the hidden but underlying causes* of what is and what can be and what is brought about.

Initial developments include (1) nurses' expressed insights about and their agreement about why persons require and can be helped through nursing, *the proper object of nursing,* and (2) in accord with this object, nurses' expression of a *generalization* about what nursing is and what nursing should be. From such broad generalizations about nursing, development is movement, which results in the emergence of detail about the conceptualized entities, with higher and higher levels of integration of emerging structures and features that reveal speculative and practical details of nursing.

Five Stages

Five stages of development of the practical science nursing are identified (Figure 8-3). Each stage is understood as a development of different kinds of knowledge within the domain and boundaries of nursing established by nursing's identified proper object and subject matter. This object, as previously expressed, is understood as a person's subjectivity to health-associated deficits for engagement in self-care or dependent-care.

General Features of the Stages

The five suggested stages of development of nursing science are based on two assumptions: (1) there are populations requiring nursing and (2) nursing is

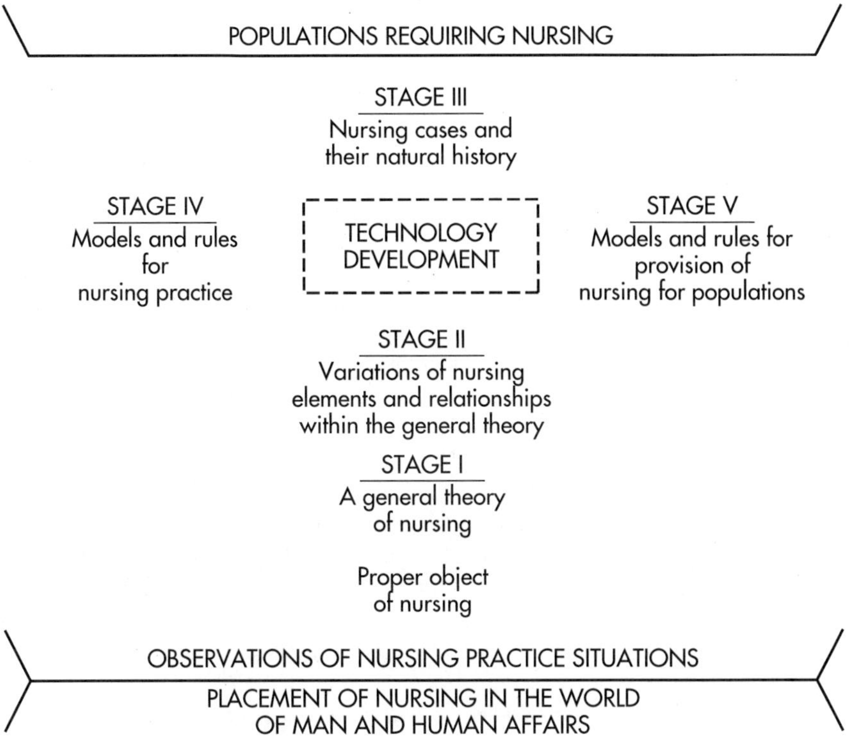

POPULATIONS REQUIRING NURSING

STAGE III
Nursing cases and
their natural history

STAGE IV	┌─────────────┐	STAGE V
Models and rules	│ TECHNOLOGY │	Models and rules for
for	│ DEVELOPMENT │	provision of
nursing practice	└─────────────┘	nursing for populations

STAGE II
Variations of nursing
elements and relationships
within the general theory

STAGE I
A general theory
of nursing

Proper object
of nursing

OBSERVATIONS OF NURSING PRACTICE SITUATIONS
PLACEMENT OF NURSING IN THE WORLD
OF MAN AND HUMAN AFFAIRS

Figure 8-3 Stages of understanding nursing.

recognized and occupies a place in the world of human affairs. The stages (I-V) noted in Figure 8-3 move from the generalizations expressed for stage I to the development of the conceptual elements and the demonstration of relationships among elements of the generalization in stage II to the identification, naming, and description of the features and relationships among features of situations in which persons require nursing, including the history of their development, in stage III to the formulation of models and rules of practice for the provision of nursing to individual and multiperson units in stage IV and for populations in stage V.

Description of Stages

The stages are described as follows:

- *Stage of generalizations* about nursing's proper object, the description and explanation of the nature and features of nursing as a health service, and the results sought through nursing. This stage expresses in specific terms the human focus of nursing, nursing's domain, and boundaries and begins the identification of the subject matter of nursing.
- *Stage of validation and development* of the *conceptual elements* within the generalization about what nursing is; demonstration of relations among the conceptual elements; uncovering the nature and substantive structure of the

conceptual elements and their articulation with facts and theories from non-nursing fields of knowledge.

- *Stage of investigation and description of concrete situations* in which persons who required nursing then received nursing (nursing cases); identification and naming of the patient variables, the enduring and characterizing features of nursing cases; identification of the human and environmental factors that can condition the values of the variables and the range of values of patient variables that can result from such conditioning; development of models of nursing cases; development of classifications of nursing cases.
- *Stage of development of models and general principles of nursing practice,* using the variables of nursing cases and the human unit being served by nurses—an individual, a dependent-care unit, a residence unit including families or other types of multiperson units. Practice models and rules of practice set forth principles to guide the diagnostic processes to determine the values of patient variables and relationships between them under some range of conditions and circumstances. Practice models identify conditions that allow positive movement in patient variables or conditions that are indicative of regressive change. Values of patient variables and their interrelations may give rise to particular requirements for nurse-patient interaction. Nursing prescriptions for regulation of specific values of patient variables and total or partial design models for systems of nursing care become parts of nursing practice models.
- *Stage of identification and description of nursing cases by common features of the patient variables* that distinguish them from other nursing cases. These operations distinguish subgroups or subpopulations within the totality of the instances of persons who sought or received nursing or are seeking or receiving nursing. At times subpopulations as identified here are referred to as populations. Looking at persons who require nursing from the viewpoint of common features provides the basis for making inferences about appropriate nursing diagnostic, prescriptive, and treatment modalities; common features of nursing system designs; kinds of nursing results sought; and the values of nursing agency that would qualify nurses to provide care or consultation.

Developments in stages II through V have their foundations in the generalizations expressed in stage I. Without these most general foundations, there is no basis for developmental movement to identify structures and processes that reflect greater and detailed complexity. Nurses' failure to recognize that nursing has a proper object and to appreciate the functions of a valid general theory of what nursing is and what nursing should be account in part for the undeveloped state of nursing science.

Given the foundations described for stage I, developments in the other four stages may be emerging concurrently or sequentially as theorists and scholars continue developmental work. In fact, all stages of understanding nursing in order to develop nursing science may be in process during the same period.

Technology Development

In addition to the developments expressed, there is a continuing need in nursing and other practice fields for the development, formalization, and validation of technologies essential for effective nursing practice. A *technology* is defined as an application of scientific knowledge to the practical purposes to be achieved in a field. In related fields, for example, nursing and medicine, a technology developed in one field may be used by persons in a related field. For example, some technologies for measuring cardiac and circulatory functioning are used by physicians and nurses; other measuring technologies, however, are used by medical specialists and specialized technicians. At times, technologies may be developed and be used productively without a rationale of why they work.

Nurses develop technologies in the course of their practice of nursing, often without recording them or verbally communicating them to other nurses for further development and validation. Nursing technologies include those related to human interaction and communication, as well as to the observational, diagnostic, and regulatory operations of nursing practice. The following edited listing of types of technologies required for nursing practice was developed in 1969[8] and appeared in a modified form in the first edition of this book.

1. Technologies or processes through which interpersonal, intergroup relations are brought into existence and maintained as long as such relations are essential for achievement of nursing and nursing-related goals in specific types of practice situations.

2. Technologies of human assistance through which help or service is rendered by one person to another. The reasons for the requirements for help and for the matters about which persons need help determine the characteristics of assisting processes.

3. Technologies of individual personal care, which is self-administered by adults and administered by them to infants and children. When such care has as its goal positive health and when it has a base in scientifically derived knowledge, it is referred to as *therapeutic self-care.*

4. Technologies for appraising, changing, and controlling human integrated functioning, with emphasis on physiologic or psychological modes of functioning in health and disease. These are technologies based in medical science.

5. Technologies to bond persons together in therapeutic relations (relations from which flow positively therapeutic results), which contribute to the maintenance of personal integrity and development, despite disease and disability.

6. Technologies for bringing about and controlling the position and movement of persons in their physical environments.

7. Research methods and techniques necessary for the initial and continuing formalization of the named practice technologies, their validation, and the establishment of their validity and reliability for use under specified conditions and circumstances. Rules would be expressed for conditions of use in nursing practice situations.

The work of developing and formalizing the technologies and techniques of nursing practice is not adequately attended to by nurses. Whenever a practice technology is developed, it should be formalized to the degree possible at the time and validated through use and through research. Rules for use under conditions encountered in nursing practice should be formulated, expressed, and communicated within the profession.

Summary of Stages of Development

Figure 8-3 presents suggested stages of development of self-care deficit nursing theory within a frame of practical science. The figure includes features of the prescience phase of nursing's development as a field of knowledge and inquiry, stage I.

The stages of development of self-care deficit nursing theory and developments within various stages have characteristics of a normative model of nursing, reflecting what nurses ought to know and what they ought to bring about. The historical model of nursing was deficient because it represented the nurse role in terms of tasks to be learned and performed, it did not define the domain and boundaries of nursing, it underplayed the role of the professional nurse with respect to nursing's contribution to health care, and it did not contribute to nurses' development of honest regard for themselves as therapeutically trained persons. The five suggested stages of development of the practical science nursing reflect but deviate to some degree from the traditional stages represented for the development of sciences, namely, (1) the stage of natural history, which is largely descriptive of what is the case; (2) the stage of normative thinking, which is what ought to be the case; (3) the stage of science proper, which is the stage of explanation and validation of hypotheses; and (4) the stage of application.

The nursing profession should be concerned not only with nurses and their practice of nursing but also with the practical science of nursing. This science can be developed and formalized only through the activity of nurses with the talents and interests of nursing scholars, theorists, researchers, and developers, who at the same time may be nursing practitioners or teachers of nursing or may work closely with practitioners.

IDENTIFICATION AND NAMING OF THE NURSING SCIENCES

As a conclusion to this chapter on the practical science of nursing, two sets of speculative or theoretical nursing sciences are suggested—namely, nursing practice sciences and foundational nursing sciences (see Box on p. 175). The work of development and validation of the self-care deficit theory of nursing and its conceptual constructs has resulted in an accumulation of subject matter,* as well as insights about its organization and structuring from a practical science perspective. The isolation, naming, and description of the two sets of

---

*See Chapters 2, 7, and 10 to 13.

Speculatively Practical Nursing Science

Nursing Practice Sciences

Wholly Compensatory Nursing
Partly Compensatory Nursing
Supportive-Developmental Nursing

Foundational Nursing Sciences

The Science of Self-Care
The Science of the Development and Exercise of Self-Care Agency in the Absence
  or Presence of Limitations for Deliberate Action
The Science of Human Assistance for Persons with Health-Associated Self-Care
  Deficits

Applied Nursing Sciences
Basic Non-Nursing Sciences

| Biologic | Medical | Human | Environmental |

---

sciences are based on my understanding of the nature of the practical sciences, on my knowledge of the organization of subject matter in other practice fields, and on my understanding of components of curricula for education for the professions.

Nursing Practice Sciences

These sciences—wholly compensatory nursing, partly compensatory nursing, and supportive-educative or developmental nursing—define and explain three practice fields in nursing. Each of the **nursing practice sciences** supplies an organizing framework for bringing together the essential features of nursing practice through which nurses generate systems of nursing care. Essential features of nursing practice include the following: the nature and extent of the deficit relationship between the patient variables therapeutic self-care demand and self-care agency; valid methods of assisting; patient and nurse roles in the production of care to achieve the nursing results of knowing and meeting patients' therapeutic self-care demands and regulating the development or exercise of self-care agency by the patient; the values of nursing agency demanded for nurses able to provide safe and effective nursing; and the time-place demands for the provision of nursing. These practice sciences also provide rules for the diagnostic, prescriptive, and production operations of nursing. These operations extend to identification of those personal and environmental factors, basic conditioning factors, that are stable or are active conditioners of the patient variables. Each of the nursing practice sciences also provides the framework for integration of relevant societal factors (see Chapter 4) and interpersonal factors (see Chapter 5).

The content elements and some relationships for the three nursing practice sciences are shown in schematic form in Figure 8-4. The essential natures of the content elements are the same for each of the three nursing practice sciences. Content elements for these sciences differ according to the nature and extent of the self-care deficits of the members of the population who are the objects of concern of each science. In Figure 8-4 the subject of dependent-care is not addressed. Separate models could be developed.

Foundational Nursing Sciences

Three speculatively practical sciences are identified as foundational or supporting sciences for the nursing practice sciences. The **foundational nursing sciences**

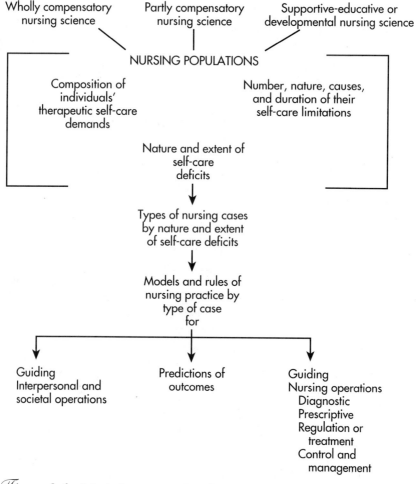

Figure 8-4   Schematic representation of content elements of three nursing practice sciences.

offer descriptions and explanations of self-care, including therapeutic self-care demands, the development and exercise of self-care agency, and the nature and limits of human assistance for persons with self-care deficits.

The characterizing features of the three foundational nursing sciences, including areas of content, are shown in the Box below and those on p. 178. These sciences also are relevant to understanding dependent-care.

The three named foundational nursing sciences supply the foundations for understanding and for making required observations, judgments, and decisions in nursing practice situations. These sciences are narrower and more specialized than the nursing practice sciences. They are speculatively practical in nature but closer than the practice sciences to the detailed observations and judgments that nurses must make in nursing practice situations.

Basic Sciences

Basic to understanding and developing both the *nursing practice sciences* and the *foundational nursing sciences* are sciences outside the domain of nursing identified as **basic sciences.** In their provision of nursing care, nurses select facts, points of theory, models, and hypotheses from these sciences and use them in the intellectual processes of initial and continuing development of the practice and foundational nursing sciences. These sciences basic to nursing include biologic sciences, medical sciences, human sciences, and environmental sciences. Medical sciences are included because nurses use both foundational and applied medical sciences in their work. Basic sciences also serve in the formation of nursing's applied sciences. The *physiology of universal self-care requisites* is an example of an undeveloped but much needed applied nursing science.

Characterizing Features of the Science of Self-Care

Name of Science: A. Science of self-care

Type of Science: Speculatively practical with practically practical content elements

Reality Focus or Proper Object: Persons in human societies continuously producing systems of self-care

Major Content Areas:

I. Self-care, its nature and function

II. Self-care agents and their powers to know and meet their demands for self-care of a therapeutic quality

III. Self-care requisites, nature, and functions; types; formulation and expression

IV. Therapeutic self-care demand, a constructed entity; its components; process of construction

V. Self-care practices and self-care systems; variations by individuals, families, culture groups; variations by available resources

Characterizing Features of the Development and Exercise of Self-Care Agency

Name of Science: B. Science of the development and exercise of self-care agency

Type of Science: Speculatively practical with practically practical content elements

Reality Focus or Proper Object: The human powers activated and evidenced by persons when they perform the investigative, judgment, decision-making, and production operations of self-care

Major Content Areas:

I. Modeling the structure of self-care agency; identification of types of powers and capabilities necessary for all forms of deliberate action, with specific adaptations for self-care

II. Development and exercise by periods of the life cycle; conditioning factors affecting development and those affecting exercise; individual and group variations

III. The operability and adequacy of the self-care agency of individuals in time-place localizations; criteria for measuring operability and adequacy; the concept of self-care deficit

IV. Personal factors and other restricting factors affecting individuals' activations and exercise of their developed powers of self-care agency

V. Processes for the continuing development of self-care agency throughout the life span

Characterizing Features of the Science of Human Assistance for Persons with Health-Associated Self-Care Deficits

Name of Science: C. Science of human assistance for persons with health-associated self-care deficits

Type of Science: Speculatively practical with practically practical content elements

Reality Focus or Proper Object: Persons with demands for engaging in self-care that they are unable to know or meet because of action limitations associated wtih their health states or health care requirements

Major Content Areas:

I. Nature, causes, duration of self-care deficits

II. Types and degrees of dependence resultant from nature and extent of self-care deficits; types of and individual variations in interdependence and interaction; factors conditioning interpersonal relating and interacting

III. Modalities of human assistance or helping methods; conditions that ensure validity of selection and use; processes for use and results sought through use of each modality or combination of modalities

IV. Roles and role-sets associated with use of the assisting modalities; helping systems generated by use of the modalities; physical and psychological effects on persons in their role fulfillment in use of assisting modalities

V. Care and caring dimensions of human assistance for persons with health-associated self-care deficits

Nurses' mastery and use of basic sciences is a feature of their education for nursing. It is in this area that technical preparation for nursing differs in a major way from professional entry education.

Mastery of the sciences basic to nursing is an essential qualification for nurses who practice in highly complex nursing situations. This includes situations in which technologies for regulation of patient variables are undeveloped or, if developed, lack high degrees of validity or reliability.

SUMMARY

Nursing examined from the perspective of a human practical science is very complex. Nursing's complexity, when grasped, can be a challenge to nurse scholars, theorists, and researchers and to nursing practitioners and teachers, or it can be a reason for turning away from the wholeness of nursing science. Whatever the effect on the individual nurse and however a nurse elects to use his or her talents, it is imperative to develop and maintain a vision of the whole of nursing science and know about how his or her endeavors fit into the whole.

References

1. Wallace WA: *The modeling of nature, philosophy of science and philosophy of nature in synthesis,* Washington, DC, 1996, Catholic University of America Press.
2. Maritain J: *The speculative order and the practical order: the degrees of knowledge,* translated from the French ed 4, under the supervision of Gerald B. Phelan, New York, 1959, Charles Scribner's Sons.
3. Wallace WA: *Being scientific in a practice discipline: from a realist point of view, essays on the philosophy of science,* ed 2, Lanham, Md, 1988, University Press of America.
4. Simon HA: *Sciences of the artificial,* Cambridge, Mass, 1969, MIT Press.
5. Argyris C, Putnam R, Smith DMc: *Action science,* San Francisco, 1985, Jossey-Bass, p 4.
6. Notes taken by DE Orem during the presentations of James Dickhoff and Patricia James, "Theory about nursing theories" and "Researching research's role in theory development," respectively, at the Symposium on Theory Development in Nursing, October 7, 1967, Frances Payne Bolton School of Nursing, Case Western Reserve University, Cleveland, OH.
7. Orem DE, editor: Nursing Development Conference Group: *Concept formalization in nursing: process and product,* ed 2, Boston, 1979, Little, Brown.
8. Orem DE: The levels of education and practice, *Alumnae Magazine of the Johns Hopkins Hospital School of Nursing:* 68:2, 1969.

CHAPTER 9

Health and Health Care

Nurses accept nursing as one of the health professions. They accept what they do in nursing as contributory to the personal health and well-being of individuals and to the health of populations in societies throughout the world. Health care is of increasing sociopolitical interest in advanced and developing societies. Ensuring the provision of essential health care to all members of societies is viewed as necessary for the general welfare and happiness of people and for maintaining and developing their productive capacities. As members of the health profession of nursing, nurses must not only have a comprehensive and dynamic understanding of health but also be able to use these understandings in their provision of nursing to individuals and groups. As nursing practitioners, nurses must understand how the nursing systems of care they produce articulate with systems of care produced by other health professionals for the health care of individuals, groups, or populations.

SECTION A: HEALTH

HEALTH AND NURSING

Within the framework of the self-care deficit theory of nursing, the health of individuals is understood as a factor, *a basic conditioning factor* that affects the values of their therapeutic self-care demands and their self-care agency, the patient variables of the theory. Health in the sense of a basic conditioning factor is related to other characterizing features of individuals, such as developmental state and culture (see Fig. 8-2). Nurses must deal not only with health-relevant data about individuals but also with features of their states of health as interactive with other personal factors. In concrete nursing practice situations, nurses work with the health state data of individuals not only from a *patient variable perspective* but first, foremost, and continuously from the perspective of the concrete *person* who is the nurse's patient and who is in a particular state of health, desirable or undesirable. The health state of nurses' patients affects not only the technological features of their care but also the interpersonal and societal dimensions of their nursing.

Developing insight about health is not a simple matter. The lexiographic definition of *health* as state or condition of structural or functional wholeness or integrity of living beings is rejected by some nurses, especially by nurses with inadequately developed insights about the unitary nature of human beings. Two questions must be addressed by nurses and others who search for understanding of the meaning of health when the term is used as a descriptor of humankind. Health does not connote an independent entity. In its traditional use, health is associated with the nature of living things and their natural features. The questions to be answered by each nurse are (1) What are my perceptions of the nature of human beings and their natural features? and (2) In light of these perceptions of human beings, what information must I have or obtain and reflect upon to make judgments about the health of an individual(s) at a specific time under prevailing conditions? Because there is always a judgment when the term *health* or *healthy* is used as a descriptor of a person, a plant, or animal, there must be informative data upon which the judgment is based.

UNDERSTANDING HEALTH

Health and *healthy* are terms used to describe living things—plants, animals, human beings—when they are structurally and functionally whole or sound. Individual human beings are said to be healthy or unhealthy. The same words are used to describe parts of the body, physiologic mechanisms, control of emotional reactions, and mental functioning, as well as attitudes and motives. Individuals evaluate their own states of integrity or wholeness, appraising each day, or sometimes more frequently, whether they feel well or sick. They also make judgments about the health of others with whom they have direct or even indirect contact. These evaluative judgments imply that individuals have ideas of what health means, at least to them, as well as ideas of the evidence needed to judge that a person is healthy or unhealthy.

In light of the complexity of human functioning and its relationships to environmental elements and conditions, the term *health* has considerable general utility in describing the state of wholeness or integrity of human beings. However, temporary indispositions, such as not feeling well today, having a brief illness, or being injured, do not necessarily place the individual in the unhealthy category. Some structural and functional changes do not seriously interfere with human integrated functioning or else interfere with it in a circumscribed fashion. For example, a healthy child or adult with a fracture of an extremity may feel well though not structurally or functionally whole because of the break in the bone and the limitations of movement. Individuals in this state would be referred to as "injured and disabled" rather than as "sick" or "in poor health." However, any deviation from normal structure or functioning is properly referred to as an absence of health in the sense of wholeness or integrity.

Human beings are distinguished from other living things by their capacity (1) to reflect upon themselves and their environment, (2) to symbolize what they experience, and (3) to use symbolic creations (ideas, words) in thinking, in communicating, and in guiding efforts to do and to make things that are beneficial for themselves or others. Health, then, must include that which makes a person human (form of mental life), operating in conjunction with physiologic and psychophysiologic mechanisms and a material structure (biologic life) and in relation to coexistence with other human beings (interpersonal and social life). The meaning of the term *health* changes as views about people's human and biologic characteristics change.

Members of the health professions realize that they should be concerned with health in relation to integrated human functioning, including the contribution of their roles to its attainment. Health professionals must have knowledge from a number of different fields if they are to use and develop health sciences and health technologies that are valid in bringing about the kinds of changes in human beings that move them toward, rather than away from, a state of wholeness, a state of human integrity. With the extension of the term *health* to include psychologic, interpersonal, and social aspects of living, as well as the commonly emphasized physical aspect, the health professions are beginning to recognize that, ideally, health is the responsibility of a society and its individual members and not of any one segment of that society.

The physical, psychologic, interpersonal, and social aspects of health are inseparable in the individual. For example, consider a mother of several small children who has learned that she has tuberculosis. Her husband is employed full-time in a local factory, and the family lives in a crowded apartment in a large city. Her income from a part-time job has been important in providing some of the essential family needs. Her medical treatment, in addition to drug therapy, requires a prescribed amount of rest, a nutritious diet, and fresh air. The family's socioeconomic situation will affect the mother's ability to have the care she needs to arrest the tuberculosis. Her concern for her family and herself, in turn, will affect her mental state and thus her ability to rest and to participate in her own therapy. The maturity of the husband and wife, their creative abilities, the availability of resources, and the support received from family members, friends, neighbors, and persons in the helping professions will affect the well-being of the family. The abilities of the husband and wife to cooperate and to coordinate their efforts toward designing and producing a system of effective self-care for the wife that is integrated with dependent-care systems for the children and the husband's self-care system will be a determining force in providing restorative health care for the mother and primary preventive health care for the children and father.

Adversity in the form of ill health, scarcity of resources, or widespread disaster brings human suffering. But adversity may also bring people increased understanding of themselves and others. People who suffer adversity often reveal the human qualities of courage, patience or self-possession, and willingness to give of oneself to others.

The hypothetical example illustrates in a general way that various aspects of human functioning are interrelated. Accepting that an individual is a unity, an integrated whole, is often difficult, perhaps because the sciences split up humanity; that is, they focus on different aspects of human structure or functioning to develop bodies of knowledge about human beings. Lay persons and some health workers tend to think of the individual human being as having one part called a *body* and another part called a *mind,* with the two parts interacting. A more acceptable image is that a human being is a unity that can be viewed as functioning biologically, symbolically, and socially.

Deliberate action by adults to maintain a state of health for themselves and their dependents involves the components of self-care discussed in prior chapters. Self-care as action requires a base of education in the home, at school, and from practical experiences in self-care. Self-care is only one aspect of healthful living, but without continuous self-care of a therapeutic quality, integrated human functioning will be disrupted. Good health habits are essential in maintaining health, but the ability to change old habits to meet new requirements may be as essential. Education in self-care, not just training in self-care practices, is necessary for the development of knowledge, skills, and positive attitudes related to self-care and health. Children, adolescents, and young adults have interests in health and health care. All too frequently, adults with whom young people have contact are unable, unwilling, or uninterested in providing adequate help. In modern society parents and other educators should be concerned with what can be done to enable children to learn to direct themselves toward a state of integrated functioning and well-being that would promote human dignity and beauty even in illness and disability.

Health as a State

Dictionaries as well as the World Health Organization, an agency of the United Nations, use the term *state* in defining health. Human health or well-being is defined as "the state of being whole or sound." Although the word *health* is especially used to refer to the state of being free from "physical disease or pain," it is also used to refer to "soundness of mind and soul." The World Health Organization emphasizes that health is a state of physical, mental, and social well-being and not merely the absence of disease or infirmity. To conceptualize health, it is necessary to explore the term *state* in relationship to being sound or whole.

The term *state* applied to people is defined as the way a person reveals his or her existence. State is applied in a very general fashion to well-defined conditions of persons that are considered as a whole without specification or analysis of components, for example, the states of being calm or anxious, asleep or awake, acutely ill, debilitated, or depressed. *State* is also defined as a compound state. The term *state* is appropriate when observations upon which to judge a person's health are expressed as a set of determined values of specified human characteristics that simultaneously reveal some aspects of the person's existence. The specified characteristics are worked with as a compound entity (a vector) having a definite number of components, which, when taken together as a set, describe the state of the person or his or her natural features at a particular time.

Examples of the use of the term *state* in the health field in the sense of compound state include taking the vital signs of temperature, pulse, respiration, and blood pressure and considering these together as an index of the state of selected vital processes. The component parts of and the findings of a complete or partial physical examination can be considered a compound entity useful in specifying an individual's health state to some desired completeness[1] (pp. 30-31). At times it is necessary to monitor events or seek evidence of characteristics during a particular period to have knowledge of (1) the actual frequencies of the occurrence of events and (2) their determinate probabilities[2] (pp. 82 and 86).

The term *sound* means possession of full vigor and strength and the absence of signs of disease and morbidity. The term *whole* means that nothing has been omitted, ignored, or lessened. These terms, when used together in regard to health, signify human functional and structural integrity, absence of genetic defects, and progressive integrated development of a human being as an individual unity moving toward higher and higher levels of integration[2] (pp. 476-484). Each human being as a complex unity is often described as having physical, psychic, and intellectual characteristics that become more highly integrated with progressive development. It is obvious that health, defined as a state of being sound or whole, is an ideal state of human perfection that includes continuing human development. It is also obvious that bodies of accumulated knowledge about humankind are necessary for making determinations of the health states of individuals. Furthermore, time-oriented norms are required if judgments are to be made about structural, functional, and genetic integrity at various stages of human development. Some **health state indicators** are presented here.

A person's general appearance is often the basis used for making judgments about the person's health state, for example, making the judgment that this or that person appears to be in good or poor health or that his or her health has improved or worsened. A scientific appraisal of an individual's health state requires that the term *state* be used in the compound sense. This approach necessitates that persons with the requisite knowledge search out the sets of human characteristics that will be useful in specifying health state to some desired completeness. Within the health field, biologists and physicians have contributed substantial bodies of knowledge about the physical aspects of human health. Norms have been established and approaches to determining anatomic, physiologic, genetic, and psychophysiologic components of the health state have been developed and refined (including specifying the kinds of information needed, data-gathering techniques, and rules for inference).

Psychic and intellectual components of an individual's health state viewed in the compound sense include (1) inner experiences, (2) behaviors and conduct (deliberate action) that can be observed in interpersonal and group situations, and (3) solitary endeavors. Concepts of mental health are not as firmly structured as those of physical health. Physical examinations, psychologic tests, and subjective information elicited from individuals about their behavior in interpersonal and group situations are used as means for obtaining information as a basis for making judgments about mental or psychic health states. The development and use of these means is apportioned among a number of disciplines.

Health workers, including nurses, obtain and use information that describes and explains selected aspects of human structure and functioning. For example, nurses use information obtained and expressed in terms of the disciplines of physiology and pathology in making judgments about self-care needs and capabilities of patients. Nurses are responsible for defining the components that describe health states of individuals and the quality and quantity of information about these components that are sufficient for nursing purposes. To deal with the many kinds of information obtainable about human developments and structural and functional states, some nurses and other health workers use the concept of "field," as Kurt Lewin defined it with respect to the life space of an individual or group[3] (pp. xi and 45). Field theory is essentially a method useful in analyzing relationships and organizing information. Those who use this approach must identify and describe the component parts of the field (the vector) that they are examining.

When health is described as a state of being whole and sound, it is necessary to link human growth and development to human structure and functioning. A person's state of growth and development changes over time. At a specific time, a person exhibits a degree of structural and functional integrity according to his or her stage of development. Genetic factors can affect the development as well as the structural and functional integrity of individuals.

For nursing purposes, it is more practical (1) to recognize that at any one time an individual has reached a particular stage of development, which means that certain developments have occurred or are occurring and that specific developments are or are not in accord with established norms and (2) then to attend to the person's functional and structural integrity. For this reason and for purposes of this text, health state and developmental state are considered as separate entities. Nurses often *assume* that the developments of a person of a particular age are in accord with norms, for example, accepting the mature appearance of an individual as a basis for the judgment that he or she is mature. If a nurse *observes,* for example, that an individual cannot read or write, the nurse begins to examine various developments (e.g., cognitive developments) in order to know how to help the person understand and deal with meeting his or her requirements for care.

For practical reasons, members of the various health professions must be able to take an approach to the health of individuals that will enable them to fulfill their purposes as health professionals in the social group. Ideally, members of the health professions view persons for whom they provide care as complex unities but view components of the health states of individuals from the perspectives of their own disciplines. This means that they know the meaning components have for their own specialized work.

Throughout life, individuals tend to learn that some combination of components usually serve them well as an index of their health state. Persons with certain diseases and those under certain forms of medical diagnosis or therapy must learn to collect data as a basis for judging their own human functioning. Learning to determine and determining what combination of components will serve as an index of health state may be a part of the patient role in health care situations. Nurses should seek information about how patients perceive their own health states and the meanings they attach to these states or to various components.

Positions About Health and Well-Being

In this text the terms *health* and **well-being** refer to two different but related human states. *Health* is used in the sense of a *state* of a person that is characterized by soundness or wholeness of developed human structures and of bodily and mental functioning. *Well-being* is used in the sense of individuals' perceived condition of existence. Well-being is a state characterized by experiences of contentment, pleasure, and kinds of happiness; by spiritual experiences; by movement toward fulfillment of one's self-ideal; and by continuing personalization. Well-being is associated with health, with success in personal endeavors, and with sufficiency of resources. However, individuals experience well-being, and their human existence may be characterized by features of well-being even under conditions of adversity, including disorders of human structure and functioning.

Conceptualizations of health and well-being are related to points of view about human beings. These points of view should be made explicit for purposes of understanding human health and well-being.

Nurses in their writings express a variety of ways of viewing human beings. Emphasis is placed on the unity of human beings, on human beings as psychosomatic unities, on human beings as being greater than the sum of their parts, on human beings as open systems, on human beings as having various modalities of functioning, and on human beings as persons. Some nurses, as well as others in the health field, tend to search for an all-encompassing way of viewing human beings and their health states. For nursing purposes it may be more effective to consider human beings from more than one point of view. The Nursing Development Conference Group held the position that in nursing there are practical advantages to viewing human beings as *persons,* as *symbolizers* and *agents,* as *organisms* and as *objects* subject to physical forces[4] (pp. 122-123). (See Chapter 6.)

The view of human beings as *persons* subsumes the views of human beings as agents and symbolizers and organisms. However, for practical purposes one or more of these views can be taken at different times without considering all that characterizes human beings as persons.

Before taking this or that view of human beings, it is a safeguard to posit that each human being, like other living things, is a *substantial* or *real unity* whose parts are formed and attain perfection through the differentiation of the whole during processes of development. The unity of living things stands in distinction to the unity of artifacts.

Because human beings have discernible parts (for example, arms, legs, stomach, lungs, functional systems such as urinary system or neural circuits or neuroendocrine system), it is essential to recognize them. Each developmentally differentiated structure or functional system can be studied as an existent entity with its own operations, with relations to other differentiated parts and to their operations, and to the unitary functioning of individuals who coexist in a world with other human beings. If there is acceptance of the real unity of individual human beings, there should be no difficulty in recognizing structural and functional differentiations within the unity.

Two points of view about human beings that afford considerable meaning to states of human health and well-being are that of human beings as *persons* and that of the *structural and functional differentiations of human beings.* Both are considered briefly.

The point of view of human beings as persons is moving rather than static. It is the view of personalization of the individual, that is, movement toward maturation and achievement of the individual's human potential. This process of coming to be a person involves individuals in communications with their worlds; in action; in the exercise of the human desire to know, to seek the truth; and in the giving of themselves in the doing of good for themselves and others. Personalization is not a condition of individuals but a task in process while they live in coexistence with others.

Personalization proceeds as individuals live under conditions favorable or unfavorable to human developmental processes. Individuals learn to set their goals and choose among many goals as they move toward maturity. The process has two intertwining aspects. There is striving by individuals to achieve the potential of their natural endowments for physical and rational functioning while living a life of faith with respect to things hoped for, and there is striving to perfect themselves as responsible human beings who raise questions, seek answers, reflect, and come to awareness of the relationship between what they know and what they do. *Self-realization* and *personality development* are terms used at times to refer to the process of personalization.

Individuals coming to view themselves as self-care or dependent-care agents, their exercise of responsibility for and engagement in self-care or dependent-care, and their deliberate engagement in action to develop or redevelop the capabilities for self-care and dependent-care are facets of the process of personalization. These facets of personalization relate to fulfillment of the potential of individuals for regulating their functioning toward soundness or wholeness within an existent potential and to their experiencing of well-being.

Some psychologists speak of persons who have progressed along the path of personalization to a high degree of maturity as *mentally healthy* and view *psychologic maturity* and *intellectual maturity* as components of maturity proper. The signs of a mature or maturing person are accepted by these psychologists as signs of *mental* or *psychic health;* philosophy, the humanities, psychology, and theology are helpful in the development of insight about human beings as persons.

The second view of human beings that focuses on structural and functional differentiations within the unity that is a human being is the view that has been developed by various human and life sciences. These include the sciences of genetics, biochemistry, biophysics, human anatomy, and human physiology with its various branches, psychology, psychophysiology, and social psychology. These sciences organize validated knowledge about human structures and functions at a range of levels of differentiation and integration, including their ranges of variation by age and other factors. The medical science of pathology and its various branches structure knowledge about disorders of human structures and human functions.

The detailed approaches of the human and life sciences are coalesced and organized by the identification and naming of modalities of functioning. This process is accomplished in a number of ways. For example, bodily functions are distinguished from mental functions; organic, psychic, and intellectual functioning are specified sometimes with more specific differentiations or with additional differentiations such as psychosocial functioning. An individual's state of health, when *state* is used in the *compound sense,* can be investigated along one or more of these dimensions. For example, a routine complete physical examination is an investigation of organic functioning, and various types of psychologic tests are used to investigate psychic functioning. The particularized self-care requisites of individuals and their prescribed therapeutic self-care demands are regulatory of one or a number of modalities of human functioning toward soundness or wholeness of functioning of individuals.

Nurses' use of knowledge in practice situations about specific structural or functional aspects of the human existence of their patients, because it is knowledge of parts and not the whole, demands asking and answering a number of questions: Are other functions affected? Will they be affected? Can the effects of particular structural disorders or levels of functioning on the life and well-being of the individual be projected? How will efforts to regulate this aspect of functioning affect other aspects of functioning and the state of well-being of the patient? Nurses should understand that the two represented views of human beings are related and that nurses should develop facility in the use of both views in practice situations.

The represented positions about human health and well-being and the described views of human beings are not attempts to answer questions about the nature of health or the nature of humankind. They are expressions of insights useful in nursing and in health care of all types.

SECTION B: HEALTH CARE

Understanding nursing as health care demands that nurses develop and use insights about variations in the health states and health care requirements of individuals and members of populations. Up-to-date knowledge of societal and community provision for health care is also required. Ways of providing health care may be institutionalized or emerging.

Kinds of health care and ways for providing it vary from society to society and in some instances from one segment of society to another. The kinds and quality of health care in particular places vary over time. Changes are brought about to conform to advances in knowledge; to more realistic and valid perceptions of the health care requirements of individuals, families, and populations; to the education and availability of health care workers; and to the financial and material resources available for health care and health care education.

Two major influences on the adequacy and availability of health care in any community are (1) the prevailing means and the adequacy of means used to finance health care and (2) the characterizing features and geographic distribution of populations and subpopulations. The critical feature, however, is the fit between the kind and the amount of health care needed by people and the health care services available to them and used by them. Availability is understood as having both geographic and financial features. Health care services may be available in communities but not used or inadequately used by the people.

NURSING AS HEALTH CARE

Every nurse must be qualified to design and provide nursing to adults or children who have demands for nursing assistance. As a helping art, nursing is the complex ability to accomplish or to contribute to the accomplishment of a person's usual and therapeutic self-care by compensating for or aiding in overcoming the physical or psychic conditions or disabilities that cause the person (1) to be unable to act, (2) to refrain from acting, or (3) to act ineffectively in self-care. From the viewpoint of the patient, nursing care is always something received; it is personal assistance or help from a person who is qualified and able to help. From the viewpoint of the nurse, however, nursing care is help effectively given. It is help that facilitates regulation of a patient's functioning through meeting the therapeutic self-care demand as well as movement by the patient under enabling conditions toward fulfillment of responsibilities for self-care.

Nursing and Health

The points where nursing converges on individuals because of their states of health were expressed in the previous section. The proper object of nursing and the self-care deficit theory of nursing (the hypothesized model of what nursing is and should be) expresses the points of convergence.

There are five critical points of articulation of nursing with persons' health state features. The points of articulation are expressed in terms of *how* persons' general states of health, or some feature(s) of health state, *condition* what persons can or should do to regulate their own or their dependents' functioning and development. *Condition* is used in the sense of to affect, modify, or influence. The five points of convergence of nursing and health are expressed as follows:

1. Persons' engagement in or failure to engage in self-care or dependent-care and their action limitations that are associated with health state or health-related factors
2. The conditioning effect of health state features on the values of universal and developmental self-care requisites (e.g., fluid intake) adjusted to an existent health condition (as well as other factors)
3. The conditioning effect of health state features on the means to be used in meeting self-care requisites (e.g., giving fluids by intravenous infusion to persons in deep coma)
4. Health state conditions and features that give rise to (a) health-deviation self-care requisites (e.g., control experiences of pain associated with bursitis) and (b) health-deviation self-care requisites associated with medical diagnostic and treatment measures (e.g., take medication as prescribed for relief of pain)
5. The effects of health state features on the integrity of specific human capabilities, dispositions, and enabling powers essential for engagement in self-care (e.g., loss of tactile sense in fingers)

The foregoing points of convergence of persons' health states and nursing are expressed within the frame of reference of self-care deficit nursing theory. The five points can be coalesced under the patient variables therapeutic self-care demands and self-care agency or dependent-care agency. These are objective focuses of nursing and subject to fluctuations in their elements. Types of conditioning effects of health state expressed in items 2, 3, and 4 all affect constituent elements of persons' therapeutic self-care demand. Items 1 and 5 express how persons' self-care agency is or can be affected by health state. This overview of the relations of features of persons' health states to the patient variables specific to nursing is supplemented by details in later chapters.

Understanding nursing as health care requires understanding of self-care, the elements and internal structure of persons' therapeutic self-care demands, and the power or agency of persons to engage in self-care and dependent-care. Self-care has been described as deliberate action that enables the individual to survive in a variety of states of well-being or health or to move from one state to another. The person who has self-care agency and activates it can be said to be a *regulator.*[1] Such a person is a good regulator if his or her self-care actions bring about internal and external conditions necessary to maintain life processes and environmental conditions supportive of life processes, integrity of human structure and functioning, and human developmental processes.

Self-care actions are deliberately performed; they can be reproduced from one time to another, and they are selected and performed with the goal of keeping internal and external conditions constant according to some standard. The universal, developmental, and health-deviation self-care requisites are expressions of the types of regulatory actions that should be performed by self-care or dependent-care agents. Identification and description of self-care requisites of individuals or populations supply nurses, other health workers, and the public with what is important and what is wanted with respect to regulation. The calculation of an individual's therapeutic self-care demand provides information about regulatory actions, which would ideally be performed because of the known values of selected health state components and the probability of constancy or change in these values.

Information about the values of health state indicators (characterizing features) and the probabilities attached to their values allows nurses to make judgments about the current and projected effects of these indicators on the individual's performance of self-care operations. Furthermore, such information provides nurses with knowledge about conditions that require use of particular helping methods to meet self-care requisites and to regulate the exercise or development of self-care agency. Nurses should also seek information about the stages of cognitive and moral development of individuals whenever they are significant for the development of the constituent parts of self-care agency and for their exercise in performing self-care operations. One broad index of health (including development) is an individual's view of self as a self-care or dependent-care agent and the freedom with which the individual accepts and acts with responsibility in matters of self-care or dependent-care.

The impending birth of a child, a construction worker's hospitalization after a fall from a building, a young man's paralysis sustained in an automobile accident, or a mother's prolonged illness are a few examples of some of the health-related situations in life that require the assistance of nurses in helping an individual or family compensate for or overcome the limitations in self-care activities imposed by an existing health situation. The goal in nursing, like the goal in all other health services, is to achieve movement toward integrity of functioning for individuals or groups, sick or well, when they need help. Commonly heard expressions describe quite clearly, if not in scientific terms, what is meant by health goals: "to stay well," "to get well," "to be cured," "to get stronger," "to get back to work," "to get over my nervousness," "to regain the use of my hand," "to have a healthy baby," "to have my child able to run and play again," and "to be able to live like other people again." These and similar expressions, heard many times a day by health care workers, describe the health goals sought by and for patients. They are associated with a movement of the patient away from abnormalities and the restriction of normal human activity resulting from disease, injury, or unsound relationships toward a goal of normalcy or wholeness. Health results sought for patients also may mean stabilizing the condition of a patient who is chronically ill or easing the suffering of the patient who is dying.

The provision of health services has become increasingly complex with the broadening concept of health, with advances in the sciences and in technology, and with the increasing numbers of health care workers and supportive and administrative personnel. Achieving health results for individuals, families, and communities within health services as now organized is costly and often inefficient for the providers as well as the seekers and receivers of service. Financing health services, availability of services needed, quality of health care provided, communications among health workers, and coordination of services are some of the problem areas. Both the public and organized health services must become more involved in finding solutions to problems in the delivery of health services in order to avoid serious breakdowns in service, to provide service when and where it is not presently available, and to improve the quality of service when needed. Nurses must continue, and in some instances begin, to assume their part in this effort. To do this, nurses must be able to differentiate their focus in health care situations from that of physicians and other health care professionals.

The Nursing Focus Versus the Medical Focus

Healthy adults perform many of the universal components of self-care without direct help. They feed, wash, dress, and perform many health-related actions themselves, including seeking medical care when they recognize the need for it. These and other activities usually become a fixed part of daily living and are scarcely noticed. The sick or injured adult, however, may find that he or she is unable to accomplish usual self-care tasks. The universal components of self-care may have to be modified because of an individual's health situation. The person may have little or no knowledge about the new care components that are required because of illness or injury. The person requires nursing assistance, and the nurse contributes to his or her well-being by providing that assistance. The following example demonstrates the **nursing focus** and the part the nurse shares with others in achieving health results for patients.

> A man has sustained serious burns of the face, neck, chest, and arms. He is suffering considerable pain, and certain movements intensify his pain. He is very ill. Some of his body tissues have been destroyed; he is extremely anxious about his condition; he fears disfigurement, disability, and even death. He does not question his hospitalization, his need for medical care, or his wife's

continuous presence. He accepts without question the ministrations of the attending doctors and nurses, including the pain they may unavoidably cause him as they care for him. The doctors and nurses know their roles in assisting him. They have learned what they must do for him and how to do it most effectively through initial and continuing specialized education and training. This knowledge includes medical knowledge of burns and treatment techniques; a background knowledge of anatomy and physiology, chemistry, microbiology, pharmacology, nutrition, psychology, and sociology; and experience in observing and working under the supervision of experienced doctors and nurses caring for burn patients.

The focus of the nurse's activities in this example is the man with burns who requires assistance to prevent further deterioration of his health and to recover and return to his normal or a near-normal way of life. But the doctor has the same focus for his or her activities. What then is specific to the nursing objectives for the patient? First, one must look closely at the interests shared by doctor and nurse. Both see the patient as a human being—as a person who is unique, who has rights and responsibilities for self and others, who has motives and values, and who has a way of life that has been disrupted by the accident and present states of illness and dependency. Both see the patient as they see other human-beings—as a rational living being, vulnerable to disease and injury, but with great capacity to combat disease and injury, to recover, or to adjust and find ways for compensating for lost abilities and to be courageous.

The doctor's special interests in this situation are the patient's life processes as they have been disrupted as a result of the burns. They may be further disrupted by improper or careless treatment, by invading microorganisms resulting in infection, and by failure to support the patient psychologically and help sustain the will to live during the initial and critical phase of his illness and in the recovery phase when disfigurement must be faced. The doctor is specially prepared to evaluate the physical and psychophysic aspects of the patient's condition and progress and to prescribe appropriate therapeutic measures to prevent or alleviate complications that may develop.

The nurse's special interest is the continuing therapeutic care the patient requires. The nurse is concerned with the universal components of self-care, now modified by the burns and their effects upon the man's integrated functioning, and with all the health-deviation components of care that may arise as a result of the burns. The nurse assists the patient on a continuous basis with his personal care, which he can no longer manage for himself, and sustains him during the periods of great suffering and mental stress resulting from his pain and fear.

The nursing focus takes into account both the medical point of view and the patient's point of view. The doctor's prescribed measures for the treatment and control of the patient's condition will have been instituted promptly as a part of the patient's continuing care, as have other measures designed to aid the doctor in diagnosing and instituting early treatment to prevent complications. The doctor requires information about the physiologic and behavioral state of the patient during the time he or she is not present to observe them. Continuing observation and recordings of the patient's condition throughout each day are important components of therapeutic care made necessary by the patient's specific health situation. The nurse must be alert to the patient's condition to adjust care to immediate needs, including the possibility of a need for immediate or emergency medical care because of a worsening of the patient's condition.

Recognizing an emergency situation and securing immediate medical assistance are important components of self-care that the patient in the example can no longer manage. They necessarily become part of the nursing focus. The patient may not be aware of the need for observation and may not even be able to recognize the need for emergency medical assistance. The nursing focus, from the patient's point of view, requires recognition and acceptance by the nurse that it is the patient who is living with burned tissues, that it is the patient who must cope with the effects of physiologic changes and of fear and pain on his personal integrity. The patient perceives the situation and thinks about the future. He imagines what it may be and is afraid. A nursing focus is unrealistic if it does not take into account how the patient views and is personally affected by his illness. The nurse's acceptance of the patient's point of view is essential if the patient is to be assisted through nursing to live with his illness and disability, to cooperate with those who assist him, and above all to be motivated to direct his energies toward recovering a normal or near-normal state of health.

Parts of the Nursing Focus

There are six components of a nursing focus. These components include the physician's perspective of the health situation, the patient's perspective of the health situation, and four central patient components: (1) state of health, (2) health results sought, (3) the therapeutic self-care demand, and (4) present abilities and disabilities to engage in self-care. The parts of a nursing focus and their interrelationship are shown in Figure 9-1.

Each of the six components is in itself complex. Both the physician's medical perspective of the patient's health state and health care needs and the patient's perspective of his or her health situation should be seen as encompassing all or parts of each of the four central patient components. The four patient components are complex and interrelated. Both physician and nurse contribute to the identification and delineation of these components, which require securing and validating information about the patient's health state and health-derived care requirements. The patient's health state not only gives rise to requirements for health care but also affects the patient's ability to engage in self-care activities.

One foundation for the basic design of a system of nursing for a patient is determined by identifying and describing the nursing focus for the patient. The parts of the nursing focus and their interrelationships are the elements from which the nursing design is formed. The design changes as the components change; for example, as a patient's health state improves, the health-deviation self-care requisites may decrease and self-care ability increase, thus increasing the patient's self-care activities and decreasing the number of care activities that nurses perform for the patient. Identification and description of the six

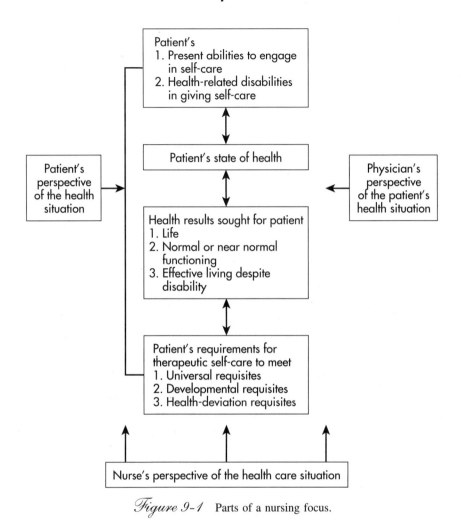

$\mathcal{Figure}\ 9\text{-}1$ Parts of a nursing focus.

components of the nursing focus and their interrelationships for individual patients make explicit the *health dimension of nursing* for each patient. This information serves to guide the nurse in maintaining a nursing perspective on the patient that is defined in health terms.

In developing a nursing perspective, the components of the nursing focus become the guides for nursing action to the degree that the nurse understands each component, acquires time-specific information relating to it in nursing situations, and is able to interpret this information and attach nursing meaning to it. Consider a healthy adult woman who has sustained a fracture of a lower extremity and is immobilized in a cast. The patient is unable to do many things for herself because of her lack of mobility. The nursing focus in this situation should consider the patient's lack of mobility in its relationship to her general state of health and the health results sought. It will be clear to the nurse, in the light of nursing knowledge, that nonuse of the fractured extremity is both a component of the patient's therapeutic self-care and the underlying cause of the patient's inability to perform other usual self-care measures. It will also be clear that, objectively, the health results sought are (1) protection of the injured extremity and healing of the fracture, (2) a return of the normal functioning of the extremity, and (3) the patient's recovery of mobility. The health results sought, however, are in turn directly related to and depend on the patient's age, general state of health, nutritional state, and physiologic capacity for forming the new bone growth necessary to the healing of the fracture. (The physiologic capacity for forming new bone tissue is frequently reduced in aged or undernourished patients.) The physician may view the patient's health situation primarily from an orthopedic point of view, with a primary concern for the effectiveness of the method of immobilization used and other aspects of the therapeutic regimen to promote healing. The patient may be primarily concerned with the effects of the fracture—pain, discomfort, disability, disruption of activities—and with the probable duration of the treatment.

When nurses enter nursing relationships with patients, they must distill from the mass of patient characteristics those that are relevant to the nursing focus. Nurses do not ignore the irrelevant factors but view them in light of the influence they may exert on the factors that determine the specifications for nursing action. Further, nurses must keep in mind that the nursing focus for a patient may be either relatively stable or undergoing continuous change. In the earlier example of the patient with severe burns, the nursing focus probably would require adjustment from hour to hour or even more frequently during the critical periods of the patient's illness. The frequency of change in both the physician's perspective and the patient's perspective during these critical periods would necessarily affect the nursing perspective as well. Changes in the nursing perspective probably would occur less frequently after stabilization of the patient's condition, but the nurse would need to know and understand how change in one component of the nursing focus would affect the other components. For example, if there is a sudden and dramatic improvement in the condition of the patient who is burned or if he suffers a sudden relapse and becomes comatose, his requirements for therapeutic care and his ability to engage in self-care would change dramatically. The sudden change in one component of the nursing focus (the patient's state of health) may set off a chain reaction in all the other components that would make it essential for the nurse to completely revise the nursing focus for the patient.

The nursing focus is also the index or key in estimating the complexity of a nursing situation and thus in determining the kinds of nurses (e.g., level of education and training) that will be needed to meet the patient's requirements for nursing care. The complexity of a nursing situation is determined by (1) the rapidity of change in the components of the nursing focus, (2) the elements of the components, and (3) the number and kinds of relationships between the components. The complexity of a nursing situation is increased whenever the nursing focus is not clear-cut or obvious, for example, a situation in which the patient is critically ill but the reasons for the illness are unknown. A clear-cut or obvious nursing focus is one that can be validly established by means of readily available information about the components and their relationships.

The ability to develop and maintain a valid nursing focus in nursing practice is directly related to the nurse's educational preparation and experience. The mark of the expert in nursing is the ability to see a health care situation from a nursing perspective and to recognize personal capabilities and limitations in establishing and maintaining a valid nursing focus. Because of their educational preparation, some nurses are not prepared to design, establish, and maintain a valid system of nursing for a patient without the supervision of a nurse with advanced preparation and experience. These same nurses, however, may be qualified by their educational background and well prepared to work in cooperation with another nurse, or they may be prepared to care for a patient in keeping with a design preestablished and maintained by another qualified nurse (see Chapter 15).

PURPOSES OF HEALTH CARE

There are ways in common use for expressing the broad purposes of health care, that is, what is being sought for individuals with reference to their states of health. These are health maintenance, health promotion, primary prevention, secondary prevention, tertiary prevention and rehabilitation (considered as part of tertiary prevention). These purposes and the kinds of health care required to achieve them are interrelated. There are different ways of viewing these relations. The position expressed here is that health maintenance and health promotion are the most general of the named purposes and that the purpose expressed in terms of prevention and rehabilitation contribute to the attainment of health maintenance and health promotion (Figure 9-2). Health workers who operate with

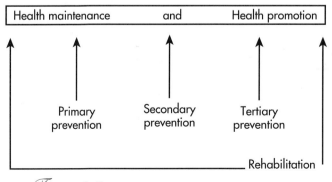

Person in a Described Health State

| Health maintenance | and | Health promotion |

Primary prevention   Secondary prevention   Tertiary prevention

Rehabilitation

Figure 9-2   Health care purposes and relationships.

prevention as their overriding purpose may see health maintenance and health promotion care as parts of prevention.

Health maintenance and health promotion are valid purposes for persons whose states of health have known characterizing features marked by some degree of stability. Features may be overt general states, for example, *being well, being critically ill,* or as one or a set of specific features of health state as expressed in the medical diagnosis "patient has experienced a myocardial infarction." The three forms of *prevention* are for persons who either are subject to or have experienced untoward health state occurrences. For example, *individuals exposed to persons with measles* who have not had measles and who have not been adequately immunized are subject to *contracting measles* as contrasted with individuals *suffering from measles.* Rehabilitation involves persons in becoming major contributors to their own required regimen of health care directed to achieve functional restoration, improvement, or compensation. It is important for nurses and other health professionals to keep in the forefront of their awareness that health care is for persons as individuals and as members of populations and subpopulations.

Health Maintenance and Health Promotion

The terms *health maintenance* and *health promotion* are in common use in the health care field. Health professionals are expected to know their meaning and how to achieve these purposes within the frames of reference of their own disciplines. For students, however, appropriate questions are: What is health maintenance? What is health promotion?

Health maintenance as a purpose to be achieved and as a form of health care is valid under certain conditions. These include (1) general and specific features of persons' health states are known; (2) untoward features of persons' health states (for example, disordered pancreatic functioning as in diabetes mellitus) are subject to regulation or control, and regulation or control regimens are effectively pursued; and (3) there is knowledge of the limits of regulation and control for untoward health state features and knowledge of the signs of deterioration of human functioning. Health maintenance care always includes effective meeting of persons' therapeutic self-care demands. Therapeutic self-care demands always include primary prevention measures and may include secondary and tertiary prevention care measures. Health maintenance care always includes periodic or continuous evaluation of general health state and of specific health state features by physicians who are generalists or specialists, or by other recognized and qualified health professionals. Health maintenance care has as its focus sustaining a person in his or her existent dynamic functional state without worsening of its general or specific features.

Health promotion has as its focus movement of individuals to improved general states of health or to improvement of specific structured or functional features of health state. Health promotion is based on a known or presumed human potential for improvement. Improved nutritional status, musculoskeletal fitness, and enhanced respiratory functioning express some common goals of health promotion. Other goals include improved ability to control stress-producing emotional states, self-image adjusted to existent human structural and functional features, and overcoming of prejudices. Health promotion presumes a baseline of health maintenance care and adds to it movement to a more humanly appropriate level of functioning.

The purposes of health maintenance and health promotion often merge in the design and provision of health care for individuals and members of populations. Their meaning is enhanced by insights about the three levels of preventive health care including rehabilitation.

Prevention

Prevention, as described in Leavell and Clark[5] (pp. 14-38), is based on (1) knowledge of the natural history of human health disorders, (2) knowledge of the combination of causes of specific disorders of human structure and functioning, and (3) an identified rational basis for methods of intercepting or counteracting causative factors before the onset of a disease or at some period after its onset. **Preventive health care** thus requires knowledge of specific interferences with normal human structure and functioning at various stages of the life cycle in particular environments.

Systems of preventive health care recognize three levels of prevention: primary, secondary, and tertiary. *Primary prevention* is appropriate before the onset of disease and is directed to the *maintenance and promotion of integrity of structure and functioning* and the *prevention of specific diseases*. *Secondary prevention* is appropriate after the onset of disease and is directed to the *prevention of complications* (disease that occurs concurrently with other disease) and of *sequelae* (disorders of structure or function that follow or are caused by an attack of a disease) and *prevention of prolonged disability*. *Tertiary prevention* is appropriate when there is disability with a demand to function in society with limited human capacities. It is directed toward bringing about *effective and satisfying human functioning in accord with existing powers for human functioning*. (Refer to works in preventive medicine for detailed explanations of these levels of prevention.)

Requirements of individuals for the three levels of preventive health care vary with age, state of development, health state features, and external environmental conditions. Care at the primary level of prevention is a requirement of each individual throughout life. With the onset of disease or when a person is disabled, there will be requirements for care at the secondary and tertiary levels of prevention. Each person in a health care situation can be viewed, therefore, as having one of the following kinds or combinations of preventive health care requirements:

- Care at the primary level of prevention
- Care at the primary and secondary levels of prevention
- Care at the primary and tertiary levels of prevention
- Care at the primary, secondary, and tertiary levels of prevention

These four kinds of health care requirements have meaning for nursing because of their implications for life, health, and effective living on the part of the patient and the health care role responsibilities that each level of care specifies for patients, health workers, and others who provide care and services. They further impose demands for specific attitudes, knowledge, and skills on the part of patients, health workers, or others who provide care and services.

REQUIREMENTS FOR HEALTH CARE

Health care is based on systems of knowledge about human development and functioning and on practices with some demonstrated value in promoting health or in preventing, curing, or regulating disease. Concepts descriptive of systems of *preventive health care* are useful in unifying the meaning of health, disease, and health care for individuals. For this reason, prevention is the concept used as the means for presenting and interpreting variations of health care requirements and their meaning in nursing situations. Each level of prevention is considered, and some implications for nursing are made explicit.

Health Care Requirements at the Primary Level of Prevention

Requirements for health maintenance and promotion and disease prevention are specified in relation to what is known about (1) human structure and functioning and (2) specific diseases or interferences with the normal human condition. The effective meeting of the universal self-care requisites adjusted to age, environmental conditions, and the individual's health and developmental state is health care at the primary level of prevention.

The adult has a major instrumental role in health care at the primary level of prevention because it is a continuous requirement. When the person is young, aged, ill, unknowing, or unskilled, the role of agent for meeting that person's universal and developmental self-care requisites should be taken by a responsible and qualified adult. The nurse may be this adult or may help another adult fill the role competently. The physician's or dentist's role is that of diagnostician in periodic health examinations, prescriber of preventive therapy (for example, diet adjusted to age), or instrumental agent in giving preventive therapy (e.g., specific preventive therapy after exposure to but before the onset of a specific communicable disease). The community role in health care at the primary level of prevention is a large one and relates to control of environmental conditions and adequacy of essential resources. It provides health services in the form of education to prepare individuals and families to fulfill their personal care roles. It also provides private or public health services to protect individuals from a specific disease or to help them with problems of health maintenance and promotion.

General rules to guide nurses in identifying some of the nursing dimensions of health care requirements at the primary level of prevention include the following:
- Every individual under nursing care has health care requirements at the primary level of prevention.

- Universal self-care and developmental self-care, when therapeutic in quality, constitute health care at the primary level of prevention. They include practices to maintain and promote health and development and to prevent specific diseases. Practices to promote health are based on rationales of resources and conditions essential for survival and development and for normalcy of structure and functioning. Practices to prevent specific diseases are based on rationales of how to prevent or interrupt relations between causative agents of disease and factors in patients or the environment that together establish the conditions necessary for the disease to develop.
- In assisting individual patients, nurses are able to select and use or guide patients to select and use methods for meeting self-care requisites that promote and maintain health and development and prevent specific disease. Methods are properly adjusted to the factors of age, health, individual modes of functioning, and environment.
- Nurses apply factual information about the patient, the environment, and the patient's lifestyle and routine of daily living in their selection or use of universal and development self-care practices at the primary level of prevention. Health care at this level should be incorporated into each patient's system of daily living and be a permanent part of it (Appendix A).
- Nurses assist patients in health care directed to the goals of health maintenance and promotion and disease prevention with an awareness of the essential role of the patient or a responsible adult in the continuous provision of this level of preventive health care.

Health Care Requirements at the Secondary and Tertiary Levels of Prevention

Requirements for (1) prevention of complicating diseases and adverse effects of specific diseases and prolonged disability through early diagnosis and treatment (secondary prevention) and (2) rehabilitation in the event of disfigurement and disability (tertiary level of prevention) are specified in relation to what is known about the nature and effects of specific diseases, valid methods of regulating disease, and the human potential for living with and overcoming the disabling effects of disease. Health-deviation self-care of a therapeutic quality includes practices at either or both of these levels of prevention.

Health care at the secondary level of prevention is accomplished through accurate diagnosis and effective treatment at the onset or in some later stage of a disease. Periodic health examinations; accurate observations of signs and symptoms of health disorders by patient, family, or nurse; and the selection of further health care as indicated by observed signs and symptoms facilitate early diagnosis and treatment when adequate health services are available. Case finding in public health practice also facilitates early diagnosis and treatment.

During the course of a disease, health care requirements and the instrumental role of the patient as self-care agent vary with the effects of the disease and with the methods of diagnosis and treatment used. Health care is effective at the secondary level of prevention if (1) the disease is cured, the pathologic process arrested, or the effects of the disease kept under control; (2) complicating diseases are prevented; and (3) the dissemination of the causative agents of the disease is prevented.

Rehabilitation, as previously indicated, requires deliberate action on the part of the patient and health workers to adapt or adjust functioning to compensate for or overcome disorders that restrict human functioning in specific ways. Rehabilitative health care varies with the nature and the effects of the disorder, including the stage of the life cycle when the condition occurred. It also varies with the methods used for determining the extent of the disorder, patient's remaining functional capacity, and the techniques used to enable the patient to function effectively with some degree of satisfaction. This level of health care requires a belief in the human potential to overcome functional disorders and disability, effective techniques for determining functional loss and remaining functional capacities, and effective restorative or compensatory techniques. It also requires willingness on the part of the patient, the family, health workers, and communities to work toward the goal of rehabilitation. Many types of specialists and provision for special education, recreation, travel, and work must be available on a community basis. This level of preventive health care is effective whenever an individual is able to live or is making progress in enhanced well-being and in living as an active member of a community.

General rules to guide nurses in identifying the nursing dimensions of situations in which patients have requirements for the secondary or tertiary levels of preventive health care include the following:

- Persons who suffer from disease or disorders of health or their effects have health care requirements at the secondary or tertiary levels of prevention that are specific to an active disease and its continuous dynamic effects or to a state of disfigurement or dysfunction.
- Health-deviation self-care (Chapter 10), when therapeutic in quality, is health care at the secondary or tertiary level of prevention. It has the form of self-care measures to regulate and prevent adverse effects of the disease, prevent complicating diseases, prevent prolonged disability, or adapt or adjust functioning to overcome or compensate for the adverse effects of permanent or prolonged disfigurement or dysfunction.
- In assisting individual patients, nurses must be able to use and to guide patients in the use of medically prescribed or endorsed measures of diagnosis, treatment, and rehabilitation to be incorporated into self-care, including adjustments of universal and developmental self-care requisites to the health and disease state of the patient.
- Nurses gather and apply factual information about the patient, including results of medical evaluations that specify level of functioning measured against norms for healthy individuals in the patient's age-group as well as medical orders, environment, lifestyle, and routines of daily living.
- Health care at these levels becomes a temporary or permanent part of a patient's daily life.
- Nurses assist patients in health care directed to the goals of secondary and tertiary prevention with the awareness that the role of the patient as responsible

instrumental agent in health care varies not only with age but also with the nature of the disease and its effects. It also varies with the measures and techniques of diagnosis, treatment, and rehabilitation used in health care, their effects on the patient, the resources and services available to the patient, and his or her state of readiness to give or manage self-care with or without guidance and supervision.

CLASSIFICATION OF NURSING SITUATIONS BY HEALTH FOCUS

Because the same totality of things, persons, or situations may be classified in more than one way, it is necessary to consider the methods of establishing classifications. For example, if one has a box of red and yellow beads and if some of these beads are round and the others square, the beads may be grouped according to color or shape. The groupings are red beads and yellow beads when classified by color and round beads and square beads when classified by shape. If some red beads and some yellow beads are round and others square, then it is possible to group them according to both schemes of classification by placing red ones into separate groups of round and square beads and yellow ones into similar groups.

Classification is useful not only in organizing information or facts but also in serving practical purposes. In practical endeavors, considering each of the varying factors (e.g., color and shape of the beads) is necessary whenever the variations have an effect on the desired result. For a very simple example, consider that the red and yellow beads in the box are to be used in making two necklaces of the following design: beads of the same color, alternating round and square beads. Both color and shape must be considered in the planning. The number of round and square beads of each color for making two necklaces of specific lengths must be determined. The size of the beads and the number of beads available are other relevant considerations. Arrangement of the beads into color groups and of each color group into two shape groups would facilitate making judgments about the number of beads available as well as stringing the beads. This simple example of the beads illustrates how classifications are developed in terms of characteristics and how useful classification is in identifying and naming things and in accomplishing a task or a series of tasks. To function effectively, nurses require knowledge of both the **health and helping aspects of nursing situations.** A classification system that would assist nurses in understanding the health aspects of nursing situations is presented.

A person in need of nursing care can be described from a health perspective with reference to (1) the presence or absence of disease, injury, disability, or disfigurement; (2) the quality of general health state described in the general sense as excellent, good, fair, or poor or in terms of the values of sets of selected characteristics that together define the person's health state; and (3) the life-cycle-oriented events and circumstances that indicate current changes and existing needs for health care. These dimensions of health, when accurately described for a patient, indicate appropriate health care goals, specify the kinds of health care required, and may also indicate the kinds of obstacles to self-care that are present or could be present. A classification system based on these dimensions of health is suggested, and seven groupings of nursing situations according to the health focus of the situation are proposed. The suggested variations in each group identify subgroups. The classification is generally useful—that is, not just useful to nurses. It is essentially a classification of *health-care situations* from which inferences about the nursing aspects of health care can be made.

- **Group 1.** The health focus is oriented to events and circumstances in relation to the *life cycle* that give rise to anatomic, physiologic, or psychologic changes associated with periods of growth and development, maturity, parenthood, aging, and old age. General health is within the range of excellent to good.
- **Group 2.** The health focus is oriented to the process of *recovery* from a specific disease (e.g., measles) or injury (e.g., a fracture of the pelvis resulting from a fall) or to overcoming or compensating for the effects of the disease or injury. Permanent *dysfunction, disfigurement,* or *disability* may or may not be present or expected. General health is within the range of excellent to good to fair.
- **Group 3.** The health focus is oriented to *illness or disorder of undetermined origin,* with concern for the degree of illness, specific effects of the disorder, and effects of specific diagnostic or therapeutic measures used. General health is within the range of good to fair.
- **Group 4.** The health focus is oriented to *defects of a genetic or developmental nature,* or the *biologic state of the premature infant,* or the *low-birth-weight* infant. The state of general health may be affected by the direct or indirect effects of the defect or the biologic state.
- **Group 5.** The health focus is oriented to *regulation through active treatment of a disease or disorder or injury of determined origin,* with concern for the degree of illness; the specific effects of the disease, disorder, or injury; and the specific effects of the therapeutic measures used. Temporary or permanent disfigurement or disability may or may not be present or expected. The state of general health is or may be affected by direct or indirect effects of the disease, disorder, or injury.
- **Group 6.** The health focus is oriented to the *restoration, stabilization, or regulation of integrated functioning.* A vital process may have stopped or be seriously disrupted; in a newborn infant, breathing may not have started.
- **Group 7.** The health care focus is oriented to the regulation of the effects of processes that have disrupted human integrated functioning to the degree that quality of life is gravely affected or that life cannot long continue. Rational processes may be disturbed or relatively unaffected.

VARIATIONS IN HEALTH CARE AND NURSING

Because of differences in health focus, each of the seven groupings of nursing situations indicates requirements for different kinds of combinations of health care directed to one or more of the goals of preventive health care. For example, in nursing situations with a life cycle focus, the requirement for health care is at the primary level of prevention with the goals of maintaining and promoting health and preventing specific diseases and injuries. Awareness of these goals guides nurses as well as other health workers in the selection of measures of care and assistance for individuals or groups within specific environments.

In the descriptions that follow, health care goals and health care needs are specified and variations and indicated for each health focus. It should be understood that although the life cycle orientation to health care represents a type of nursing situation, in nursing practice the guides suggested for care with this focus are used along with guides for each of the other six situations, because every person is in one of the phases of the life cycle. The life cycle focus validates and provides the base for both universal and developmental self-care requisites. Health-deviation self-care requisites are associated with groups 2 to 6. The helping focus of nursing must be linked to the health care focus (Figure 9-3). The linking of the helping and health focuses in nursing practice is mediated by patient variables, therapeutic self-care demand and self-care agency, and the relationship between them.

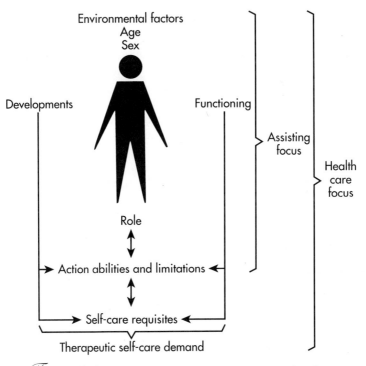

Figure 9-3 Two focuses of nurses in health care situations.

Life Cycle

In a nursing situation in which the health focus is oriented to the life cycle, the care is designed for promoting and maintaining health and for protecting against specific diseases and injuries. Environmental conditions and internal changes connected with intrauterine growth and development, infancy, childhood, adolescence, and maturity and related events and conditions such as pregnancy, menopause, and aging determine the specific kinds of health care that will be needed.

A nursing case of this type is one in which the patient's behavior indicates well-being rather than illness and in which there is evidence that the patient is in good to excellent health. The general health care needs would include:

- Periodic health evaluation to determine the normalcy of the patient's growth, functioning, and development and the quality of general health
- Health maintenance and promotion adjusted to the specific phase of and events in the patient's life cycle and to general health
- Protection against environmental factors, with specific concern for growth and development
- Assistance to the patient and the family in assuming appropriate roles in continuing health care through self-care

When the health focus is oriented to the life cycle, therapeutic self-care consists primarily of meeting the universal and developmental components of self-care adjusted to age; to sex; to the conditions of puberty, pregnancy, menopause, and aging; and to environmental factors. The self-care limitations of the patient arise from age or from lack of knowledge, skills, or essential resources.

Types of nursing cases with the life cycle focus include cases in which the specific health focus is on (1) normal growth and development of infants, children, and youth; (2) the continuing psychologic and intellectual development of the adult; (3) pregnancy in girls, young women, and older women; and (4) the anatomic, physiologic, and psychologic changes of middle age and advanced age. The four general kinds of health care appropriate for the life cycle orientation would be adjusted to specific demands represented by the four types of nursing cases. The four types of cases require that a nurse have knowledge of growth and development as related to the phases in the life cycle; validated health care practices in the area of primary prevention; cultural practices related to infant or child care and to adolescent and adult life, family living, sexual and marital relations, and prepartum, intrapartum, and postpartum care; social and economic forces affecting the individual and family; and the influence of physical, biologic, and social agents in the environment on individual, family, and community health. The life cycle focus, including its specific types of cases, is inherent in the health focus of the other five groups of cases. In a sense, it may be considered the core of any type of nursing situation.

Recovery

Recovery from disease, injury, or a functional disorder is the focus of health care. Medical treatment for the disease or injury has been instituted and has been effective in cure or regulation. Vital functions are stabilized. The characteristics of the medical therapy and its effects on the individual and the residual effects of the pathologic process prescribe the needs for health care.

Specific cases within group 2 would be instances in which complete recovery is expected with no residual defect or disability, cases in which there will be a permanent structural or functional defect through loss of or defect in an organ or a part of the body, and cases in which a functional disorder is regulated by continuous therapy. Cases may also vary as to the degree of illness; there may be normal functioning, except for the affected structures or functions or degree of illness experienced. Health care needs would include:

- Continued control of the recovery process through medical evaluation to determine the presence of sequelae and complications, the progress in recovery, and the effectiveness of disease regulation
- Continued medical therapy and self-care specific for the cure or regulation of the disease, injury, or functional disorder and its effects
- Specific protection when needed and possible to prevent sequelae and complications, defect, or disability resulting from the disease, injury, or functional disorder or from care measures
- Early detection and medical diagnosis of complications with prompt treatment
- Rehabilitation of the patient including the patient's self-image in the event of disfigurement, including loss of body parts or temporarily or permanently impaired functions
- Health maintenance and promotion and specific protection from the actual or possible effects of the disease, injury, or functional disorder on general health and growth and development
- Assistance to the patient and the family in assuming appropriate roles in health care, including self-care as related to the overall health care needs

In nursing cases of the group 2 type, therapeutic self-care would include care measures related to and derived from the disease process or functional disorder and measures derived from and related to medical diagnosis and therapy. Universal and developmental self-care requisites would require adjustments, not only to age and sex and environmental factors but also to the effects of the disease or injury and to the prescribed medical therapy. Self-care limitations may be caused by the effects of the disease process, the therapy used, the lack of necessary knowledge and skills, or a lack of resources.

Illness of Undetermined Origin

In group 3 health care is organized around signs and symptoms, degree of illness, and the need for medical diagnosis of the disease or disorder causing the signs and symptoms. A nursing case of this type is one in which the patient is suffering from a disorder with evident signs and symptoms and is either seriously ill and incapacitated, moderately or mildly ill, or functioning normally except for the presenting signs and symptoms of the disorder. The unknown causes of the signs and symptoms indicate that medical diagnosis and health evaluation are the principal health care needs. The health care needs would include:

- Prompt medical diagnosis of the nature, causes, and effects of the disease or disorder
- Alleviation of symptoms through medical therapy and self-care measures with precautions for not masking symptoms
- Prompt treatment and other protective care to prevent further structural or functional impairment or permanent defect and disability
- Health maintenance and promotion required as a result of the nature of the signs and symptoms, the degree of illness, and actual or possible effects on the patient's general health
- Assistance to the patient and the family in assuming appropriate roles in continuing health care, including self-care

The nursing aspects of group 3 situations would be similar to those of group 2 situations. Participation in health evaluations and medical diagnostic measures could be a major component of self-care in group 3 situations because the undetermined nature of the disorder would be a major concern that would affect both self-care and nursing.

Genetic and Developmental Defects and Biologic Immaturity

The health focus is oriented to the care and treatment of patients with structural and functional defects or a state of immaturity present at birth. The defects may be hereditary or congenital. Immaturity may be a consequence of a premature birth or associated with low birth weight or other factors. Health care is oriented to making adjustments and adaptations necessitated by the defect or undeveloped state and to supplying the environmental conditions necessary to support life, facilitate integrated functioning, and contribute to present and future normalcy in daily living.

The characteristics of each structural or functional defect or behavioral disorder would determine how human functioning and daily living are impaired. For example, an infant with a cleft palate presents a different requirement for health care than does an infant with an inborn error in metabolism (in which certain biochemical processes necessary for health and integrated functioning do not occur). Both the nature and the extent of the effects of specific defects— for example, a cleft lip as compared with a cleft palate—on life, health, and effective living must be considered. Health care requirements in group 4 would include:

- Continuous health care (including provision of a therapeutic environment) to achieve the adjustments and adaptations the patient needs for support of life processes and integrated functioning
- Continuous health evaluation to determine the effects of the defect, behavioral disorder, or biologic state on general health, growth, and development and functioning

- Continuous diagnosis to determine the extent and the effects of the defect or disorder, indications for forms of therapy, forms of therapy instituted, and the effects of therapy
- Specific protection against complications or extension of present impairments into more disabling limitations
- Rehabilitation of patient or parents of patient as indicated
- Health maintenance and promotion and specific protection from actual or possible effects of the defect or disorder on general health, growth, and development and functioning
- Assistance to the patient and family in assuming appropriate roles in continuing health care, including self-care

Nursing care is focused on contributing to the necessary adaptations and adjustments required as a result of the defect or biologic state and for maintaining essential environmental conditions. Rehabilitation may be of great importance in cases of this type. In some instances, major adjustments in family life are required. When defects are extensive and affect self-direction and behavioral control or mobility, provisions for continuing care within or outside the family setting are necessary.

Cure or Regulation

Health care in the form of active treatment for the cure or regulation of the effects of an injury, or disease, or functional disorder, including behavioral disorders, may be required during any period of a patient's life cycle. Major variations within this pattern relate to (1) the nature and extent of the injury and its effect; (2) the manner in which the disease or disorder manifests itself, including presenting signs and symptoms; (3) whether vital functions are stabilized or not stabilized; and (4) the degree of illness.

The following factors should be considered: Are the effects of the condition localized or generalized? Is the disease acute or chronic? If it is chronic, is it in an acute phase or in a phase of remission? Can the disease be cured? If not, can it be regulated with continuous therapy? Is some degree of regulation possible when the disease process is progressive and cannot be cured or entirely controlled? Is palliative and symptomatic therapy required? Health care requirements would include:

- Continuous care and medical therapy to cure or regulate the disease process or the functional disorder, to heal injured tissues, to alleviate symptoms, and to prevent disability
- Therapy to stabilize or to protect vital functions and integrated functioning
- Continuous control through evaluation of the progress of the disease process, the disorder, or the progress of recovery from the injury
- Specific protection to prevent complications or the extension of present effects of the disease, disorder, or injury that might result in disability
- Early diagnosis and prompt treatment of complications
- Health maintenance and promotion of general health, growth, and development
- Care to assist the patient in coping with suffering and disability when present

- Rehabilitation
- Assistance to the patient and family to assume appropriate roles in continuing health care, including self-care

The nursing aspects of the cure or regulation type of situation range from relatively simple to extremely complex. The specific symptoms, the degree of illness, the prognosis, the effects of the disease process on vital functions and integrated functioning, the amount and type of stress, and the form(s) of medical diagnosis and therapy and the effects of these measures determine the kind and amount of self-care required by the patient. Self-care and nursing care are adjusted according to the changes in the patient's health state and to changes in medical diagnosis and therapy.

Stabilization of Integrated Functioning

In this type of case, health care is oriented to stabilization and control of the vital processes that have been disrupted by disease processes or by injury or by impaired respiratory and cardiac functioning at birth. Variations in the individual case should be identified. What is the extent to which integrated functioning has been affected? Has an injury or its effects directly involved vital organs or affected integrated functioning? Is there immediate danger of death? Can any degree of control be established? If there is suffering, what is its nature and degree? Is the patient aware of the probable effects of the condition on life and health? Is there an anticipation of death or an uncontrolled fear of death? Whether the patient is an infant, child, adolescent, or adult is of great importance in nursing patients in this category. General health care requirements would include:

- Immediate institution of therapy to initiate, restore, or stabilize and support vital functions and facilitate integrated functioning
- Continuous control through nursing and medical evaluation to determine the degree of functional deviation in the life processes and to adjust or institute therapy as required
- Nursing care and medical therapy to alleviate distressing symptoms and relieve suffering
- Nursing care and medical therapy to prevent complications, to diagnose them early, and to institute prompt treatment
- Assistance to the ill or injured patient and family to sustain themselves in their suffering and to assume appropriate roles in the health situation
- Care to enable a dying person and the family to face the reality of death

Quality of Life is Gravely and Irreversibly Affected (Group 7)

Nursing is the essential health service for persons whose quality of life is gravely and irreversibly affected because of serious disruption of integrated functioning. Medical supervision, rather than active medical care, is required except in emergency situations. Care is directed to overcome obstacles arising from the effects of pathology to meet the universal self-care requisites. In many situations, the major focus is on meeting universal self-care requisites particularized for the conditions and circumstances under which persons live. Developmental self-care requisites would be concerned with learning how to live with some degree of effectiveness and satisfaction under the disrupted and abnormal conditions of human functioning. Health care requirements would include:

- Effective nursing management of patients and their environments
- Continuing medical supervision and active medical care as required
- Continuous effective meeting of the universal self-care requisites
- Finding ways and means and their use in supporting patients' development, for example, finding new ways of communicating, management of fear, and feelings of despair or rejection
- Continuous symptom management
- Appropriate assistance to family members (and to patients when appropriate) to help them understand patients' functional states, including the stability or instability of their states, their roles in care, and realistic planning for care in the present and the future
- Continuing support to patient and family to enable them to sustain themselves and to have a measure of security

In situations in which the quality of life is gravely and irreversibly affected because of the effects of disease and injury, nurses work with patients and their families, are in communication with physicians, and collaborate with other health workers about goals being sought. The provision and maintenance of a safe and developmental environment form an essential aspect of health care.

Terminal Illness (Group 7)

Health care is frequently oriented to the comfort and security of those who are in the terminal stages of illness. Care is directed to the control of persistent pain (if present) and to the regulation or control of other distressing symptoms (e.g., anorexia, dyspnea, frequency of urination, depression). Patients suffer increasing weakness and total distress.[6] Variations result from the natural history of the disorder, the types of symptoms experienced, and the methods used to regulate symptoms. The aims of health care are to enable individuals with a terminal illness to live as themselves, to understand their illness and how to participate in care, to approach death in their own particular way, and to be with family, friends, and health care workers in an environment of security and trust. General health care requirements would include:

- Effective medical management of the terminal illness
- Active medical treatment as advisable
- Continuous regulation of presenting sets of symptoms
- Continuous effective meeting of the universal self-care requisites
- Assistance directed to control of feelings of despair or rejection
- Assistance to the patient and family to understand the patient's illness and its projected outcome, and their roles in care and in preparation for the future
- Continuing support to patient and family to enable them to sustain themselves and to have a measure of security

• Development of care measures to support the patient at the time of death and ensure that family members know what help to secure and how to secure it

In situations of terminal illness, nurses ideally function with patients and family, physicians, paramedical personnel, and priests, ministers, or rabbis to institute and maintain a developmental environment for patients and all persons involved in their care.

SOCIETAL AND COMMUNITY PROVISIONS FOR HEALTH CARE

The health states of members of a society or a specific community vary in time and by members' places of residence. The way of life of a people and their states of health and well-being are positively or negatively affected by stability or change in physical or biologic environmental conditions; availability of life-sustaining resources of water, food, shelter, clothing; and by social, cultural, and political conditions and change. The way of life of a people also is affected by the knowledge that they have acquired and found to be effective in guiding their efforts to maintain themselves in satisfactory functional states. This includes knowledge about sanitation, essential resources and management of ill health and injury, including recognition and treatment. Some knowledge of healthful living, health and illness, and health care practice becomes a part of the general culture; other knowledge is acquired through specialized education and training.

In societies there is need for two levels of health care services that are enabling for ensuring the positive health and well-being of the people. One level of care serves populations and subpopulations. The other level of care serves individuals, families, and community groups. Populations are served by public health professionals and prevention programs. Health care requirements of individuals, families, and community groups are met through the service provided by members of the health care disciplines, such as medicine, nursing, and clinical psychology. State and local public health services now provide some of these services.

Public Health and Prevention for Populations

Public health is a discipline of knowledge and practice. Its object is the prevention of disease, the support of life processes, the promotion of physical and mental health, and human efficiency for populations. Prevention with a population focus is the work of public health practitioners. This is in contrast to preventive health care for individuals and families practiced by physicians, nurses, and other health care providers.

Public health practitioners have knowledge and skills not only in the discipline of prevention but also in epidemiology and biostatistics. Epidemiology is concerned with the occurrence and distribution of states of health and the occurrence and distribution of disease, defect, disability, and injury in populations. Biostatistics is an essential tool in the expression and analysis of demographic data about populations, in epidemiological research, and in the appraisal of population-focused prevention programs. Qualified public health professionals also may be qualified physicians and nurses who can bring knowledge from their own fields to bear in the practice of public health.

In brief, public health practitioners continuously seek information that is descriptive and explanatory of the health-relevant features of populations and their environments. They develop programs of preventive health care with health promotion features for populations at risk from specific human or environmental factors. They act to control and eradicate communicable disease. Ensuring the safety and adequacy of resources consumed by people and environmental safety are other concerns.

The World Health Organization, national, state, and local departments of health, and health visitors in villages work to provide preventive health programs for the large or small populations under their jurisdictions. Professional organizations such as the American Public Health Association also foster research and development in areas of preventive health care. Some national and international organizations are interested in research and preventive health care with respect to specific health conditions, for example, respiratory illness, cardiac disease, cancer, genetic defects, and mental health. Many services provided by governmental jurisdictions inside or outside departments of health, such as water purification, building codes and building inspection, and sewage disposal, also are essential for or contribute to the public health. Provision of shelter, food supplies, and meals for those in need are preventive health care measures, as are programs of early childhood education.

Health Care for Individuals and Families

In societies today a major concern of people and governments is the provision and availability of health care for individuals and families. Along with this concern there is growing recognition of the importance of primary preventive health care for individuals and families, both for public health and for the control of health care costs. One outcome is a growing worldwide movement to ensure that individuals and families have access to what are called **primary health care** services.

The connotations of primary health care are not clear-cut. However, features of this care make it *primary for people* and not just primary in the sense of primary prevention health care. Historically in the United States the family physician, physicians and nurses in general medical clinics in hospitals, and public health nurses served as primary care agents. Today there is movement toward formal recognition and organization of primary care services.

The following are some conclusions reached about the common features of effective primary care services. Primary care services are geographically and financially available to individuals and families—children as well as men and women. Such services provide periodic examinations to determine health states of individuals, involve individuals and families in exercising their responsibilities for health care, and ensure that persons participate in development and planning for their own individualized programs of care. Program purposes include health maintenance and health promotion as well as primary, secondary, and tertiary prevention as required.

Primary health care agents should be prepared to recognize in clients or patients overt signs of structural or functional disorders (physical or psychic), the presence of risk factors, and premonitory signs of pathologies such as stroke. Primary care agents refer clients to specialists in clinical medicine or nursing or other fields in accord with the features of clients' health disorders or health care problems. Primary care services should include access to dental care service and to specialized nutritional assessment and guidance. Existent and developing primary care services may provide some but not all of the foregoing features of care.

In the United States, primary care practitioners include both physicians and nurses. Physicians who practice primary care include family care practitioners and practitioners of general internal medicine and general pediatrics. Nurses include those qualified as nurse practitioners, as well as advanced clinical practitioners of nursing for individuals or families. Health care for individuals and families from the perspective of primary health care necessarily includes the availability of the services of physicians who are specialists in internal medical or surgical subspecialties. These physicians may work in association with clinical nursing specialists who serve the same populations.

Other health care services available or required in communities include hospitals with care facilities and programs for persons with life-threatening injuries, requirements for surgery or rehabilitation, and acute illnesses—physical or psychic. Convalescent care, nursing home care, hospice care, and home care services are also important services in many communities. After use of such services, individuals return to their primary care agents.

In some communities in the United States many of these services are either provided by or arranged for by organizations named health maintenance organizations. HMOs may be governed and operated by insurance companies or medical centers or by companies for their own employees. Individuals and families apply for and become members of health maintenance organizations. They must meet the financial arrangements for membership and select a plan for specific health care services.

Primary care services also are provided by physicians and nurses who maintain their own offices. Other primary care physicians and nurses function in joint practice with colleagues, some offering clinic-like services. In some places, nurse-managed primary care clinics make essential contributions to the positive health and well-being of communities.

There is a growing movement for employing organizations to offer wellness programs for workers. These programs are additions to traditional occupational health programs that take into account prevention of hazards specific to occupations.

Managed care is service provided for persons who are members of health insurance programs that offer what is referred to as *managed* or *comprehensive care*. The central focus of service to members is represented as continuing preventive health care from a primary care physician in accord with age and existent health care requirements of individuals. According to needs, referrals are made to, for example, medical specialists, hospitals, or home care programs. After specialized health care, members return to the primary care physician, who may function in his or her own office or in an HMO facility. These movements are arranged for and followed up by persons who are titled patient care coordinators who serve to coordinate the care of members in all settings through which they move.

Established standards are used to assess client progress within the various health care services. Standards are specific to health disorders of clients and are medically derived standards based on progress expected from specific forms of medical therapy. Allowances are or should be made for individual differences.

Managed care is also used with reference to particular forms of care, for example, medical care and nursing care. In such situations nurses must understand the relations between nursing care and medical care. Nurses must be able to differentiate progress from a nursing point of view from progress from a medical point of view. Results sought from nursing must be known, and differences from the results sought from medical care understood.

In summary, the provision of health care services for individuals and families continues to be a problem of availability and financing. The qualification and willingness of health workers to practice preventive health care are of considerable importance.

NURSING AS HEALTH CARE, A CONTINUATION

Nursing may be one of a number of health services needed by and provided to persons with health care requirements. The mix of health services being provided, the essential relationships among the services and the individual, and the combined contributions of the services to the health of an individual or a group constitute the health care system. From a service perspective, persons who seek and are provided with health care services have the *role* of consumer and purchaser of an available service. From the perspective of their relationship to the actual providers of care, they are in the *patient role*. In the role of consumer and purchaser, people pay for what they receive through taxes, third-party payments, or direct payment. In the role of patient, individuals should be helped to actively participate in their health care to the degree that their health and developmental states permit.

Nurses seek information to describe why an individual has sought and received health care. Two questions are suggested as guides in securing information: (1) Why and from whom did the patient seek (is the patient seeking) health care? (2) Why and by whom was the patient accepted (is the patient being accepted) as a recipient of health care? The *subjective measures* of a person's need for health service include (1) state of satisfaction or dissatisfaction with his or her own structure and modes of functioning; (2) judgments about what is normal and abnormal, tolerable or intolerable; and (3) judgments about existing abilities to cope with the effects of perceived disorders of structure or functioning. Adults and older children have data on how they now appear, function, and feel to compare with their state at some previous time. In making these judgments, individuals use two sets of norms: what is usual or "normal" for them and cultural norms about what is "normal for the group," which may or may not be based on scientific knowledge.

To provide nursing that is relevant to a patient's health care requirements, a nurse must be able to define his or her *nursing role,* including *role relationships* to the patient and to other health workers. Role definition requires awareness of the general dimensions of a patient's health care situation. It is a task that nurses perform at the time they enter health care situations and periodically thereafter. The seven groups of nursing situations organized according to differences in health care focuses and the general formulations of health care needs for each group can be used as an aid to the nurse's role definition.

This definition is of *role content* with respect to patients' health care requirements. But nurse role must also be defined in terms of nurses' relationships to patients that arise from patients' requirements for personal help because of the nature and extent of their health-related self-care deficits (the inadequacy of their self-care agency for knowing and meeting their therapeutic self-care demands). This personal help is provided through the instrumentality of methods of helping (Chapter 3) selected and used by nurses.

To define their own roles and the roles of their patients, nurses require more than information about patients' health states and health care requirements. Required information includes patients' patterns of daily living, available resources, and self-care agency and therapeutic self-care demands. This information is essential whenever patients have or are taking on an active role in knowing and meeting their therapeutic self-care demands.

To aid nursing students in learning to acquire this information, a three-part form for obtaining a *nursing history* from a patient is made available in Appendix A. This nursing history seeks information from patients about changes they have perceived in their therapeutic self-care demands, their development and exercise of self-care agency, and conditions and patterns of living and routines of self-care. The goal of taking such a nursing history is to explicate for nursing purposes the self-care aspects of a health care situation from a patient's perspective.

Nursing students should be aware of the reasons for and importance of taking nursing histories of patients. They must be able to differentiate the content of a nursing history from the content of a medical history. Nurses are accustomed to seeking information from physicians' medical histories. They are not accustomed to taking nursing histories that provide essential information for nurses and may provide useful information for physicians and other health care workers.

A nursing history is one tool for use in nurses' search for knowledge to define patients' roles in health care situations. It is but one aspect of the professional function of nursing diagnosis that is considered under the practice of nursing.

However, taking a nursing history can be an early exercise in the clinical education of nursing students.

SUMMARY

Nurses practice in a wide variety of health care situations. When nursing is effective, nursing results contribute to the accomplishment of the broad purposes of health care for populations, individuals, families, and community groups. Nurses must develop and continuously refine their dynamic concepts of health and nursing. Articulation of nursing with health states of persons nursed can be understood only within the frames of reference provided by the expressed proper object of nursing and by a valid general theory of nursing. One test of the validity of a general *theory of nursing* is its usefulness in pointing to articulations of nursing with persons' general health states and health state components. The self-care deficit theory of nursing meets this test as it provides five points of articulation with health states of persons nursed.

The commonly accepted purposes of health care and features of health care to attain these purposes are basic to nurses' understanding of and communication about nursing as health care. The description of nursing situations by their health care focuses and the related outlining of variations in health care and nursing requirements by situational focuses serve an orienting purpose for nursing students when they enter clinical nursing situations.

Up-to-date knowledge of societal and community provisions for health care help nurses to know how they and their nursing endeavors fit with health care situations, both from organizational and health care practice perspectives. Establishment of nurse role and patient role in health care situations is a nursing function.

The various sections of this chapter should be supplemented by students' use of authoritative references that provide detail about the topics presented. The selective reading of public health and medical journals as well as nursing journals is a scholarly practice of nurses that contributes to increasing understanding of the health care requirements of populations, individuals, and families.

References

1. Ashby WR: *An introduction to cybernetics,* London, 1965, Chapman & Hall, pp 195-218.
2. Crowe FE, Doran RM: *Collected works of Bernard Lonergan. Insight: a study of human understanding,* Toronto, 1992, University of Toronto Press, pp 82, 86-87, and 476-484.
3. Lewin K: *Field theory in social science, selected theoretical papers.* Cartwright D, editor: New York, 1951, Harper Torchbooks, pp xi and 45.
4. Nursing Development Conference Group, Orem DE, editor: *Concept formalization in nursing: process and product,* ed 2, Boston, 1979, Little, Brown, pp 122-123.
5. Leavell HR, Clark EG: *Preventive medicine for the doctor in his community,* ed 3, New York, 1965, McGraw-Hill, pp 14-38.
6. Saunders C: *The management of terminal illness,* London, 1967, Hospital Medicine Publications, p 14.

PART III

Variables of Nursing Systems

CHAPTER 10

Therapeutic Self-Care Demand: A Patient Variable

This chapter continues the development of the *theory of self-care* expressed in Chapter 7. In this development, knowledge with structure and content is provided for the proposed *foundational science of self-care* identified in Chapter 8. The knowledge also contributes to further development of the theory of *self-care deficit,* which postulates relationships between *therapeutic self-care demands* and the *powers of self-care agency* of individuals. Attention is directed in the first section to the term *therapeutic self-care demand* and the conceptualized entities that are its referents and its sources.

221

THE CONCEPT AND THE TERM

The term *therapeutic self-care demand* was introduced by the Nursing Development Conference Group in 1970. Before the formalization of the concept and the introduction of the term, *action demand* and *self-care demand* were terms used to refer to the *amount and kind of self-care* that persons should have. The process of formalization of the concept consumed a period of 3 years. The details of this process of formalization are recounted in "Dynamics of Concept Development" in *Concept Formalization in Nursing: Process and Product* (pp. 149-155).[1]

The analysis of nursing case data enabled group members to arrive at the understanding that the action demand for self-care for an individual is separate from the abilities of individuals to engage in self-care. It also became evident to the group that the stimulus for performing measures of self-care did not always arise within patients and that demands, whether of internal or external origin, did not always appear to be productive of therapeutic results. Nursing case analysis also led to the recognition that self-care demands were associated with the health states of individuals and also with the need for rehabilitation of the self-concepts of individuals under nursing care. This is the beginning recognition of the conditioning relationship between the self-care requisite components of a self-care demand and the identifiable human and environmental factors descriptive of persons.

The results of case analysis led the group members to use the terms *self-care demand* or *demand for therapeutic self-care.* Formalization of the concept of therapeutic self-care demand was also facilitated by contributions to the group by nurses qualified in speciality areas. Nurses in three specialty areas developed statements about the proper objects and the subject content of their nursing areas. The statements implied relationships between functional states of members of the populations served and what nurses in specialty areas do. This conveyed the idea that members of populations served had discernible demands for care with features common to the population.

At this stage of formalization of the concept **therapeutic self-care demand,** the following insights were components of the thought processes of group members:

1. Therapeutic self-care demand is an entity separate and apart from persons' engagement in self-care.
2. The recognition of the need and the stimulus to engage in specific measures of self-care may have an origin in external sources as well as internal sources.
3. What nurses do for patients in specialty areas of nursing practice implies relationships with the functional states of members of the populations served.
4. The individual who uses the term *therapeutic self-care demand* conceptually constructs a cluster of related conceptualized entities. The clustering of the elements that serve in construction of the concept results from insights about

a range of types of elements and not about a single concrete datum or cluster of data about an element.

5. Therapeutic self-care demand is a difficult concept to master and to use with conceptual consistency.

Structure and Derivation of the Concept

Therapeutic self-care demand is a *structure of formulated and expressed courses of action or care measures* that must be performed to generate action processes, using the technologies (means) selected to meet—that is, fulfill—the regulatory goals (functional or developmental) of known existent and emerging self-care requisites of individuals. Technologies selected to meet each known requisite should have known degrees of validity and reliability. The regulatory function of each self-care requisite is known, and the values at which it should be met are particularized—that is, personalized—for individuals before the selection of technologies.

Figure 10-1 shows the totality of care measures that is the therapeutic self-care demand for meeting self-care requisites identified as 1, 2, and *n* requisites. The figure also shows the correlatives, entities that imply or complement one another, that serve in the design of processes that generate the courses of action, the care measures to meet each self-care requisite. Courses of action to meet a single self-care requisite or a number of self-care requisites cannot be understood or judged as valid in the absence of knowledge of the correlations expressed in the figure. In the figure, specific self-care requisites expressive of regulatory goals correlate with human functions to be regulated, technologies (means) correlate with self-care requisites and courses of action, or care measures correlate with technologies in use. Both self-care requisites and technologies are shown to correlate with the human and environmental factors named *basic conditioning factors*. The model representing the structures of a therapeutic self-care demand and the sources of its derivation is based on models of deliberate action and action systems.

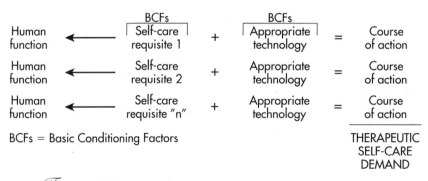

Figure 10-1 Components of therapeutic self-care and their sources.

Summary Statements About the Concept

The term *therapeutic self-care demand* stands for a complex theoretical concept that is an essential conceptual component of the theories of self-care, self-care deficit, and nursing system. The concept is theoretical because it has its origins in the self-care deficit theory of nursing and derives meaning from the subsidiary theories of self-care, self-care deficit, and nursing system. The concept is complex; it must be constructed by nurses in concrete nursing practice situations through a process of investigation and judgment making to determine (1) the kind and number of self-care requisites with specific regulatory functions to be achieved, (2) the known processes and valid technologies through which each self-care requisite can be met, and (3) the action sequences or courses of action (care measures) through which technologies are made operational in the process of meeting each self-care requisite.

Nurses must be dynamic in their knowing and be proficient in the use of developed intellectual and perceptual skills to engage in the complex process of calculating persons' therapeutic self-care demands. Their knowing must extend to types of self-care requisites, and variations in them, to valid and reliable technologies for meeting self-care requisites, and to factors that condition the values at which requisites should be met, condition the validity of technologies, or set up obstacles to meeting requisites, as described in Appendix C.

Therapeutic self-care demands are specific to individuals in their time-place situations. However, persons characterized by comparable age, developmental state, health state, or other basic conditioning factors have common components to their therapeutic self-care demands. Changes in persons' therapeutic self-care demands are associated with the nature of their characterizing **basic conditioning factors.** Some basic conditioning factors that characterize individuals, such as health state, may be relatively stable or in a state of rapid change. For example, persons in intensive care units are often characterized by an absence of stability in those human structural and functional features that define their health states, with rapidly changing values of their self-care requisites and their therapeutic self-care demands.

Every individual at every stage of development has a therapeutic self-care demand. Therapeutic self-care demands are constant features of persons under nursing care. Because the constant feature is subject to variation in individuals from one time to another, it is known as a *patient variable.*

Meeting self-care requisites constitutes the reasons for engagement in self-care, and the technologies for meeting self-care requisites produce the structural and content components of therapeutic self-care demands. For these reasons, nurses should have extensive knowledge of self-care requisites. Development of content specific to self-care requisites is presented in the following two sections.

SELF-CARE REQUISITES, DEVELOPMENTS 1958 TO 1995

Self-care requisites are formulated insights about actions to be performed by or for individuals that are known or hypothesized to be necessary in the regulation

of individuals' human functioning and development. The beginning formalization of the idea of self-care requisites occurred in 1958 in work performed and
published for the U.S. Department of Health, Education and Welfare, Office of
Education (pp. 48-53).[2]

In describing situations of personal health in a chapter on nursing situations,
"some major requirements for personal health" were identified. Fifteen requirements were described, five requirements each for physical health, mental health,
and emotional health. Factors to be controlled and reasons for the exercise of
control were identified. In some instances basic conditioning factors that affected
the value at which a requirement should be met were named. The following is an
example from *physical health:* "Food, water and air in accord with the nutritional
and energy requirements of the person derived from age, activities and the
particular situation of health" (pp. 51-52).[2]

The ideas expressed in 1958 in the requirements for physical, mental, and
emotional health can be identified in later expressions of universal and
developmental self-care requisites. The three types of self-care requisites
identified in Chapter 3—universal, developmental, and health-deviation—are
described.

Universal Self-Care Requisites

Universally required goals to be met through self-care or dependent-care have
their origins in what is known and what is validated or in process of validation
about human structural and functional integrity at various stages of the life cycle.
Eight self-care requisites common to men, women, and children are suggested.

1. The maintenance of a sufficient intake of air.
2. The maintenance of a sufficient intake of water.
3. The maintenance of a sufficient intake of food.*
4. The provision of care associated with elimination processes and excrements.
5. The maintenance of a balance between activity and rest.
6. The maintenance of a balance between solitude and social interaction.
7. The prevention of hazards to human life, human functioning, and human
   well-being.
8. The promotion of human functioning and development within social groups in
   accord with human potential, known human limitations, and the human desire
   to be normal. *Normalcy* is used in the sense of that which is essentially human
   and that which is in accord with the genetic and constitutional characteristics
   and talents of individuals.

These eight requisites represent actions that bring about the internal and
external conditions that maintain human structure and functioning, which in turn
support human development and maturation. When it is effectively provided,
self-care or dependent-care organized around universal self-care requisites

---

*Constituents of foods that human beings need are referred to as nutrients. These include proteins and
the amino acids of which they are composed, fats and fatty acids, carbohydrates, minerals, and
vitamins. Water is also a constituent of many foods.

fosters positive health and well-being. The Box on page 227 presents general actions for meeting these eight requisites. The results of meeting each of them contribute in different ways to health and well-being, as specified by their regulatory functions.

The maintenance of sufficient intakes of air, water, and food provides individuals with the materials required for metabolism, energy production, and constancy of body fluids. The provision of effective care associated with elimination processes and excrements should ensure the integrity of these processes and their regulation, as well as effective control of the materials eliminated. The maintenance of a balance between activity and rest controls voluntary energy expenditure, regulates environmental stimuli, and provides variety, outlets for interest and talents, and the sense of well-being that comes from both. The maintenance of a balance between solitude and social interaction provides conditions essential for developmental processes in which knowledge is acquired, values and expectations are formed, and a measure of security and fulfillment is achieved. Solitude reduces the number of social stimuli and demands for social interaction and provides conditions conducive to reflection; social contacts provide opportunities for the interchange of ideas, acculturation and socialization, and the achievement of the human potential. Social interaction is also essential to obtain the material resources essential to life, growth, and development.

Prevention of hazards to life, functioning, and well-being contributes to the maintenance of human integrity and, therefore, to the effective promotion of human functioning and development. The promotion of human functioning and development (promotion of normalcy), in turn, prevents the development of conditions that constitute internal hazards to human life and to human functioning and development. It also promotes conditions that lead individuals to feeling and knowing their individuality and wholeness, to cognitional objectivity, and to freedom and responsibility as human beings.

One aspect of the development of areas of knowledge about the universal self-care requisites is the explication of relationships among them. For example, the requisites *prevention of hazards* and *promotion of normalcy* must be related to each of the other six requisites, as illustrated in Figure 10-2, in relation to maintenance of a sufficient intake of air, water, and food. Caregivers can inquire as to how requisites for prevention of hazards and promotion of normalcy articulate with the other six requisites by seeking answers to questions in the following series.

Three questions for investigation are suggested for the requisites' maintenance of sufficient intakes of air, water, and food.

- What is a sufficient intake of air, water, and food under known or hypothesized internal and external conditions? For example, should water and food intake be adjusted under conditions of heat stress and, if so, how?
- What hazards, if any, may be associated with meeting each of these requisites for the intake of materials? How can identified hazards, such as the presence of noxious substances in inspired air, water, or food, or food intakes that are not sufficient, be eliminated or controlled?

General Sets of Actions for Meeting the Eight Universal Self-Care Requisites

1. Maintenance of sufficient intakes of air, water, food
   a. Taking in that quantity required for normal functioning with adjustments for internal and external factors that can affect the requirement or, under conditions of scarcity, adjusting consumption to bring the most advantageous return to integrated functioning
   b. Preserving the integrity of associated anatomic structures and physiologic processes
   c. Enjoying the pleasurable experiences of breathing, drinking, and eating without abuses
2. Provision of care associated with eliminative processes and excrements
   a. Bringing about and maintaining internal and external conditions necessary for the regulation of eliminative processes
   b. Managing the processes of elimination (including protection of the structures and processes involved) and disposal of excrements
   c. Providing subsequent hygienic care of body surfaces and parts
   d. Caring for the environment as needed to maintain sanitary conditions
3. Maintenance of a balance between activity and rest
   a. Selecting activities that stimulate, engage, and keep in balance physical movement, affective responses, intellectual effort, and social interaction
   b. Recognizing and attending to manifestations of needs for rest and activity
   c. Using personal capabilities, interests, and values as well as culturally prescribed norms as bases for development of a rest-activity pattern
4. Maintenance of a balance between solitude and social interaction
   a. Maintaining that quality and balance necessary for the development of personal autonomy and enduring social relations that foster effective functioning of individuals
   b. Fostering bonds of affection, love, and friendship; effectively managing impulses to use others for selfish purposes, disregarding their individuality, integrity, and rights
   c. Providing conditions of social warmth and closeness essential for continuing development and adjustment
   d. Promoting both individual autonomy and group membership
5. Prevention of hazards to life, functioning, and well-being
   a. Being alert to types of hazards that are likely to occur
   b. Taking action to prevent events that may lead to the development of hazardous situations
   c. Removing or protecting oneself from hazardous situations when a hazard cannot be eliminated
   d. Controlling hazardous situations to eliminate danger to life or well-being
6. Promotion of normalcy
   a. Developing and maintaining a realistic self-concept
   b. Taking action to foster specific human developments
   c. Taking action to maintain and promote the integrity of one's human structure and functioning
   d. Identifying and attending to deviations from one's structural and functional norms

Maintenance of a sufficient intake of:

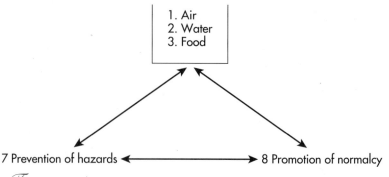

Figure 10-2 Interrelations of some of the universal self-care requisites.

- In meeting these three requisites for material intakes, can normal functioning and development be promoted and, if so, how (e.g., the institution and maintenance of patterns of food consumption based on a knowledge of the nutrients in consumed food, not just on habits and preferences)?

To be effective, the provision of care associated with elimination processes and excrements requires answers to the following:

- What are the elimination patterns of individuals? Are current patterns congruent with former patterns?
- What care practices or care measures are associated with acts of elimination and the disposal of excrements?
- Do the identified elimination patterns or the care practices (or lack of them) in and of themselves constitute hazards?
- What hazards, if any, are associated with preparation for or engagement in elimination under the individual's internal and external conditions?
- What constitutes the norm for elimination for an individual? If elimination patterns are now outside the norm, can normal functioning be brought about, and how can this be accomplished?
- What care practices related to acts of elimination and disposal of excrements would benefit individuals and the social group?

The provider of care in relation to maintaining a balance between activity and rest and a balance between solitude and social interaction would need to answer the following questions:

- What constitutes a balance between rest and activity and between solitude and social interaction under prevailing internal and external conditions?
- What kinds and degrees of rest and activity or solitude and social interaction constitute a hazard under existing conditions?
- What kinds and degrees of rest and activity or solitude and social interaction can be expected to maintain human structure and promote human functioning and development in relation to the human potential and its

limits, and at the same time be in accord with the interests, desires, and talents of the individual?

Caregivers would need to answer the following questions with respect to the association between prevention of hazards and promotion of normal human functioning and development:

- What hazards to human life, functioning, and development exist in the individual's environment or pattern of living?
- What will happen to an individual if a hazard is not eliminated or controlled?
- What patterns of action should individuals develop and exercise in order to become aware of or prevent or control hazards?
- What individual interests, values, and actions with respect to known hazards are causing conditions that impair human structure and functioning or are obstacles to normal human functioning and development?

Four questions may guide inquiry about requisites for maintenance of normalcy:

- What internal or external factors are suggestive of or positive indicators of specific requisites for the promotion of normalcy with respect to (1) individualization and personalization and (2) human functioning described psychologically, cognitively, or biologically?
- Can these requisites be phrased in a way that can be understood and serve as a guide in the selection of care measures?
- What courses of action would be effective and possible under existent or predicted conditions?
- Are individuals involved in programs to attain some personalized or group goals that are hazardous to personal well-being, health, or life?

Meeting the universal self-care requisites through self-care or dependent-care is an integral part of the daily living of individuals and groups, but such actions tend to become separated from the fabric of human life when certain conditions predominate. These conditions include (1) contamination of air, water, and food with noxious materials; (2) scarcity of food and water; (3) conditions that adversely affect the work, recreational, educational, and religious activities and the daily living patterns of human groups; and (4) illness, defects, specific pathology, and disability of social group members. Under such conditions, individuals and the group as a whole focus attention on these self-care requisites and may act to bring about conditions under which they can be effectively met.

Each of the eight universal self-care requisites from either a qualitative (kind) or a quantitative (amount) perspective or both becomes differentiated for individuals or groups in relation to differences in age, gender, developmental state, health state, sociocultural orientation, and resources. The varieties of practice within culture groups and the range of practices individuals use reflect not only long-term adjustment to environmental conditions but also the kind and amount of knowledge that has been acquired, is transmitted, and is put to use with respect to these universal requisites for care.

Developmental Self-Care Requisites

Initially these requisites were subsumed under the universal self-care requirements. They have been separated out to emphasize their importance and because of their number and diversity.

Human development can be studied in terms of its various dimensions that have been the subject of investigation in a variety of fields. There is a growing literature on the organic dimensions of growth and development; the psychic dimensions, including cognitional and affective development; and the personal dimension expressed in terms of personality and character formation and mental health. The associations among these developmental dimensions are also objects of inquiry. Human development should be understood as a flexible, dynamic process involving occurrences, events, and functioning in each individual existing unity that is a man, woman, or child.*

The identification, formulation, and expression of developmental self-care requisites are difficult. Differences as well as associations among the dimensions of human development must be assumed, as well as the unity of the individual. Developmental self-care requisites are relevant to initial formation of human structural, functional, and behavioral features of individuals and their dynamic movement toward increasingly higher and more complex and intricate levels of organization and functioning.

Expression of developmental self-care requisites is complicated by the different bodies of knowledge to be mastered in order to understand the dimensions of human development and to isolate the factors that promote and regulate it at various stages of the life cycle. Stages of the life cycle and associated conditions and circumstances must be recognized. The commonly recognized life cycle stages with developmental events and occurrences are:

1. The intrauterine stages of life and the process of birth
2. The neonatal stage of life when an individual is (a) born at term or prematurely and (b) born with normal or low birth weight
3. Infancy
4. The developmental stages of childhood, including adolescence and entry into adulthood
5. The developmental stages of adulthood
6. Pregnancy in either childhood or adulthood

Each individual develops as a separate, unique person in society. Conditions and resources that promote the natural development of individuals vary within families, communities, and whole societies. Each individual throughout his or her life experiences internal and external conditions that can adversely affect development. And each individual at certain stages of development becomes personally involved in his or her development and movement to maturity. At other stages of the life cycle (stages of intrauterine life, infancy, and childhood),

---

*Lonergan's *Insight*[3] presents a philosophic treatment of development. This may be helpful toward understanding the various dimensions of human development and the relations among them (pp. 476-504).

developmental requisites can be met only by dependent-care agents, parents, or others. In light of these considerations, three sets of developmental requisites are suggested for consideration and for determination of their usefulness in practice situations. The sets are identified as provision of conditions that promote development, engagement in self-development, and prevention of or overcoming effects of human conditions and life situations that can adversely affect human development.

Provision of Conditions That Promote Development

These are requisites that are met by dependent-care agents in the early stages of the human life cycle. When older children and adults are subjected to disasters, seriously ill, or in states of fear and anxiety, persons in helping roles (disaster workers, family members, nurses) may need to provide the following conditions:

1. Provide and maintain an adequacy of materials, such as water and food, and conditions essential for development of the human body at stages when foundations for bodily features are laid down and dynamic developments occur, and at later stages.
2. Provide and maintain physical, environmental, and social conditions that ensure feelings of comfort and safety, the sense of being close to another, and the sense of being cared for.
3. Provide and maintain conditions that prevent both sensory deprivation and sensory overload.
4. Provide and maintain conditions that promote and sustain affective and cognitional development.
5. Provide conditions and experiences to facilitate beginning and advances in skill development essential for life in society, including intellectual, perceptual, practical, interactional, and social skills.
6. Provide conditions and experiences to foster awareness that one possesses a self and of being a person within the world of the family and community.
7. Regulate the physical, biologic, and social environment to prevent development of states of fear, anger, or anxiety.

Engagement in Self-Development

These requisites are ones that demand the deliberate involvement of the self in processes of development.

1. Seek to understand and form habits of introspection and reflection to develop insights about self, one's perception of others, relationships to others, and attitudes toward them.
2. Seek to accept feelings and emotions as leading, after reflection on them, to insights about self and about relationships to others, to objects, or to life situations.
3. Use talents and interests in preparing for and in maintaining and supporting engagement in productive work in society.
4. Engage in clarification of goals and values in situations that demand personal involvement.

5. Act with responsibility in life situations in accord with one's role or roles and with a developed or developing self-ideal.
6. Seek to understand the value of positive emotions in development of "firm emotional dispositions" that "give rise to the habits we call virtues." Positive emotions and action impulses include the desire to know; variations of human love, love of beauty, joy of making and doing, mirth and laughter, religious emotions, happiness"[4] (pp. 311-330).
7. Seek to understand that negative emotions and action impulses are experienced when conduct is in discord with one's life goals and self-ideal. Negative emotions include guilt and guilt feelings, states of guilt, and unconscious conflict[4] (pp. 294-299).
8. Promote positive mental health through deliberate efforts to
   a. function within a veridical (reality) frame of reference
   b. function to bring about and maintain order in daily living
   c. function with integrity and self awareness
   d. function as a person in community
   e. function with increasing understanding of one's own humanity*

Interferences with Development

Throughout the life cycle there is need to have knowledge of events, conditions, and problems that adversely affect human development at the various stages of the life cycle. Developmental requisites express two goals:

1. Provide conditions and promote behaviors that will prevent the occurrence of deleterious effects on development.
2. Provide conditions and experiences to mitigate or overcome existent deleterious effects on development.

The conditions and problems referred to include
   a. Educational deprivation
   b. Problems of social adaptation
   c. Failures of healthy individuation
   d. Loss of relatives, friends, associates
   e. Loss of possessions, loss of occupational security
   f. Abrupt change of residence to an unfamiliar environment
   g. Status-associated problems
   h. Poor health or disability
   i. Oppressive living conditions
   j. Terminal illness and impending death

These conditions and problems do not constitute an exhaustive list. In some nursing situations, the kinds of problems named may be a central focus of care; in other situations, the results of the problems are considered a qualification on action within the particular situation. For example, the developmental problem of

---

*The five features of positive mental health were developed by D.E. Orem and E.M. Vardiman.

"failure of healthy individuation" may provide a central, organizing focus for nursing action in some child nursing situations. By contrast, the arrested cognitive development of an adult, associated with "educational deprivation," may be accepted as a qualification on action because it is not likely to change during the duration of a nursing situation. Nurses move to help patients learn and develop personally, regardless of their stage of cognitive development, but the methods used will be selected in light of the stage of operational knowing the patient has achieved. The following excerpt from descriptive materials about one ember of an adult ambulatory population exemplifies this nursing approach.

> Mr. M. is a 66-year-old diabetic who has never been to school, who thinks very concretely, who cannot read, who can distinguish colors but not name them, and who has fairly good motor ability. Recently he was asked to begin testing his urine at home and the nurse began teaching him. Content had to be broken into small units and presented slowly. After two sessions Mr. M. did learn to test his urine and repeated demonstrations by him at subsequent clinic visits indicate that he continues to do it accurately. As a result the clinic staff can be certain that they have accurate information about test results. Mr. M. is extremely pleased at having learned to do this and views this as an important *self-development*. During his last clinic visit he said to me, "You know, I've had this diabetes 4 years now and nobody ever did as much for me till I got tied up to this nurse. She done more for me in this time and now I know more than I did before" (p. 789).[5]

Health-Deviation Self-Care Requisites

These self-care requisites exist for persons who are ill or injured, have specific forms of pathology including defects and disabilities, and who are under medical diagnosis and treatment. Obvious changes in human structure (edematous extremities, tumors), in physical functioning (difficult breathing, limited movement of a joint), or in behavior and habits of daily living (extreme irritability in relations with others, sudden changes in mood, loss of interest in life) focus a person's attention on himself or herself. These changes may raise questions. What is wrong? Why is this happening? What should I do? Family members and friends may also ask the same questions when they observe these obvious deviations from health. Changes that occur subtly and gradually are not detected as quickly as those that appear suddenly and dramatically. When inability to focus attention or attend to oneself is part of the disease process (for example, a cerebral accident), manifestations of the pathology may be noted first by family members or co-workers. When a change in health state brings about total or almost total dependence on others to sustain life or well-being, the person moves from the position of *self-care agent* to that of *receiver of care*. Parents also experience a similar change in position when a child's health deviation demands care that exceeds their capacities as *dependent-care agents*. Evidence of health deviations leads to demands for determining what should be done to restore normalcy. In modern society, this would be expressed as a demand for medical diagnosis and treatment. Seeking and participating in medical care for health deviations are self-care actions.

Health deviations may bring about feelings of illness or of not being able to function normally. These feelings, which are related directly or indirectly to the nature of the health deviation, influence what the person may choose to do. Disease processes may also be functional in individuals and may not be accompanied by feelings of illness. The localized or generalized effects of disease or injury are related to feelings of illness. For example, a person with a simple fracture may feel well despite some discomfort, but a person with a "cold" may feel quite ill. In either situation, a disease or injury is something to be lived with and lived through, in that disease and injury have some duration over time. The duration varies with the nature of the disease or injury. Some diseases terminate only with death, whereas others are brought under control by biologic processes with or without human intervention using medically derived measures. The characteristics of health deviations as conditions extending over time determine the kinds of care demands that individuals experience as they live with the effects of pathologic conditions and live through their duration.

Disease or injury affects not only specific structures and physiologic or psychologic mechanisms but also integrated human functioning. When integrated functioning is seriously affected (severe mental retardation, comatose states, autism), the individual's developing or developed powers of agency are seriously impaired either permanently or temporarily. Conditions that limit physical mobility, even when such limitations are severe, may be less disruptive of integrated human functioning than emotional and mental disorders. Extreme limitations of physical mobility or sensory deprivation as in total blindness may lead to emotional and mental problems, which, if unresolved, can interfere with human integrated functioning. Whenever health deviations result in disfigurement or disability, there is a demand for specialized medical and nursing assistance to prevent further deviations in human functioning.

Self-care requisites arise not only from disease, injury, disfigurement, and disability but also from medical care measures prescribed or performed by physicians. Medical care measures may modify structure (surgical removal of organs) or require behavioral modification (control of fluid intake). Pain, discomfort, and frustration resulting from medical care also create requisites for self-care to bring relief. Some medical care measures introduce hazards into a person's life situation. For example, the possibility of dependence on prescribed drugs and the risks attendant on anesthesia and major surgical intervention are real problems. The use of these measures necessitates protective care measures. The specific techniques of medical diagnosis and treatment used produce particular self-care requisites. Nurses must know and be alert to these results and requisites.

This analysis of health-deviation self-care has shown that in abnormal states of health, self-care requisites arise from both the disease state and the measures used in its diagnosis or treatment. Understanding these types of self-care requisites requires a foundation of knowledge in medical science and medical technology. Modern medical advances require nurses to be well grounded in pathology and in various medical technologies if they are to effectively assist individuals with health-deviation self-care. If persons with health deviations are to become competent in managing a system of health-deviation self-care, they must be helped to apply relevant medical knowledge to their own care.

There are six categories of health-deviation self-care requisites:

1. Seeking and securing appropriate medical assistance in the event of exposure to specific physical or biologic agents or environmental conditions associated with human pathologic events and states, or when there is evidence of genetic, physiologic, or psychologic conditions known to produce or be associated with human pathology

2. Being aware of and attending to the effects and results of pathologic conditions and states, including effects on development

3. Effectively carrying out medically prescribed diagnostic, therapeutic, and rehabilitative measures directed to preventing specific types of pathology, to the pathology itself, to the regulation of human integrated functioning, to the correction of deformities or abnormalities, or to compensation for disabilities

4. Being aware of and attending to or regulating the discomforting or deleterious effects of medical care measures performed or prescribed by the physician, including effects on development

5. Modifying the self-concept (and self-image) in accepting oneself as being in a particular state of health and in need of specific forms of health care

6. Learning to live with the effects of pathologic conditions and states and the effects of medical diagnostic and treatment measures in a life-style that promotes continued personal development

Exercise

Exercise to Assist in Learning to Obtain Information About Dependent-Care Systems for Children and Adults

1. Select a friend who is the responsible adult or one of the responsible adults providing continuing care for a child in the family. Make sure the person is willing to answer questions about giving care.
   a. Ask the person to tell you about how he or she cares for the child. Tell the person that you are interested in the components of care as they are understood by persons who are involved in giving care. Ask the person to proceed by telling you what he or she does.
   b. Record what the person tells you, attending to the person's focus (1) on care to meet the universal, developmental, and health-deviation self-care requisites and (2) on what is said about the child's role in care.
   c. Ask questions if necessary to get a description of the care provided.
   d. As a conclusion, ask the person how he or she feels about being in the role of caregiver.
2. Follow the same procedure for a person providing care for an adult member of a family or a household.

Care measures to meet existent health-deviation self-care requisites must be made action components of individuals' systems of self-care or dependent-care. The complexity of self-care or dependent-care systems is increased by the number and kinds of health-deviation requisites that must be met in specific time frames.

As previously indicated (see Figure 10-1), values of self-care requisites as well as technologies for meeting them are conditioned by factors (basic conditioning factors) such as age and developmental states of individuals. It is important to recognize that health-deviation self-care requisites have their origins in *health states of individuals* and in *health care system factors*. The health states of individuals, however, affect or condition if and how existent health-deviation self-care requisites can be met.

The development of knowledge descriptive and explanatory of self-care requisites from 1958 to 1995 is summarized:

1. The regulatory functions of self-care requisites are described.
2. Self-care requisites are expressed as actions to achieve regulatory goals.
3. Self-care requisites are recognized as the source of action components of therapeutic self-care demands and systems of self-care.
4. Three types or categories of self-care requisites are identified, described, and named: universal, developmental, and health-deviation types of self-care requisites. Specific requisites within each of the three types are identified and described as actions with regulatory purposes.
5. Subsidiary goals to be attained to meet the regulatory purposes of each universal and developmental self-care requisite are formulated and expressed.
6. The need for identification of relationships between and among requisites is identified, noting that the universal self-care requisites "to prevent hazards" and "to maintain normalcy" are related to all other universal types of self-care requisites. This need is not confined to universal types of self-care requisites.
7. Questions are formulated about each universal type of self-care requisite. The answers should yield information required to ensure effectively meeting each requisite.
8. There is an unequal development of knowledge for the three types of self-care requisites. The least organized development is for health-deviation types of requisites.

SELF-CARE REQUISITES, CONTINUED DEVELOPMENTS 1996 TO 2000

During the years 1996 to 2000, efforts were directed by three interested persons* to review the work that had been done to describe and explain self-care and self-care requisites. Following the review, we decided to focus on the refinement

---

*Mary J. Denyes, Gerd Bekel, and Dorothea E. Orem constituted this work group. They were members of the Orem Study Group, a voluntary association of nurses concerned with continuing development of self-care deficit nursing theory.

and further development of content descriptive and explanatory of *self-care requisites.* This decision was based in part on insights that led to the judgment that a science of self-care could and should be developed as a theoretically practical *foundational nursing science.* Five areas of the proposed science were formalized and developed to greater or lesser degrees: self-care, self-care agency, self-care requisites, therapeutic self-care demands, and self-care practices and self-care systems.

This judgment was based on recognition that a science of self-care has as its *object of study*—that is, its *reality focus*—the enduring systems of self-care produced by or for men, women, and children from birth to death through the deliberate performance of care measures and care sequences in time and over time. Why are such care systems a constant and enduring reality in human groups? What do such care systems effect in individuals or in their environments? What are the constituent elements of these self-care systems or dependent-care systems? What are these constituent elements designed to bring about, and what is their derivation? The answer to those questions were known to the members of the study group. Their decision to focus on self-care requisites recognized that the deliberate action systems of self-care have their origins and their reasons of being in existent and emerging self-care requisites with their specific regulatory functions.

With recognition that self-care systems produced by or for individuals and the therapeutic self-care demands on which they are based change in time and over time, possibilities for such changes were understood to be associated with self-care requisites. These possibilities included (1) changes in the frequency with which each existent self-care requisite should be met, (2) elimination of self-care requisites because their regulatory functions are no longer required, (3) increase in the kinds and number of self-care requisites, and (4) changes in the qualitative and quantitative values of existent self-care requisites. These possibilities for changes in self-care systems emphasized the importance of further development and refinement of the already expressed self-care requisites, as well as the need for explication of the conditioning effects of factors descriptive of persons and their environments on persons' self-care requisites.

These conditioning factors shown in Figure 12-1, as noted in Chapter 8, bring descriptors of persons as individuals into the frame of reference of self-care, therapeutic self-care demand, and self-care systems. Existent values of factors descriptive of persons in their life situations that condition existent self-care requisites or give rise to new requisites help nurses understand the movement from a theoretically practical mode of thinking to a practically practical mode of thinking. Existent values of these basic conditioning factors in concrete life situations can and do change the values at which universal and developmental self-care requisites should be met, give rise to new self-care requisites, and affect the technologies or means that have validity in meeting self-care requisites.

Refinement of the Expression of a Self-Care Requisite

The study group focused attention on the identification of regulatory results sought in the expression of one self-care requisite. The universal self-care requisite selected for refinement was expressed originally as "maintain an adequate intake of water." The question raised by this expression is: Adequate for what? or What are the physiologic requirements that it should be adequate to meet? The reformulated requisite is expressed in the box below.

In addition, the process necessary to attain the regulatory results sought was formulated and expressed. Four constant aspects or subprocesses of the process were identified as follows:

1. Ensuring the availability of the resource water, its safety, and readiness for its intake
2. Having knowledge of and maintaining awareness of the quantity of the required intake of water
3. Taking water into the body
4. Determining adequacy of water intake

The importance of the formulation and expression of the parts of the process of "maintaining an adequate intake of water" rests in the recognition that not one but at least four different types of deliberate action sequences must be formulated and expressed as the therapeutic self-care demand is constructed. These action sequences, when performed in concrete life situations, meet the self-care requisite and fulfill its regulatory function, all things being equal. It is recognized that the critical and essential feature is "taking water into the body" to supply what is known to be needed. This is, of course, dependent on having the resource water and the willingness to consume it. This example makes clear how content is identified and structured as the expressions of self-care requisites are refined, their regulatory function is identified, and the **processes for meeting self-care requisites** are formulated and expressed.

Premise: Water is Essential for Life

The Requisite: Maintain an intake of water adequate to:

A. Keep concentrations of water constant in the blood plasma, tissue fluids, and intracellular fluids by balancing water intake with water loss through all channels of elimination.

B. Prevent, alleviate, or control disturbances of water concentration in body fluids—blood plasma, tissue fluids, and intracellular fluids—by using technologies with known or presumed validity and reliability that have become parts of the common culture or are within the domain of medical practice. In the absence of such technologies, advanced practitioners in medicine and nursing must proceed by using the most advanced knowledge in the search for ways to prevent, alleviate, or control disturbances.

Another Example of Refinement of Expression of a Universal Self-Care Requisite

There are three universal self-care requisites that require intake of material substances, namely, the requisites to maintain adequate or sufficient (what is needed) intakes of air, water, and food. A refined expression of the requisite for food is expressed in Chapter 3, and the requisite for water in the preceding section of this chapter. A refined expression of the requisite "maintain an adequate intake of air" is presented in the box below.

With this universal self-care requisite, the method of air intake is the natural continuing process of breathing. The resource required is atmospheric air with that amount of oxygen found in air at sea level or below 12,000 feet. The deliberate actions, courses of action prescribed in a therapeutic self-care demand, include courses of actions, care measures to (1) prevent interference with breathing and hence with pulmonary ventilation, (2) maintain self (or others) in environments where the composition of air and the availability of air meet physiologic requirements, and (3) be or become aware of conditions, circumstances, or disorders that interfere with pulmonary ventilation and take action to regulate or control the obstacles or interferences.

Obstacles to meeting this universal self-care requisite are identified in Appendix C. Knowledge of some obstacles may be parts of the common culture, as are the means for their regulation or control. Other obstacles are associated with health state features—that is, with structural or function pathologies—and may require medical regulation or control.

A Health Deviation Self-Care Requisite with Expressed Elements of Its Therapeutic Self-Care Demand Component

Health deviation self-care requisites, as indicated by their name, have their origins in health state features that express human functional or structured disorders and methods for their regulation or control. The requisite now described has its origin in a human disorder that is named *bronchial asthma,* a condition that affects breathing and lung ventilation. The condition is one of a number of conditions that interfere with meeting the universal self-care requisite to maintain a sufficient intake of air. The description shows the complexity of this health-deviation self-care requisite and the number of subsystems within the process of meeting the requisite.

A generalized expression of the health-deviation self-care requisite, focused on control of the occurrence of bronchial asthma and regulation of its effects, is

---

Requisite

Prevent interference with the natural process of breathing to ensure inspiration of air sufficient to maintain pulmonary ventilation with air that has a partial oxygen pressure consonant with air at sea level or below 12,000 feet.[6]

presented in the following box. This generalized health-deviation self-care requisite cannot have its regulatory purposes achieved without the performance of five formulated and expressed constituent parts of the process of meeting the generalized requisite. The subsystems of the process, are identified as follows:

1. Patients accept themselves as having periodic attacks of bronchial asthma and learn to understand and fulfill their responsibilities for maintaining or restoring adequate pulmonary ventilation during pending attacks and attacks in process.

2. Patients secure and maintain the position of patient in relation to specialized health care professionals (physicians, nurses) who have the knowledge and skills to diagnose the nature and severity of their asthmatic attacks, instruct them in making observations and reporting, prescribe therapeutic measures and regimens, and help them learn to manage themselves and their environment and perform care measures to restore and maintain adequate pulmonary ventilation.

3. Patients make observations of the occurrence of respiratory difficulties, their nature, the time and sequence of occurrences and their duration, their severity, and the prevailing relevant internal conditions (e.g., respiratory infection) and external conditions (e.g., exposure to extreme cold) at the time of occurrence; on the basis of this information, they make judgments about the initiation, progress, and severity of the attack; the preferred regulatory care to be instituted, and the probable outcome if appropriate care is instituted.

4. Patients make a decision to perform and perform the selected regimen of therapeutic care after assembling the medications and equipment required,

---

The Health-Deviation Self-Care Requisite: Control the Occurrence of and Regulate the Effects of Bronchial Asthma

Maintain or bring about pulmonary ventilation by preventing or controlling the pathologic processes known as bronchial asthma that result in experienced respiratory difficulty by engaging in self-care regimens with some known effectiveness in:

1. Reducing swelling and inflammation of the smaller bronchioles (airways to the alveoli of the lung) to prevent them from being blocked by swelling or by the production of excess mucus or the leaking of fluid from blood vessels

2. Preventing or controlling anxiety that may aggravate respiratory difficulty

3. Avoiding, eliminating, or minimizing exposure to allergens, irritants, and other inspired materials or those internal conditions (triggers) that can activate immune cells produced in the body that are associated with inflammation of airway tissues

---

The source for the features of the pathology expressed in these statements is "Medical Essay—Asthma," Supplement to *Mayo Clinic News Letter,* February 1996, Mayo Foundation for Medical Education and Research, Rochester, MN.

with understanding of the value of the selected regimen of care in preventing an impending attack or in controlling an attack in progress. When respiratory difficulties are severe and may be life-threatening, they immediately place themselves under emergency medical care. Family members and associates, when informed, can assist.

5. Patients make observations of respiratory functioning and the severity and duration of asthmatic symptoms once a therapeutic regimen has been instituted for either prevention or control of an attack. They report to health care professionals as appropriate.

These five subsystems lay out the broad dimensions of the process to be followed by persons in meeting this expressed health-deviation self-care requisite in time and over time as long as the condition prevails. An example of the actions and action sequences within one subsystem or part of the process, the first one named, is developed and expressed to demonstrate what action sequences or care actions are required to fulfill it.

Subsystem 1: Accept themselves as having periodic attacks of bronchial asthma and learn to understand and fulfill their responsibilities for maintaining or restoring adequate pulmonary ventilation during pending attacks and attacks in process. To fulfill this subsidiary requisite, they must:

a. Maintain an awareness that as persons with bronchial asthma they are responsible for acting effectively before or during attacks in maintaining or restoring their pulmonary ventilation, including securing professional health care.

b. Reflect upon how they know that they are having an asthmatic attack and isolate in their thoughts their specific experiences and ways they know to represent and describe them.
   Tightness of chest
   Wheezing, coughing
   Shortness of breath
   Occurrences when breathing is very difficult
   Other

c(1). Become able to express what they experience (symptoms), their severity, sequence of occurrence, and their duration in order to represent their condition and experiences to health care professionals.

c(2). Seek help as needed from physicians and nurses to assist them in learning to describe their symptoms accurately and to make judgments about the severity and meaning of their attacks; learn the sources of authoritative written materials that will help them fulfill their responsibility for care.

d. Learn to work and work cooperatively with their families and with health care professionals to understand and learn to carry out prescribed regimens of therapeutic self-care.

e(1). Reflect upon and seek information about how their condition of bronchial asthma and its associated care can or should affect their usual routines of self-care and daily living, including those universal types of self-care requisites that need special attention and adjustment; for example, maintain a balance between activity and rest; prevent hazards to life, health, and well-being; maintain normalcy.

e(2). Learn how to effectively integrate new care elements into their routine systems of self-care and daily living.

   f. Reflect upon what they now do and what they should do to fulfill their self-care responsibilities associated with bronchial asthma to prevent attacks or control their harmful effects.

The six courses of action (a through f) constitute a protocol to be learned and followed, to be made operational, by persons who want to be responsible self-care agents.

Nurses who accept the five named parts of the process for meeting the requisite can assist persons under nursing care to identify the courses of action to be performed to fulfill the goals. This form of assistance to persons who have bronchial asthma or their families enables them to learn the components of their therapeutic self-care demand associated with this specific health-deviation self-care requisite.

SELF-CARE SYSTEMS, THERAPEUTIC SELF-CARE DEMANDS, AND SELF-CARE REQUISITES

As previously described, **self-care systems** are concrete entities in human society. As deliberate action systems, they come into existence and go out of existence as actions and **action sequences** are performed during the production phase of self-care. What endures over time are the effects produced by the actions. Self-care systems reflect (1) what self-care agents, dependent-care agents, and nurses *know* about the components of the therapeutic self-care demands of persons for whom care is provided and (2) and the **care measures** they are *able* and *willing to perform* at the time self-care systems are under production.

Care agents must have or acquire knowledge of existent and emerging self-care requisites and the processes for meeting them for self-care systems to be therapeutic in achieving the regulatory results of universal, developmental, or health-deviation self-care requisites. Health professionals, as well as the public, recognize that some components of persons' self-care systems produce harmful rather than therapeutic results. The examples of this are numerous and well known.

Preventive health care in nursing or in other health care fields should, to be effective, focus on helping persons accept themselves and develop themselves as responsible self-care agents. Acceptance and recognition of oneself as self-care agent should be part of the self-concept of every individual. Education to achieve this should begin in childhood. Nurses and other health professionals should be able to identify evidence for the presence or absence of this component in the self-concept of persons under their care.

There is a second focus to preventive health care, namely, helping persons under care understand why care sequences or care measures are prescribed for them. Patients want to know this as indicated by questions such as: What is this for? Why should I do this? What will this do for me? What results should I look for? The relationship between care measures in self-care systems and the regulatory results sought through their performance must be clearly set forth in terms of the nature of existent or emerging self-care requisites. Nurses must know the nature of existent and emerging self-care requisites; their values at specific times because of the conditioning influences of factors such as age, developmental state, and health state; the processes for meeting them; and the methods, means, or technologies through which each part of the process can be met and that in turn generate the action sequences or care measures that constitute parts of patients' therapeutic self-care demands.

The two results sought through effective nursing are to know and meet patients' existent or emerging therapeutic self-care demands and to regulate the exercise or development of patients' powers of self-care agency. These results cannot be achieved by nurses who are not continuously developing their knowledge of self-care requisites, including how advances in science and technology can affect both the regulatory results sought and the processes for their achievement, or by nurses who do not know and are unable to express the relationship between a prescribed type and number of care measures and the self-care requisite(s) from which they are derived. Nurses who do not understand self-care requisites and the processes for meeting them tend to function in a task-oriented frame of reference.

The work of reformulation of self-care requisites has provided a number of guidelines for nurses to follow in the formulation and expression and in the analysis of already expressed self-care requisites. The guidelines aid in making explicit the reasons for and the results sought through the performance of care measures or action sequences that constitute components of persons' therapeutic self-care demands. The following suggestions are offered for consideration:

1. Self-care requisites expressed from a theoretically practical perspective should include specification of the regulatory function of the requisite, the materials or conditions that constitute the regulatory factor(s), how the regulatory factor is introduced, and associated preventive measures, if relevant.

2. Self-care requisites are expressed in an action frame of reference. The statement of a requisite provides indicators of the necessary operations, the subprocesses within the process for meeting it. The process, when formulated, includes operations to ensure the presence or procurement of the regulatory factor, the essential operations within the process through which the regulatory factor is introduced, having knowledge about the factor to be introduced (e.g., qualitative and quantitative information), and the operations of securing information about achieved regulatory results. *Regulatory factors* refer, for example, to air with the requisite partial pressure of oxygen, to water, and to food.

3. Each identified operation within the process for meeting a self-care requisite requires the use of specific means (technologies) for the execution of the

operation. The use of the selected means requires the performance of a number of action sequences, which at times can be identified as care measures. For example, water and food must be procured and prepared for intake, but this can be done in a variety of ways. The ways or means selected determine the action sequences that must be performed in the use of the particular means.

4. When isolated care measures are prescribed for persons to follow—for example, take *x* medication three times a day after meals—action should be taken by nurses (or patients) to make explicit its regulatory function by formalizing and expressing the self-care requisite with which it is associated.

5. The process for meeting each self-care requisite includes an operation through which the person who has the requisite understands and accepts its existence and his or her need for it to be met. This operation often is taken for granted and not expressed. The example of this requisite specific to bronchial asthma is a demonstration of its expression and the importance and meaning of this operation.

In addition to these five emerging guidelines for use in reformulation or initial formulation of self-care requisites, other developments of knowledge about self-care requisites from 1996 to 2000 are summarized.

1. There was continued recognition that the action components (courses of action) of the therapeutic self-care demands and the actions that comprise produced systems of self-care have their origins in existent and emerging self-care requisites and in the processes for meeting them.

2. The need for refinement of the mode of expression of self-care requisites to emphasize their regulatory purpose was illustrated through examples.

3. There was recognition that the nature of and inherent parts of the process of meeting each formalized self-care requisite is either explicit or implicit in the statement of the requisite and its regulatory purpose. The process of meeting a requisite is revealed or inferred to be a series of *subprocesses* or *operations,* each of which is directed to attain a more specific result than the expressed broad regulatory purpose of the requisite. (*Note:* In the prior section on developments of self-care requisite *subprocesses* or *operations* were referred to as *subsidiary goals.* Attention should be given to reaching an agreement about terms.)

4. The *health-deviation self-care requisite* associated with the condition *bronchial asthma,* included five subprocesses to be operationalized to fulfill the expressed regulatory purpose of this requisite. Each of the five subprocesses requires the use of valid and reliable means or technologies to achieve the goals specific to each. The selected means or technology can be put to use only through the performance of *courses of action* or *action sequences,* at times properly referred to as *care measures.* The identified *courses of action* for each of the five subprocesses become action elements (courses of action) of the therapeutic self-care demands of persons who seek to prevent or control their attacks of bronchial asthma.

5. Models of therapeutic self-care demands (see Figure 10-1) should be adjusted to include the processes and the subprocesses through which the regulatory purposes of self-care requisites can be achieved. Appropriate technologies or methods selected to operationalize each subprocess yield the courses of action or care measures that are the component parts of the therapeutic self-care demands.

6. The continued development of knowledge specific to self-care requisites has contributed to knowledge about how to formalize and express the structure and content of self-care requisites. Continued development has contributed knowledge about the complexity of the processes for meeting requisites and the kinds of action demands that are placed on persons who engage in self-care, illustrated in the examples presented. Nurses and physicians should be aware of this complexity and of the kinds of knowledge and skills required by persons if the therapeutic self-care demand is to be known and met.

BASIC CONDITIONING FACTORS, THERAPEUTIC SELF-CARE DEMANDS, AND SELF-CARE REQUISITES

As previously stated, factors internal or external to individuals that affect their abilities to engage in self-care or affect the kind and amount of self-care required are named *basic conditioning factors.* These factors were identified and have been worked with since 1958. They were named in the early 1970s by the Nursing Development Conference Group. The original listing included the first eight factors or types of factors identified below. Factors 9 and 10 have since been added.

1. Age
2. Gender
3. Developmental state
4. Health state
5. Sociocultural orientation
6. Health care system factors, for example, medical diagnostic and treatment modalities
7. Family system factors
8. Pattern of living, including activities regularly engaged in
9. Environmental factors
10. Resource availability and adequacy

The list should be amended whenever a new factor is identified.

As previously identified, the named factors condition therapeutic self-care demands in a number of ways. Some, such as age, gender, and developmental state, as well as physical environmental factors, affect the value at which a universal or developmental self-care requisite should be met. For example, the age and developmental state of an infant affect the amount, composition, and state of food given at a single feeding. Health state and health care system factors condition the therapeutic self-care demand through (1) the emergence of new self-care requisites, for example, a requisite to control or manage the experiencing of pain or (2) the requirement of changes in values at which the universal or developmental requisites would normally be met. Age, gender, and developmental state also condition the means (methods, technologies, techniques) that can be used to meet universal and developmental self-care requisites.

Health state factors and health care system factors sometimes bring about human conditions that interfere with, or constitute obstacles to, meeting universal or developmental requisites, for example, an infant's or adult's inability to swallow. Such obstacles must be overcome to meet requisites. This often necessitates the use of technologies designed for this purpose. The use of gastric tubes and gastrostomy tubes for feeding individuals who cannot take food by mouth and swallow are well-known examples (see Appendix C).

Nurses should take an objective approach to investigation of the conditioning effects of age and gender, physical aspects of development, health state, health care system factors, and environmental factors on component parts of the therapeutic self-care demands of their patients. Nurses can help patients take an objective approach to identifying the conditioning effects of such factors as nurses and patients work to calculate patients' therapeutic self-care demands. As part of such investigations, nurses should recognize the importance of patients' subjective information about self-care requisites they are aware of that are based on what they are experiencing, for example, the requisite for control or management of nausea or anxiety.

Patterns of living, sociocultural orientations, family system factors, and social environmental factors affect the therapeutic self-care demands of individuals, largely by limiting what self-care requisites and means for meeting them will be accepted and admitted as constituent components of persons' therapeutic self-care demands. For example, whenever persons' patterns of living involve habitual use of tobacco, *the self-care requisite to keep the lungs and body free of tar and other harmful substances* is an actual requisite and the *means to meet it is to stop smoking* with use of all the *care measures* needed to achieve this freedom from harmful substances. However, habitual smokers, for example, may not be able to admit the means and necessary care measures into their therapeutic self-care demands.

Sociocultural orientations of persons to health and health care, the care measures prescribed by their culture, and the care measures families will and will not accept all condition what will or will not be admitted into therapeutic self-care demands of family members. For example, the sociocultural orientations of some individuals determines the kind of protein-containing food that they will eat. Such factors require subjective approaches if nurses are to develop insights about them in concrete practice situations. It may not be enough for nurses to understand features of a common culture of a social group. They may need to know culture elements internalized by individuals and by members of families into their self-concepts and value systems.

Resource availability and adequacy affect primarily the selection of means to meet self-care requisites and the associated care measures. For example, the availability of protein-containing food and its cost determine what individuals can do about meeting the universal requisite to maintain food intake sufficient for persons living under specified conditions. Resource availability, by affecting the way in which a requisite is particularized for an individual, and the means available to meet a requisite affect the required series of care measures to be performed with respect to resource use.

CALCULATION AND DESIGN OF THE THERAPEUTIC SELF-CARE DEMAND

Calculation in this context is understood as an investigative process with elements of hypothetico-deductive reasoning. Engagement in the process is a search for answers to the question: What series and sequences of actions regulatory of human functioning and development should this individual perform (or have performed by another) within specified time frames in the interests of life, health, and well-being? The process results in the production of nursing design unit D identified in Chapter 12.

In concrete situations, calculating an individual's therapeutic self-care demand proceeds component by component. A component, a unit of a therapeutic self-care demand, becomes known from the following operations:

1. Identification, formulation, and expression of a single self-care requisite in its relation to some aspect(s) of human functioning and development. This includes particularizing the values and frequency with which it should be met, as well as the process for meeting it.
2. Identification of the presence of human and environmental conditions that are (a) enabling for meeting the requisite or (b) not enabling and constitute obstacles to or interference with meeting it.
3. Determination of the methods or technologies that are known or hypothesized to have validity and reliability in meeting the goals of subprocesses through which the requisite is met under prevailing human and environmental conditions and circumstances.
4. Laying out the sets and sequences of actions to be performed when a particular method or technology or some combination of them is selected for use as the means through which the particularized requisite will be met under existent and emerging conditions and circumstances.

The result of these operations as related to a single self-care requisite, is the laying out of the structural features of one component of a person's therapeutic self-care demand (operations 1 through 3) that determine the action features or elements of the demand (operation).

The baseline or foundation of a person's therapeutic self-care demand(s) is constituted from universal self-care requisites and developmental self-care requisites particularized for the person by age, gender, developmental stage, pattern of living, and environmental conditions and circumstances. These self-care requisites have their foundations in the nature of human beings, some features of which are common to other living things and not in the factors that condition them. Therapeutic self-care demands of persons whose states of health are within established norms for their age and developmental states have universal and developmental components. Universal components include those that are disease preventive in nature, such as requisites for immunizations for specific diseases.

For persons who are ill, injured, or suffering from specific medically diagnosed health deviations, the universal and developmental self-care requisites are particularized for persons by age, gender, developmental state, patterns of living, and environmental conditions. These factors serve as reference points for adjustments necessitated by health state factors and health care system factors, such as a prescribed medical treatment.

In laying out the structural features of specific components of individuals' therapeutic self-care demands, nurses work first to identify and formalize requisites that are essential for the maintenance of life processes (for example, the maintenance of a sufficient intake of air that meets physiologic needs), then those that prevent personal harm or injury or health deterioration, then those that maintain health or promote movement to a higher level of human functioning, and then those that contribute to a state of human well-being under existent conditions and circumstances.

Scholarly work to organize existent and validated knowledge about universal, developmental, and health-deviation self-care requisites is needed for nursing purposes. Some work has been done by teachers in programs of nursing education and by researchers. One early contribution was made through the University of Michigan project, Development of Criterion Measures of Nursing Care, which focused on adults hospitalized for health conditions treated medically or surgically. Nurses developed the criterion measures for all the universal self-care requisites and for selected health-deviation self-care requisites.

The identification, formulation, and expression of health-deviation self-care requisites must be learned by every nurse and nursing student. The process may begin with a physician's medical order for a patient under nursing care. A medical order, such as "cleanse and dress surgically-made incisions in the left leg twice a day," is a prescription of a method for meeting a self-care requisite that is unexpressed, namely, to promote wound healing in relation to the human function of maintenance of tissue integrity. In other instances nurses must move from symptoms that patients are experiencing or signs of health disorders to identification, formulation, and expression of self-care requisites and to selection of means for meeting them. In some instances nurses or nurses and patients together select the means; in other instances the need for a means to meet a requisite may require referral to the physician.

Health-deviation self-care requisites, like universal requisites, have their origins in the anatomic and functional features of human beings. Health state, considered as a basic conditioning factor for persons' therapeutic self-care demands, is viewed as an expressed formulation of an assessment of whether the anatomic features and the functioning of individuals is within or outside established norms for individuals of particular ages in particular developmental stages.

The methods or technologies that are valid in meeting health-deviation self-care requisites have their foundations in commonsense approaches, in the medical sciences, or in nursing. The methods or technologies to meet universal and developmental self-care requisites have their primary foundations in the human sciences, including the fields of human development and human behavior.

The baseline, scientifically determined values at which universal and developmental self-care requisites should be met for individuals by age, gender, and developmental state should be mastered by every nursing student. This knowledge is antecedent to practice with reference to calculating therapeutic self-care demands of individuals.

When persons are acutely ill, injured, or suffering from specific disorders of health, nurses in calculating therapeutic self-care demands focus on health state as the active basic conditioning factor and seek answers to two questions: Is this or that feature of a person's health state interfering with or an obstacle to meeting universal or developmental self-care requisites? What health-deviation self-care requisites are associated with specific features of a person's disordered state of health and with medically prescribed measures for diagnosis and treatment?

The activity elements of each component of a therapeutic self-care demand usually include three types of actions: (1) those directed to the person performing the care measure or for whom the care measure is performed, (2) those directed to required resources, and (3) those that meet the self-care requisite. Persons must accept themselves as being in need of the functional or developmental regulation expressed by the requisite and in need of the means for meeting it, must secure and prepare materials and equipment required, must prepare self as required, and then proceed to perform the actions through which the self-care requisite is met. The developed activity elements of each component of a therapeutic self-care demand are the procedures for meeting a particularized requisite.

The calculation of the therapeutic self-care demands requires antecedent knowledge of human structure and functioning, human growth and development, family life, occupational life, and preventive health care. It also requires current and historical information about particular individuals and groups. There is also a need for up-to-date information about valid and reliable processes or technologies for (1) identifying the presence and effects of factors that affect the values of self-care requisites or limit the methods that can be used for meeting requisites and (2) meeting specific care requisites. Methods for meeting self-care requisites should be examined and understood within the cultural context of social groups and within the total care systems of social group members. Some self-care or dependent-care measures in use within social groups may be effective and therapeutic, but health care professionals who are outsiders may perceive these measures as harmful, take steps to change them, and thereby harm individual social group members.

The adult gradually comes to have some understanding of his or her own self-care demands through an accumulation of day-to-day experiences, and parents often come to understand the care demands of their children in this fashion. Persons who are care agents for socially dependent individuals should be able to calculate the current and projected self-care demands of those under their care. Adolescents and adults ideally develop knowledge and skills that will enable them to calculate their own self-care demands in relation to developmental processes, to events in the life cycle, and to a range of environmental conditions that affect human functioning, human development, and general well-being. The recognition of some adverse condition in the environment or in the individual or group usually results in the need to look at the totality of the self-care requisites and to identify the methods and the courses of action that will bring a therapeutic return. Nursing professionals require highly developed specialized skills in calculating the therapeutic self-care demands for persons and groups within their defined domains of nursing practice.

Calculation of a therapeutic self-care demand has a focus on components. The design of a therapeutic self-care demand has a focus on essential and ideal relationships among components. Action components must be related in time and place frames of reference for the 24 hours of the person's day. Factors to be considered include the need to maintain a time-specific relationship between certain particularized requisites, for example, the relationship between food intake and insulin administration in persons with diabetes mellitus. Other factors include organization of components to ensure economy of time and effort and proper articulation with other activities of personal and family life.

Adjustment in design is needed each time new self-care requisites emerge or existent ones change significantly. Design requires knowledge of existent developed components of therapeutic self-care demands and their functional relatedness or independence. Self-care can be burdensome and at times overwhelming for individuals. A good design of the therapeutic self-care demand can lessen stress from performance to meet it.

VARIATIONS IN THERAPEUTIC SELF-CARE DEMANDS

Types of variations relate to composition, complexity, and stability. The therapeutic self-care demand varies according to the self-care requisites from which it is constituted. At least two variations occur, which can be identified in relation to preventive health care:

1. A primary prevention self-care demand
   a. Universal self-care requisites
   b. Developmental self-care requisites that promote development
2. A secondary or tertiary prevention self-care demand
   a. Health-deviation self-care requisites
   b. Universal self-care requisites
   c. Developmental self-care requisites (all types)

From the perspective of preventive health care (sometimes referred to as preventive medicine), the therapeutic self-care demand sets forth the kinds of continuing health care measures that (all things being equal) will prevent disease or its extension, maintain health or promote a more desirable health state, and positively contribute to the individual's human development. Meeting one's therapeutic self-care demand (or that of another) is engaging in preventive health care, which includes seeking and actively participating in the care provided by health professionals.

Calculating and meeting the therapeutic self-care demands of individuals are endeavors not adequately attended to by nurses in some nursing situations. Meeting universal self-care requisites and developmental requisites is often neglected, even in institutions where patients are supposed to receive and are charged for nursing. The theories of self-care deficit and nursing system aid nursing students and nurses in understanding the importance of knowledge and skills organized around the therapeutic self-care demands of patients.

The mix of types of self-care requisites in a therapeutic self-care demand indicates the complexity of individuals' continuous care requirements and is an index of the kinds of knowledge and the range of skills required by persons who can act to meet the demands. Self-care deficits or dependent-care deficits may arise from the composition and complexity of the therapeutic self-care demands, as well as from the health or developmental states of care recipients. Nurses need to have the diagnostic skill to identify the self-care deficits of adult patients in meeting their current or projected therapeutic self-care demands. A related diagnostic skill is that of determining the infant or child care or dependent adult care competencies of responsible adults who seek nursing for socially dependent family members. The range of therapeutic self-care demands of individuals who can benefit from nursing (a nursing population) and the range of self-care (or dependent-care) deficits of these individuals are indications of the kind and amount of nursing required. Care demands and deficits are also indicators of the kinds of abilities that would qualify nurses for practice.

Therapeutic self-care demands also vary in relation to the stability of their components. Some demands are stable over days, weeks, or months; others have no stability because their components are in constant flux. When therapeutic self-care demands of individuals are unstable and complex, the continuous presence and activities of highly skilled, experienced nurses in the governing or leadership role are required to protect the life, health, and well-being of persons under nursing care.

SUMMARY

This chapter continues the development of the concept of *therapeutic self-care demand,* contributing areas of knowledge to the theory of self-care and the theory of self-care deficit. The content of the chapter also contributes information essential to nurses in their conduct of the operations of nursing practice. The historical development of the concept therapeutic self-care demand is recounted with concern for both its complexity and its derivation.

The essential contribution of the chapter rests in the continuation of the formulation and expression of insights about self-care requisites. Types of requisites are described. The chapter makes it explicit that changes in self-care systems or dependent-care systems are associated with changes in self-care requisites. It stresses the importance of work to further develop and refine already identified self-care requisites, and to include the conditioning effects of human and environmental factors (basic conditioning factors) on the existence or values of self-care requisites and on the selection and use of valid and reliable technologies.

Examples of reformulated expressions of requisites in this chapter emphasize the necessity to include both the actions to be taken and the regulatory result to be achieved. The chapter develops the idea of the importance of recognizing that the expressed action component of a requisite conveys the idea of a process, series of actions to move from some initial set of actions to the end of a known action sequence. These sequences of different types of action or subprocesses can be identified for each formulated and expressed requisite. Technologies to meet each subprocess must be identified, and the care measures or operations for their use specified. These care measures become constituent parts of persons' therapeutic self-care demands.

The chapter concludes with a treatment of how basic conditioning factors can affect therapeutic self-care demands and with identification of types of variations in therapeutic self-care demands according to the preventive health focus of each requisite.

References

1. Nursing Development Conference Group, Orem DE, editor: *Concept formalization in nursing: process and product,* ed 2, Boston, 1979, Little, Brown, pp 149-155.
2. Orem DE: *Guides for developing curricula for the education of practical nurses,* Washington, DC, 1959, United States Government Printing Office.
3. Crowe FE, Doran RM, editors: *Collected works of Bernard Lonergan. Insight: a study of human understanding,* Toronto, 1992, University of Toronto Press, pp 476-504.
4. Arnold MB: *Emotion and personality, vol II: neurological and physiological aspects,* New York, 1960, Columbia University Press.
5. Backscheider JE: The use of self as the essence of clinical supervision in ambulatory patient care, *Nurs Clin North Am* 6:789, 1971.
6. Guyton AC: *Textbook of medical physiology,* ed 8, Philadelphia, 1991, WB Saunders, pp 402-413.

CHAPTER 11

Self-Care Agency and Dependent-Care Agency

This chapter continues the development of the theory of self-care. Its focus is the concept *self-care agency* and its relationship to the concept *therapeutic self-care demand*. Basic conditioning factors that affect self-care agency and its development in individuals are considered. These developments provide the foundations for consideration of and support for the *theory of self-care deficit*.

The need to conceptualize dependent-care agency is introduced. Nurses work with and provide care for persons with health-derived or health-related self-care deficits. Some patients of nurses are socially dependent on parents, guardians, other family members, or in some instances friends. These persons have been, continue to be, or will be responsible for the continuing knowing and meeting of

253

the therapeutic self-care demands of their dependents. How nurses work with persons in the role of dependent-care agent varies according to the legal status of the responsibility of dependent-care agents for dependents, the characteristics of dependents' therapeutic self-care demands, and the need to protect the health and well-being of dependent-care agents.

Both self-care agency and dependent-care agency are identified as human capabilities to perform specific kinds of action. The substantive conceptual structure of self-care agency is developed as a theoretical model of its internal constituents. The day-to-day engagement of persons in self-care is examined through an example, the recounting of a person's concrete experiences. The recounted experiences provide a basis for making inferences about the exercise of self-care agency by this individual in dealing with an attack of influenza. The development of self-care agency is addressed in terms of its dependency on learning, life experiences, and adequate instruction, instruction adjusted to individuals' time-specific abilities and readiness to learn. The relationships between therapeutic self-care demand as action to be taken and self-care agency as the power to take necessary action are developed. The chapter concludes with an examination of dependent-care agency.

AN OVERVIEW

The referents of self-care agency and dependent-care agency are human powers and capabilities necessary for persons to provide continuing care for themselves or for persons socially dependent on them. In the text the terms *capabilities* and *powers* are used interchangeably. **Capability** as described by Harré is "a power which can be acquired (or lost) without there being a change in the fundamental nature of the thing or material in question" (p. 278).[1] He identifies **power** as a "notion associated with agency, with the initiation of trains of events, with activity" (p. 272).[1] The possession of a power is different from its exercise. "In ascribing powers to people 'can' must be substituted for 'will' . . . whether he will or not is up to him" (p. 272).[1]

Capabilities for self-care and dependent-care are specific for the named types of human endeavor. The terms *self-care agency* and *dependent-care agency* stand for specific powers of individuals. These powers are associated with the nature of maturing and mature persons to take action voluntarily and deliberately in the achievement of desired ends or goals.

Self-care agency is the *complex acquired capability* to meet one's continuing requirements for *care of self* that regulates life processes, maintains or promotes integrity of human structure and functioning and human development, and promotes well-being. Self-care agency of individuals varies over a range with respect to its development from childhood through old age. It varies with health state, with factors that influence educability, and with life experiences as they are enabling for learning, for exposure to cultural influences, and for use of resources in daily living. Self-care agency of individuals at this time or that time is conditioned by factors that affect its *development* and its *operability*. Its *adequacy* is measured against the component parts of the therapeutic self-care demand, that is, the demand on individuals to engage in self-care (Figure 11-1).

Self-care is human endeavor, learned behavior, that has the characteristics of deliberate action (see Chapter 3 and Figure 7-3). Self-care is produced as individuals engage in action to care for themselves and to regulate their own internal functioning and development. Self-care actions engaged in over time are performed by persons in stable or changing environmental settings and within the context of their patterns of daily living. Sometimes the meeting of one's requirements for self-care rules out engagement in preferred activities. At other times, self-care is interspersed with the other activities of daily life and is not a major focus of attention. The human capability named *self-care agency,* the power to engage in self-care, develops in the course of day-to-day living through the spontaneous process of learning. Its development is aided by intellectual curiosity, by instruction and supervision from others, and by experience in performing self-care measures. It has been conceptualized as a unit because of the specific practical endeavor, self-care, to which it is directed. Self-care has form and content. The form of self-care is that of deliberate action and its phases. The content derives from the purposes to which it is directed, the self-care requisites, and the courses of action that are effective in meeting them.

The capability to engage in self-care is also conceptualized as having form and content. Self-care agency is conceptualized as including the ability to attend to specific things (this includes the ability to exclude other things) and to understand their characteristics and the meaning of the characteristics, the ability

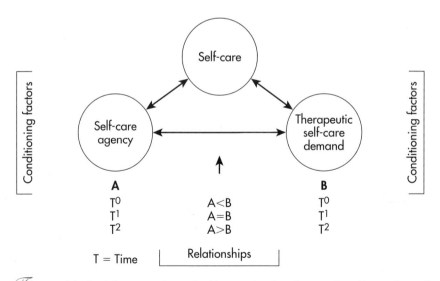

Figure 11-1 Adequacy values of self-care related to therapeutic self-care demand may vary over time.

to apprehend the need to change or regulate the things observed, the ability to acquire knowledge of appropriate courses of action for regulation, the ability to decide what to do, and the ability to act to achieve change or regulation. The content of self-care agency derives from its proper object, meeting self-care requisites, whatever those requisites are at specific moments.

Self-care agency can be examined in relation to individuals' achievements, including their skill repertoires and the kinds of knowledge they have and use, for engaging in a range of practical endeavors. It can be described in terms of *development, operability,* and *adequacy* (p. 205).[2] The *development* and *operability* of self-care agency can be affected by genetic and constitutional factors as well as by culture, life experiences, and health state. Development and operability are identified in terms of the kinds of self-care operations individuals can consistently and effectively perform. The adequacy of self-care agency is measured in terms of the relationship of the number and kinds of operations that persons can engage in and the operations required to calculate and meet an existing or projected therapeutic self-care demand. Determining the adequacy of self-care agency is essential if judgments about the presence or absence of self-care deficits are to be made.

The practice of nursing includes making a comprehensive determination of the reasons why people can be helped through nursing. An important aspect of this determination is diagnosing the abilities of an individual to engage in self-care (or dependent-care) now or in the future and appraising these abilities in relation to the person's therapeutic self-care demand. Unless self-care agency is accurately diagnosed, nurses have no rational basis for (1) making judgments about existing or projected self-care deficits and the reasons for their existence, (2) selecting valid and reliable methods of helping, or (3) prescribing and designing nursing systems.

Self-care is performed largely out of habit, but individuals who have not thought about their self-care role may need to be helped to look at themselves as self-care agents in order to understand the values to which their habits commit them and to appraise the adequacy of their self-care. Examining one's self-care habits, appraising the benefits derived from one's self-care as practiced, recognizing needs for change, and becoming knowledgeable about new self-care requisites are important for maintaining the adequacy of self-care agency. New self-care requisites resulting from changes in internal or external conditions necessitate additional knowledge, adjustments in some types of developed skills (for example, perceptual skill), and examination of one's willingness to pursue particular courses of self-care action. Persons with specific types and values of self-care requisites are important as subjects for exploratory research about the creation, use, and effectiveness of self-care practices.

Self-care agency (or dependent-care agency) is defined by capabilities ascribed to individuals. If nursing is to take place, nurses must be able to view their patients as self-care agents and to diagnose patients' or their care agents' capabilities for engagement in continuous and effective care. To do this, nurses must be able to accept individuals, families, and groups as being in specific stages of development and particular states of health and well-being. What persons can do with respect to practical affairs (including self-care) varies with age and developmental state, as well as with health state. Nurses must understand the limits of the biologic features of human beings (e.g., blood vessels), but they must also strive to understand the nature and limits of human capacities for self-care and self-management.

SELF-CARE AGENCY CONCEPTUALIZED

The formalization of the concept self-care agency occurred between 1958 and 1970. Initial insights about the human power named *self-care agency* were expressed as capabilities and limitations of individuals for engagement in self-care. Gradually, the term *self-care agency* came into use. The formalization of the structure of the concept was facilitated by the formulation of propositions about self-care agency to express current understandings. The propositions expressed critical judgments about self-care agency based on insights derived from experiences in concrete nursing practice situations or results of analyses of nursing case materials. The cognitive model for this movement is experience, understanding, critical reflection, and critical judgment. Early insights about self-care agency are expressed in the following eight propositions (p. 183).[2]

1. Self-care agency is a complex, acquired human characteristic.
2. Self-care agency is the power of an individual to engage in the operations essential for self-care.
3. The exercise by an individual of the power that is named *self-care agency* results in a system of actions directed to reality conditions in self or environment in order to regulate them, or its exercise results in a design and plan for such a system of action.
4. Self-care agency can be conceptualized as an action repertoire of an individual.
5. Self-care agency can be characterized in terms of the abilities and limitations of an individual for engagement in self-care.
6. Conditions and factors in the environment of an individual affect the development and exercise of self-care agency.
7. Persons are subject to time-sequential needs for the exercise of self-care agency.
8. Self-care agency is an estimative capability and a productive capability for self-care.

The structure of the concept was formalized as a three-part structure:

1. The self-care operational capabilities for performing estimative, transitional, and productive self-care operations
2. A set of power components enabling performance of self-care operations
3. Five sets of foundational capabilities and dispositions articulating with the power components in their relationships to operational capabilities

Historically, the movement of conceptualization was from the conceptualized self-care operations, to the foundational capabilities and disposition, and finally to the enabling power components. The structural features of the concept self-care agency are described in the historical sequence of development.

Broad Conceptual Elements: Capabilities for Self-Care Operations

The broad structure of the concept self-care agency is understood in relation to and modeled on operations specific to the phases of deliberate action, namely, estimative operations, transitional operations of reflection, critical judgment, decision making, and production operations. Thus, self-care agency is understood as developed capabilities of individuals to engage in the named **self-care operations** in order to know and meet their requirements for self-care within time and place frames of references. Figure 11-2 illustrates the power self-care agency and its broad conceptualized structure.

An identification of suboperations of the estimative, transitional, and production operations of self-care was developed to provide insight into the three operational capabilities. In describing the suboperations, the terms *self-care requisites* and *therapeutic self-care demand* are not named. They are implicit in the descriptive statements. The estimative, transitional, and productive operations and their results are identified in sequential relationships (Table 11-1).

The power and capabilities to engage in the named operations is understood as self-care agency. Actual engagement of persons in the operations within time and place frames of reference is self-care.

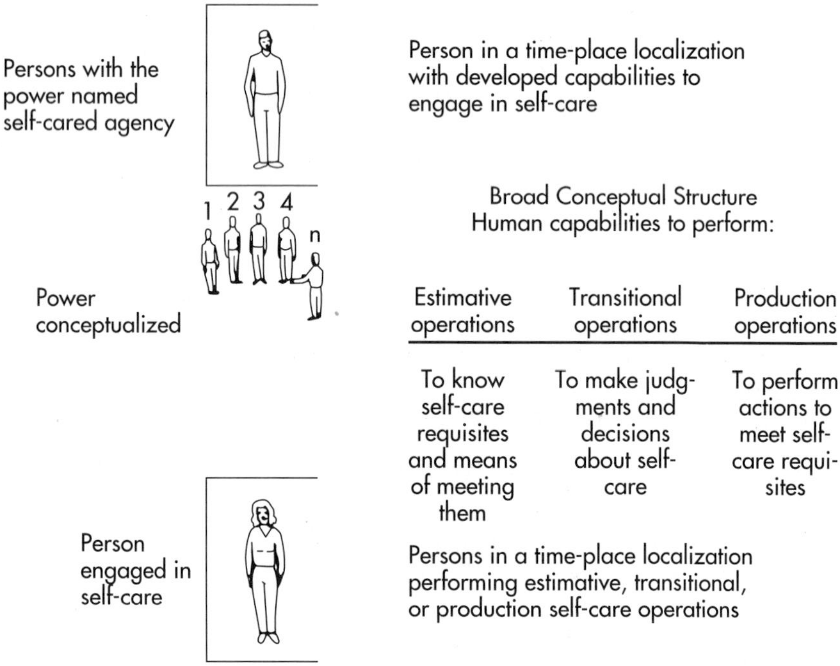

Persons with the power named self-cared agency		Person in a time-place localization with developed capabilities to engage in self-care
Power conceptualized		Broad Conceptual Structure Human capabilities to perform:
	Estimative operations	Transitional operations	Production operations
	To know self-care requisites and means of meeting them	To make judgments and decisions about self-care	To perform actions to meet self-care requisites
Person engaged in self-care		Persons in a time-place localization performing estimative, transitional, or production self-care operations

Figure 11-2 The operational structure of self-care agency.

Table 11-1 *Self-Care Operations and Results*

Operations	Results
Estimative Type	
1. Investigation of internal and external conditions and factors significant for self-care	Empirical knowledge of self and environment
2. Investigation of the meaning of characterized conditions and factors and their regulation	Experiential knowing (based in part on acquired technical knowledge) of the meaning of the existent conditions and factors for life, health, and well-being
3. Investigation of the question: How can existent conditions and factors be regulated (i.e., changed or maintained)?	Technical knowledge of what can be regulated and the means available for effective regulation
Transitional Type	
4. Reflection to determine which course of self-care should be followed	An affirming judgment that one course of self-care is preferred, or that a series of courses is preferred, or that none should be pursued
5. Deciding what to do with respect to self-care	A decision to engage in or not engage in specific regulatory self-care operations
Productive Type	
6. Preparation of self, materials, or environmental settings for the performance of a regulatory-type self-care operation	Conditions of readiness for performing self-care operations for regulatory purposes
7a. Performance of productive self-care operations with specific regulatory purposes within a time period	Knowledge that regulatory measures are in process or are completed
7b. Determining presence of and monitoring, during performance, of conditions known to affect effectiveness of performance and results	Information that conditions and factors affecting performance and results a. Are or are not present b. Are or are not under control if present
8. Monitoring for evidence of effects and results a. Desired b. Untoward	Information about events indicating that regulation is a. Being achieved b. Not being achieved Knowledge of untoward results a. Absence of b. Presence of

From Nursing Development Conference Group, Orem DE, editor: *Concept formalization in nursing: process and product,* ed 2, Boston, 1979, Little, Brown, pp. 192-193. *Continued*

Table 11-1 Self-Care Operations and Results—cont'd	
Operations	**Results**
Productive Type—cont'd	

9. Reflection to determine and confirm evidence of adequacy of performance and presence of regulatory results	An affirming judgment as related to specific self-care regulatory operations
	a. Self-care should continue
	b. Self-care should be discontinued
	  (1) To be resumed at a specific time
	  (2) Not to be resumed as related to the operations in question

10a. Decision about regulatory operations
  a. Continue action
  b. Close action
  c. Cease action but resume at a specific time
10b. Decision about estimative operations
  a. Continue to use results obtained from estimative operations (current data base)
  b. Begin a new series of estimative operations	

Some Human Foundations of Self-Care Agency

Another stage in the formalization of the concept self-care agency dealt with the question: Are there common human foundations for engagement in deliberate action, including self-care?

Understandings of group members about self-care agency were advanced by Louise Hartnett's 1968 development of a conceptualization of voluntary human action involving motor activity (pp. 135-141).[2] Two complementary models were structured to make explicit the physiologic and psychologic features of deliberate action. The psychological model of action included three articulated frames: a central veridical frame focused on persons in physical environments, a sociocultural frame focused on persons in social environments with given roles and role expectations, and a personal frame of reference focused on personal values, self-as-felt and known, ideal self, and long-range goal orientations. The physiologic model of action associates higher mental processes with sensory and motor neurologic functioning in the execution of internally and externally oriented actions. These models provided indicators for the development of the human foundation of the theoretic concept self-care agency and for its continued formalization and validation. Hartnett's models do not negate the fact that it is the person who acts. They express the complexity of deliberate human action and point the way toward expression of the foundational capabilities, dispositions, and orientations of individuals relevant to ability and willingness for performing self-care operations, as well as other forms of deliberate action.

The step of explicating the human foundations of self-care agency was formalized by Joan E. Backscheider in 1970 and 1971 in the form of a survey list of general capabilities essential for engagement in self-care. The survey list included "physical, mental, motivational, emotional, and orientative capabilities" and resulted from Backscheider's work in a nursing clinic for ambulatory adults with diabetes mellitus. Her three-pronged approach to nursing diagnosis was expressed in a 1971 article published in 1974 (pp. 1138-1146).[3] The approach included:

- Inquiry to determine regulatory goals to be achieved through self-care and the care measures to be used.
- Analyses of the foregoing to determine the estimative and production self-care operations that would need to be performed to achieve the regulatory goals.
- Inquiry to determine ability of patients to perform the action components of the estimative and production self-care operations.

The first element of the approach results in information, judgments, and decisions about components of patients' therapeutic self-care demands. The second element involves analysis of what should be done, as well as *if-then* types of reasoning: if patients are to perform x, y, z care measures associated with components of their therapeutic self-care demands, they must have X', Y', Z' developed and operative action capabilities. The third approach involves assessment of patients' action capabilities to determine the presence or absence of requisite capabilities.

Backscheider's survey list, revised in 1979 as five sets of **capabilities and dispositions foundational for self-care agency,** is shown in Table 11-2. The sets identified as *Selected Basic Capabilities* are foundational not only for engagement in self-care but also for other forms of activity. For example, persons with conditions that negatively affect sensation and perception are limited in performing estimative-type operations regardless of the object of action. The set of *Knowing and Doing Capabilities* is constituted from those that affect knowing, reasoning, and making right judgments and decisions in life situations and includes the learned skills that affect communication, as well as investigative and production types of operations. The set *Dispositions Affecting Goals Sought* expresses conditions that affect persons' willingness to look at themselves and accept themselves as self-care agents, to accept themselves as in need of particular self-care measures, or to perform certain self-care measures. The members of the set *Significant Orientative Capabilities and Dispositions* are determinants of persons' enduring habits and interests, willingness to engage in self-care, concern about health, or ability to engage in self-care.

Table 11-2　Human Capabilities and Dispositions Foundational for Self-Care Agency

Conditioning Factors and States*	Capabilities and Dispositions				
	Selected Basic Capabilities		Knowing and Doing Capabilities	Dispositions Affecting Goals Sought	Significant Orientative Capabilities and Dispositions
	I	II			
Genetic and constitutional factors	Sensation Proprioception Exteroception	Attention	Rational agency	Self-understanding Self-awareness Self-concept Self-image	Orientations to: Time Health Other persons Events, objects
Arousal state	Learning	Perception	Operational knowing	Self-value	Priority system or value hierarchy: Moral Economic Aesthetic Material Social

Social organization	Exercise or work	Memory	Learned skills	Self-acceptance Self-concern	Interest and concerns
			Reading		Habits
			Counting		
			Writing		
			Verbal	Acceptance of bodily functions	Ability to work with the body and its parts
			Perceptual		
			Manual	Willingness to meet needs of self	
			Reasoning		
Culture	Regulation of the position and movement of the body and its parts	Central regulation of motivational emotional processes	Self-consistency in knowing and doing	Future directedness	Ability to manage self and personal affairs
Experience					

From Nursing Development Conference Group, Orem DE, editor: *Concept formalization in nursing: process and product*, ed 2, Boston, 1979, Little, Brown, p. 212.

*Applicable as relevant to all sets of capabilities and dispositions.

Whenever persons under nursing care need to perform new and additional self-care measures, adjust or change currently performed measures, or resume self-care after a period of being taken care of, nurses' assessment of patients' foundational capabilities and dispositions, as suggested in the survey list, is an essential aspect of nursing practice. The sciences and disciplines of anatomy, physiology, psychology, cognitive development and functioning, psychopathology, and social psychology are some of the fields basic to understanding the capabilities and dispositions included in the survey list.

The survey list should be refined and further developed through use; it is not a complete or even an adequate development of human capabilities and dispositions foundational to self-care and other forms of action.

Power Components Enabling for Self-Care Operations

In continuing the investigation of the substantive structure of the concept *self-care agency,* the need to identify human capabilities that are empowering for engagement in the operations of self-care became evident. The reasoning process moved from the characteristics of self-care operations, as identified in the listing of self-care operations and results (see Table 11-1), to a visualization of the human capabilities needed for their performance. Estimative self-care operations are operations of inquiry that seek both empirical and technical knowledge for purposes of knowing and understanding what is, what can be, and what should be brought about with respect to taking care of self. The transitional operations of reflecting, judging, and deciding with respect to self-care matters are grounded in what individuals know about the self-care situation, their experiences and their knowledge about self-care requisites and measures for meeting them, as well as their values, self-concepts, and willingness. Productive operations are doing operations to achieve practical results demanding preparation for and performance of self-care measures, monitoring performance as well as their effects and results, and making judgments and decisions about subsequent actions.

It was concluded that the human powers enabling for performing self-care operations would be of a nature intermediate between the human functioning and human dispositions as described in the survey list and the estimative, transitional, and production self-care operations. Ten power components necessary for having the capabilities to engage in self-care operations in concrete situations were formulated and expressed (see box on p. 265). The capabilities are expressed as a single series and not in relation to the estimative, transitional, and productive operations. Figure 11-3 depicts the hypothesized substantive components of the concept *self-care agency.*

The power components have been used both in nursing practice and in research since their publication in 1979. They need refinement and continued development with respect to their own structure and to their articulation with self-care operations and foundational capabilities and dispositions.

Power Components of Self-Care Agency

1. Ability to maintain attention and exercise requisite vigilance with respect to self as self-care agent and internal and external conditions and factors significant for self-care
2. Controlled use of available physical energy that is sufficient for the initiation and continuation of self-care operations
3. Ability to control the position of the body and its parts in the execution of the movements required for the initiation and completion of self-care operations
4. Ability to reason within a self-care frame of reference
5. Motivation (i.e., goal orientations for self-care that are in accord with its characteristics and its meaning for life, health, and well-being)
6. Ability to make decisions about care of self and to operationalize these decisions
7. Ability to acquire technical knowledge about self-care from authoritative sources, to retain it, and to operationalize it
8. A repertoire of cognitive, perceptual, manipulative, communication, and interpersonal skills adapted to the performance of self-care operations
9. Ability to order discrete self-care actions or action systems into relationships with prior and subsequent actions toward the final achievement of regulatory goals of self-care
10. Ability to consistently perform self-care operations, integrating them with relevant aspects of personal, family, and community living

From Nursing Development Conference Group, Orem DE, editor: *Concept formalization in nursing: process and product,* ed 2, Boston, 1979, Little, Brown, pp 195-196.

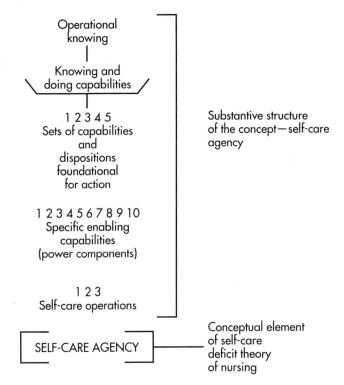

Figure 11-3 Substantive conceptual structure of self-care agency showing one set of foundational capabilities and dispositions and operational knowing as a member of the set.

PERSONS AS SELF-CARE AGENTS

As individuals engage in self-care, they exercise their developed and operational capabilities to manage themselves in their time-place localizations. They determine what self-care is required, make decisions about what self-care requisites they will meet and how they will meet them, perform the required activities, and determine their effects and results.

Self-care on a day-to-day basis is interspersed among other kinds of activities, or it is an aspect of another activity, for example, lifting or carrying a heavy object in a manner that prevents back injury or muscle strain. When persons are well, self-care is not a major concern; interests and activities are centered around personal and family life, work, and special interests. Occasionally, individuals must make choices between self-care and other activities. Parents who care for a sick child or who give up needed sleep and relaxation because of a family crisis are common examples of choices involving self-care.

Self-care is affected not only by the individual's family position and roles but also by health state. Usual activities during illness, even usual self-care activities, are disrupted, and meeting new self-care requisites may take over a large portion of a day. This is illustrated in the following self-analysis and personally recorded experiences and activities of a nursing practitioner and teacher during an attack of influenza. The recordings begin on the third day of the illness.

Saturday: Felt miserable. I knew I should see a doctor but had no energy or desire to get myself there. The thought of going seemed too much to face. Also, since I know no physician and since it is Saturday, I know I don't have the energy to hunt for one. Consulted with Joyce, a neighbor. What I was really asking was for her to motivate me to do something since I knew I would not be able to do it alone. She looked up some names and suggested that I call from her apartment.

Called the first man who handled it by telephone. He told me to treat it symptomatically (which was what I had been doing) since it is unresponsive to antibiotics. I have taken aspirin for elevated temperature, cough medicine, and hot drinks and fluids.

Up until today I felt the need to sleep a lot. Today I am not so drowsy, but my attention span is short and I have to find ways to divert myself—frequent changes of reading material, light reading only, a little knitting.

Sunday: More energy today in spurts. Felt a need to be more active with different types of things, so I repotted plants and wrapped a package. I find myself annoyed because I can't read heavier things. I keep trying, but this just increases my frustration. Read the papers thoroughly. The *Times'* crossword puzzle is good intellectual stimulus because you can put it down and pick it up and you don't have to remember anything.

Slightly nauseated today, probably from coughing. Have to watch the "quality" of fluids. Can take juices and Coke but not milk and coffee.

I am much more croupy this evening. Chest is congested. Had difficulty bringing up anything at first. In desperation I asked Joyce, who was going to the pharmacy, to bring me some tincture of benzoin [for a croup kettle]. It is good to have someone like Joyce. It makes this all seem more manageable.

Did a lot of paroxysmal coughing but finally began to cough up mucus. It is a somewhat frightening sensation. My initial reaction was to stop the coughing and not expectorate. But after doing that two or three times, I knew I had to bring it up. It's hard to do this effectively without too much distress.

Very irritable.

Monday: Soon after I got up, I took a check on the status of my symptoms. I felt better. My temperature was 98° for the first time since Thursday. I still did some paroxysmal coughing. I thought my chest felt clearer. My throat was still sore, and my ears were very stuffy. On the whole I felt I was somewhat better. I talked to two people on phone (in process of cancelling my appointments for the day), both of whom were horrified at how I sounded. This was a shock to me since I decided that on the whole there was improvement. I realized that I could not determine whether I was objectively "still bad," but I would have to trust my own assessment of improvement.

I talked to two other persons (for the same reason), both of whom had recently had flu. Both communicated anxiety by relating my symptoms to their condition. One identified with the ear stuffiness which in her case developed into otitis media. She suggested use of hot mineral oil drops. The other person said that it was urgent to drink two gallons of fluids a day, which I knew I could not do. After talking to each one, I had a very temporary reaction of feeling overwhelmed, of feeling aware of the importance of what each had said, but of being uncertain about it. I decided to try to increase my fluid intake somewhat and to observe the ear symptoms more closely.

I think my reaction to these contacts was to have my level of anxiety raised. On my own I had to devise a means of adapting and observing. If I had not been able to do this, I would have been left in a rather uncomfortable state.

My attention span is not much better today. I start but don't complete things. I need to be physically active but have limited energy.

My day has been characterized by intermittent naps and more frequent paroxysms of productive coughing. I continue to produce mucus plugs but feel better, and my chest feels clearer in between coughing spells.

One thing that is interesting is that with all this inactivity I have had no indication of muscle spasm in my back [due to muscle damage resulting from surgery]. I have only done my exercises twice since becoming ill [a set of exercises prescribed by the orthopedist]. On the recent trip to Georgia where I sat all day for two days, I very much felt the need for exercise. The level of my resistance to having to sit and to that experience may have made the exercise need greater. Sometimes at night after a long stretch of sleeping I awake with a feeling of being cramped, but my current need for physical and mental inactivity seems to override my need for physical movement. Friday I could not have done the exercises; today it felt good to do them. They were just enough.

Tuesday: Decided not to go to work today. My symptoms are gradually subsiding, and I would like to keep it that way. My energy comes in spurts, and I decided not to expend it in one long flame. I still have a stuffy ear, chest congestion, and paroxysmal coughing. I am losing creativity in dealing with them. They just exist now. My menstrual period began today, and I always have a little less energy the first day.

Eating is difficult, or more accurately, planning meals to eat. I just can't get interested in it. I have no idea how well-balanced my meals are. I eat if I become interested in food. I have taken too much prune juice. I have minor gastric disturbance and some diarrhea. I have no juice on hand except prune.

I decided to walk to the grocery store, which is one-half block away. I needed to do this to test how much strength had returned. I walked there and back with my groceries and then took a nap for an hour. I am glad I decided to stay home today.

I have begun to do some work—thinking-type. I organized the class I have to present tomorrow and am writing a report of interactions with a patient I have been seeing for four months on an outpatient basis. I feel good about getting the report written; the longer I avoided it, the longer it got. It is interesting and a good stimulation but I must stop now and go sit in a chair where I can lean back and rest.

As the nurse describes her experiences, self-care was the central focus of her daily living. Adjustment of other activities to available energy was in itself self-care action. Seeking medical care was an attempt to have a medically prescribed course of action to follow in the management of the symptoms of influenza. The nurse was able to manage her own care, but not without anxiety. She sought and received help from her friend. Unsolicited advice was perceived as relevant to a degree but also anxiety producing. The difference between the objective and subjective assessments of "how sick" she was gives insight into the importance of understanding any illness as a continuum and of the need to look for change and evaluate change over time. The statement on Tuesday, the sixth day of the illness, that the symptoms "just exist now" may be evidence of human adaptation to existing conditions and the human tendency to accept and live with a situation once its novelty is lost or when there is a decrease in the intensity of stimuli.

DEVELOPMENT OF SELF-CARE AGENCY

Self-care is learned behavior. As children grow, foundational capabilities and dispositions for engagement in forms of deliberate action, including self-care, develop. They learn what to do and what not to do in gradually widening areas of human living. They develop behavioral repertoires for taking action when various combinations of conditions and circumstances prevail in themselves or in their environments. In many cultures, children learn how to protect themselves from accident and injury. They may be admonished and learn to conform to cultural practices with respect to consumption of food and water, elimination, rest and sleep, and solitude and social interaction and to achieve normalcy within their community. Such learning results in children's development of the powers for action identified previously as **power components of self-care agency.** These power components develop in relation to performed operations through which specific decisions are made, purposes formulated, and productive actions generated.

Learning Self-Care

Learning to engage in self-care and continuous engagement in self-care are human functions. The central requisites for self-care are learning and the use of knowledge in performing externally or internally oriented sequences of self-care actions. The **self-care agent,** the provider of self-care, is open to cultural elements in the nature of known self-care requisites and ways of meeting them. Some of these elements would be known requisites and measures of care that have been integrated into the family or the general culture. Others would be elements that are medically prescribed for individuals or groups. *Medical* is used here in the sense of those systems of medicine that prevail within particular cultures and societies.

The self-care provider or agent performs actions that have either an *internal* or *external orientation.* Whether a self-care action is internal or external in orientation can be determined by observation, by eliciting subjective data from the self-care agent, or both. The internally and externally oriented self-care

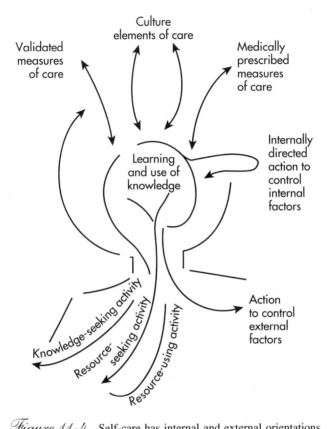

Figure 11-4 Self-care has internal and external orientations.

actions listed here provide a general index of the validity of helping methods.* The four types of externally oriented self-care actions are (1) knowledge-seeking action sequences, (2) assistance- and resource-seeking action sequences, (3) expressive interpersonal actions,† and (4) action sequences to control external factors. The two types of internally oriented self-care actions are (1) resource-using action sequences to control internal factors and (2) action sequences to control oneself (thoughts, feelings, orientation) and thereby regulate internal factors or one's external orientations (Figure 11-4).

Understanding self-care as deliberate action with internal and external orientations aids nurses in acquiring, developing, and perfecting skills needed for (1) securing valid and reliable information to describe the self-care systems of

---

*Five helping methods are described in Chapter 8 3. They are identified as acting for or doing for, supporting, guiding, providing a developmental environment, and teaching. Social support is considered to be a helping method.
†Not shown in Figure 11-4.

individuals, (2) analyzing information descriptive of self-care and dependent-care systems, and (3) making judgments about how individuals can and should be helped with respect to performing self-care operations to know and meet their therapeutic self-care demands. When the courses of action, or action sequences, of a therapeutic self-care demand are known, they can be identified and grouped according to their internal and external orientations.

Nurses must understand self-care actions classified according to their internal or external orientations with respect to their relationships to each of the five ways of helping. For example, the helping method of *doing for or acting for another* does not correlate with self-care actions, directed to the control of thoughts, feelings, and orientations. On the other hand, the method does correlate with self-care actions in which resources are sought or used in controlling external or internal factors.

Ways of determining and meeting one's self-care needs are not inborn. Broadly speaking, the activities of self-care are learned according to the beliefs, habits, and practices that characterize the cultural way of life of the group to which the individual belongs. In some cultures, a sick person assumes that he or she has displeased the spirit of a dead ancestor and will ask a shaman (a medicine man) for help in appeasing the spirit. In a scientifically advanced culture, people assume that sickness has some natural explanation, such as an infection, an indiscretion in eating or drinking, a stressful way of living, or the presence of a growth or tumor, and they will seek care from medical doctors. Keeping the body clean is a meaningless gesture in some cultures but an acceptable precaution in others. Even within scientifically advanced cultures, some groups may know more about health matters than other groups in the same society. In the more knowledgeable groups, care may be taken to meet nutritional and sanitary requirements when preparing food and to secure immunization and routine health checkups. In less knowledgeable groups, these precautions may be unknown, regarded indifferently, or rejected.

The individual first learns of cultural standards within the family. Hence, there are many variations in self-care practices. The child learns from parents or guardians, who learned from their parents or guardians. While growing up, the child learns of additional and improved ways of self-care from other persons: teachers, classmates, neighbors, friends, and playmates. When health knowledge is widespread and applied, the preventive care measures that are carried out on a community basis—water purification, sewage disposal, and regulated practices in the processing of milk and other perishable foods—provide not only community service but also education and guidance on a broader community health basis. Individuals in each community must provide the leadership, daily effort, and financial and other resources required to start and maintain these services. If there is a breakdown in community services or if services are not provided, the burden of carrying out healthful practices falls upon individuals. For example, they may be required to boil or chlorinate water after a flood or engage in these practices routinely in areas where the water supply is not safe for internal use. Some environmental hazards, such as air pollution in large cities, are relatively uncontrolled, and persons living in such areas can do little to protect themselves except by stimulating community action, remaining indoors, or changing residence.

As indicated previously, self-care requires both learning and use of knowledge, as well as enduring motivation and skill. The learning process includes the individual's gradual development of a repertoire of self-care practices and related skills. Ideally, children are helped to develop images of themselves as responsible self-care agents by gradually learning to perform care measures through which self-care requisites are met, for example, bathing, brushing teeth, looking to ensure that it is safe to cross a street, and not touching hot objects. Self-care measures executed daily tend to become integrated into the fabric of daily living, and the purposes to be achieved through use of the measures (the self-care requisites being met) may not be kept in mind. Openness to oneself and to one's environment and to known and validated self-care requisites and cultural self-care practices are prerequisites for learning as well as for engaging in continuous and effective self-care.

The individualized factors of age, developmental state, and health generally affect the self-care activities a person can perform. In addition, each adult's established pattern of responding to external and internal stimuli will affect decisions and other actions relative to self-care. Adult values and goals also affect the selection and performance of self-care actions in health or in illness. Self-care measures compatible with a person's goals and values are likely to be seen as beneficial. Their practice, however, depends on the person's judgment of whether he or she can perform the measures. The first step in the practice of self-care is answering these questions: Is it beneficial for me? Can I do it? Among adults, accepting oneself as being in particular functional and developmental states and having specific structural characteristics is another prerequisite for engaging in self-care that regulates human functional and developmental processes.*

UNDERSTANDING SELF-CARE AS DELIBERATE ACTION

Deliberate action was described in Chapters 3 and 7. The following description of self-care as deliberate action should lead to further insights about deliberate action and about the development and exercise of self-care agency.

Distinguishing Deliberate Action

Self-care and care of dependents are forms of human activity referred to as deliberate action. This means that it is purposeful goal- or result-seeking activity. It also implies that the meaning of the result sought is identified before the action is taken. This can be done at various levels of understanding. For example, adults tend to care for themselves and their dependents to sustain, protect, and promote

---

*See Nursing Development Conference Group, pp. 280-282, for Melba Anger's general ideal set of self-care actions, a model for use in working out the sets of care measures essential for meeting self-care requisites through the use of given technologies.[2]

human functioning. If adults approach care with a background of scientific knowledge, they may see results in terms of integrated functioning, as in bringing about a new metabolic balance through the controlled intake of nutrients. A person may also formulate results in terms of what he or she hopes to experience, for example, to feel better or, as related to dental hygiene, to have a "fresh" mouth or, when under dental care for a pathologic condition of the gums, to stop bleeding. Deliberate action is essentially action to achieve a foreseen result that is preceded by investigation, reflection, and judgment to appraise the situation and by a thoughtful, deliberate choice of what should be done. An adequate concept of deliberate action includes ideas to describe circumstances leading to the decision about what should be done and events and circumstances necessary to bring about the result selected. Action is deliberate when it is based on an informed judgment about the outcome(s) being sought from acting in a particular way.

Deliberate action is distinguished from physiologically and psychologically "programmed mechanisms" for responding to internal and external conditions. These include reflex activity (sneezing), instinctual urge (impulse to seek food), emotional reaction (sudden arousal of fear and movement to avoid a falling object), and feelings of pleasantness and unpleasantness (discomfort and the desire to change position after sitting for a long time). These activity patterns, however, often serve as forces motivating individuals to focus attention on present conditions and reflect on their meaning, consider the possible outcomes of various courses of action, formulate a judgment on the appropriate action, and then decide to take a concrete course of action. This can be illustrated by an analysis of the common example of individuals deliberately maintaining specific positions for medical or dental examinations or treatments despite discomfort or even pain. Knowledge of the results of moving and not moving affect the individual's decision to control position. Physiologic or psychologic mechanisms and habits will affect how long individuals can exert control over their position. Deliberate action is always self-initiated, self-directed, and controlled in regard to presenting conditions and circumstances. Human development includes learning how to take deliberate action to perform the tasks of daily living within specific environments.

The structural elements of concrete action systems, including self-care, dependent-care, and nursing systems, are discrete, that is, single actions. A discrete action (e.g., the lifting of one's hand) when taken out of its position within a sequence of actions (e.g., drinking a glass of water) may not convey the purpose and hence the meaning of the action within the particular sequence. As mentioned earlier, Talcott Parsons used the term *unit act* to refer to the smallest assembly of goal-oriented actions that make sense (i.e., convey meaning within a system of action) (pp. 44-45).[4] It is important for nurses to understand action sequences in terms of the discrete actions and unit acts from which they are constituted. For example, what kind and number of discrete actions must be performed to meet the self-care requisite "to maintain a sufficient intake of water" by taking the quantity of water by mouth that satisfies the criterion measures for being sufficient? Some examples of discrete actions include grasping a glass, holding a glass, and lifting a glass containing a known quantity of fluid.

Two examples of nurses' use of their understanding of action sequences required for meeting self-care requisites are given in articles by Backscheider (pp. 1138-1146)[3] and Pridham (pp. 237-246).[5] As previously described, Backscheider was concerned with assessment of the self-care capabilities of members of an adult ambulatory nursing population to meet their particularized self-care requisites associated with the condition diabetes mellitus. To develop a standard against which to assess the action capabilities of patients, Backscheider analyzed the action sequences involved in meeting care requisites common to the population. Pridham investigated the same nursing questions from a somewhat different perspective. Her concern was to explore and collect data as a basis for judging the self-care capabilities evidenced by a hospitalized child with diabetes mellitus who was under nursing care. The question to be answered was: What role can the child fulfill in her own self-care? Manifestation of and criteria for judging the psychologic development of the child (and factors affecting it) in relation to her self-care role were one focus of the investigation. Both of these investigations clearly point to the relationship between the (1) *demand* on individuals to consistently and effectively perform particular self-care actions in some sequence, with proper adjustments to prevailing internal and external conditions, and (2) their self-care *capabilities* at particular times in the life cycle under particular living circumstances.

Estimative and Transitional Operations

Persons who can produce effective self-care have knowledge of themselves and knowledge of environmental conditions. Before they can affirm the appropriate thing to do, they must gain knowledge of the courses of action open to them and of their effectiveness and desirability. Effective producers of self-care bring the first phase of self-care to closure by making a decision about the actions they will take and those they will avoid.

Providers of self-care require two kinds of knowledge: empirical knowledge of events and of internal and external conditions, and antecedent knowledge that aids them in making observations, attaching meaning to their observations, and correlating the meaning of events and conditions with possible courses of action. Knowledge extends to (1) internal or external conditions relevant to health and well-being, for example, stiffness and pain in the joints of the hands or feet; (2) characteristics of the conditions, for example, the degree of stiffness related to the mobility of the joints or the degree of the constancy and severity of the pain; (3) the meaning of these conditions for health and well-being, for example, that the identified conditions indicate an improvement or worsening of a diagnosed joint disorder; and (4) the beneficial or harmful results that will come about by taking one course of action in preference to another, for example, consulting the physician, resuming a prescribed therapeutic regimen that has been neglected, or using the affected parts of the body. The qualitative and quantitative requirements for empirical and antecedent knowledge are related to the number and kinds of self-care requisites; methods for meeting them; external conditions, including the location and availability of resources; and other factors.

Under a daily living routine, self-care requisites follow a normal and consistent pattern. The decisions of an adult in regard to meeting self-care requisites are "programmed" in the sense that experience A calls for deliberate action B. When a person is in ill health, however, the pattern of the therapeutic self-care demand changes. The ill person may experience new and more self-care requisites in a totally different time distribution, and more knowledge and effort may be needed to arrive at valid judgments about self-care measures. In fact, medical or nursing assistance may be necessary for the judgments to be valid.

Conflicting self-care requisites may affect decision making. For example, a need for food may be experienced at the same time that a person has received a medical order to take "no food" for some time. Making judgments and decisions about self-care must take into account time specifications and the precedence that meeting one self-care requisite takes over meeting other requisites. Environmental conditions are also relevant to making judgments and decisions about self-care. The number and nature of the inquiries the self-care provider makes about environmental conditions vary with the provider's familiarity with the surroundings. A person may be half awake yet have sufficient information to decide what he or she can and will do about being cold. In an unfamiliar place, a person may decide that being cold has advantages over changing air temperature or circulation.

Individuals must have some understanding of the meaning and value of self-care to make rational and reasonable self-care judgments and decisions. Level of maturity, knowledge, life experiences, habits of thought, and health state all affect this understanding. Knowledge of self-care measures useful in meeting self-care requisites varies with life experiences. Opportunities for learning self-care vary with families and communities. This learning process, which is continuous throughout life, is necessary for achieving understanding of self-care and being motivated to make decisions about it and to produce it for oneself and one's dependents.

Knowledge of the purposes and meaning of self-care provides the basis for appraising and attaching value to engaging in particular courses of self-care action. Factors internal to individuals—for example, extreme agitation, inexperience, or level of cognitive development—may interfere with appraisal and with judgments and decisions. External factors, such as lack of resources or extreme social pressure, also affect judgments and decisions. Nurses should understand that at times self-care decisions may be based on the meaning care activities have for significant others. For example, a person decides to follow a particular course of self-care action because it will please the family. Regardless of motive, the decision to follow a particular course of self-care action determines if and how a self-care requisite will be met.

Knowing what conditions are relevant to health and well-being and why they are relevant at various stages of the life cycle is essential for effective engagement in the investigative, judgment-making, and decision-making activities of the first phase of self-care action. Judgments may be *rational* in that they are preceded by thought about what conditions exist and what can be done. Judgments may not be *reasonable,* however, in that they are not in accord with the existing therapeutic self-care demand and existing circumstances relating to health and well-being. Both scientific knowledge and commonsense knowledge are essential in the first phase of self-care. The investigations and the ensuing judgments and decisions made in the first phase give expression to the culture of individuals and to their self-concepts as self-care agents. Some individuals hesitate or refuse to investigate conditions that are significant for self-care. Other individuals are willing to explore what exists and what is possible but have difficulty in making judgments about what can and should be done, whereas others have difficulty in making the final decision about what to do. If the first phase of self-care action does not end with a decision, phase two will not ensue.

Production Operations

Phase two begins with the decision about the course of action to be followed in relation to the specific demand or set of demands for self-care. The choice of what will or will not be done terminates the first phase of deliberate action. The choice made sets the goal for phase two because it specifies what kind of action will be taken. The questions raised by the self-care agent now include: How can I proceed in relation to my choice? What must I do? What resources do I need? Do I have them? Can I perform all the actions correctly and effectively at the time when they should be performed and for as long as they need to be performed? Will other duties interfere? How will I know if I am proceeding correctly? What rules will I follow? How will I know if I am getting the results I want? Who can help me if I need help?

The accomplishment of the various kinds of universal, developmental, and health-deviation self-care requires *expenditure of effort to satisfy the demands for care* as these demands are known and understood when action begins or as it proceeds. Effort will be demanded until specific results are achieved and as frequently as the result is required or until there is evidence that the effort is not productive. Effort is not random but deliberate. It is directed by the agent toward the result desired by following some standard technique or procedure or by adjusting action to the factors in the situation that can be changed or controlled. Attention is focused on the action performed and on evidence to be used in judging if the action is correct and if the desired result is or has been achieved. Deliberate effort should cease when the self-care agent knows that the desired result has been achieved. Effort may be withheld or changed if there is evidence that the result is not being achieved or that some other result is preferable. Expenditure of effort in self-care may not be pleasurable, and it may eliminate opportunities for other activities.

The essential condition for the expenditure of effort to meet self-care demands in specific situations at specific times is the capability to initiate and persevere in self-care to achieve desired results. This results from (1) having specific and requisite knowledge and skills, for example, knowing how to obtain dental care, how to make an appointment, and how to describe the problem; (2) being sufficiently motivated to initiate and continue efforts until results are achieved; for example, the desire to avoid loss of teeth may motivate a regimen of dental hygiene for months or years; (3) being committed to meeting particular demands for care to the degree that forgetting is eliminated or minimized and proper priority is afforded to measures of care; for example, thoughtful performance and a routine for performing prescribed dental care; (4) being able to execute the movements required; and (5) having energy and a sense of well-being sufficient to initiate and sustain self-care effort; for example, in severe illness or disability a person may be unable to care for teeth and gums. Being able to initiate and sustain a self-care effort to achieve the desired result is related to the kinds of self-care required, to external conditions, and to internal factors that affect the ability to perform deliberate actions.

Individuals may be able to initiate and persevere in self-care action to meet universal requirements if they follow routine practices but may be unable at a particular time to change old practices or to add new practices. Becoming able may involve changing one's ideas about health and illness, developing new skills, and becoming committed to new ways of proceeding. This may be very difficult for some individuals despite their knowledge that the changes should be made. Engagement in health-deviation self-care may be more difficult because abilities are specified both by the demands for care arising from the health deviation and by the medical therapy prescribed. As previously stated, specific knowledge and skills that have a base in medical science and technology are required for health-deviation self-care. Changes in medical technology have produced sometimes complicated demands for management of self-care. For example, in some kinds of drug therapy the individual may have to divide pills, take a different dose on specified days, or follow one series of doses for x days. Development of readiness to engage in health-deviation self-care may require specialized assistance. Perseverance in self-care may require assistance in the form of support and guidance.

Having some understanding of the meaning and value of self-care is fundamental to engaging in it. Some factors affecting understanding and meaning were described under the first phase of self-care. Knowledge of self-care demands and the measures to meet them is essential. Knowledge must be applied not only in the initiation of action but also throughout the performance. Knowledge must be applied to guide the performance of specific tasks and to make the practical judgments required about what to do next. Lack of skill in task performance, failure to validate judgments, or inability to make judgments adversely affect the accomplishment of self-care. Factors in the external environment—for example, availability of resources—may affect either the initiation or the continuation of self-care action.

Initiation of action and perseverance to meet self-care demands demonstrate the individual's power of agency in this form of deliberate action. Action limitation may decrease self-care capabilities and give rise to a need for assistance. Action limitations related to the individual's health state are why people need nursing.

SELF-CARE AGENCY, PRACTICAL CONSIDERATIONS

Nurses, other health workers, and the public must understand that self-care is work requiring energy expenditure, time, and resources. It cannot be done without the requisite enabling human capabilities and without knowledge of what should be done. Persons' calculated therapeutic self-care demands express the kind and amount of work to be done. Persons' capabilities to engage in self-care at particular times and places identify their abilities to do the work of self-care.

As previously mentioned, self-care agency, conceptualized as a complex of human capabilities particularized for one kind of action or work, named self-care, can be investigated in relation to its development, operability, and adequacy.

Self-Care Agency, Developed and Developing

The presence or absence of the power named self-care agency, when concretely considered, is related to the stage of development of individuals, including their development of self-direction with respect to goal selection and their physical, cognitive, and psychosocial development. Self-care agency reveals itself through evidence as the developed or developing capability to engage in the *investigative and decision-making phase of self-care* (phase one) and the capability to engage in the *production phase of self-care* (phase two). There may be an unequal development of capabilities for phase one and phase two operations because of the states of development of individuals. For example, children learn to perform and do perform some measures of self-care before learning the related investigative operations. This does not rule out young children's determinations that they want or don't want to perform this or that self-care measure. Children also make decisions that they want to learn how to perform certain care measures so that they can be the care agent with respect to aspects of required, prescribed, medical treatment measures, for example, giving themselves medication by injection.

Self-care agency can be identified if it is *developed* or is *developing*. Self-care agency at particular times reveals itself in individuals' performance of learned sequences of self-care actions to meet foreseen goals. Its appraisal requires investigations of what individuals do and do not do consistently in self-care. Self-care agency is considered undeveloped when capabilities for performing operations for both phases of self-care are not evident. This holds for infants even though their *inherent capacities for action* and *impulses to action* are operative, for example, the action impulses and the inherent action capacities exhibited in the feeding behaviors of infants. Arnold describes the feeding behaviors of infants as implying "wanting, appraising, liking, and disliking," as well as recognition that "no more is wanted," and "an impulse to stop" (pp. 54-55).[6]

Self-care capabilities that are developed and could be made operative by individuals are sometimes not exercised. This may be through deliberate choice, by forgetting, or because factors of time or place or availability of required resources do not allow for performance of self-care operations. Such situations must be differentiated from situations in which the capability for self-care of particular kinds is developed but cannot be made operational *at all* or to *some degree* because of structural or functional conditions associated with specific pathologies, states of illness, injury, and disability.

The degrees of development of self-care agency of individuals in concrete situations of daily living and in nursing practice situations can be identified for persons of various ages within the following five developmental categories (p. 205).[2]

1. Undeveloped
2. Developing
3. Developed but not stabilized
   a. in need of continued development
   b. in process of continued development
   c. in need of redevelopment
   d. in process of redevelopment
4. Developed and stabilized
   a. in need of redevelopment
   b. in process of redevelopment
   c. redeveloped and stabilized
5. Developed but declining

The development or redevelopment of self-care agency by individuals throughout their life cycles should be understood as associated with the human desire to know, the power to learn, and movement to higher and more complex stages of personal development.

Self-Care Agency, Operability, and Adequacy

Questions about the operability and adequacy of self-care agency of individuals assume some degree of development. It is recognized that self-care agency, whatever its degree of development at particular times under some human conditions and circumstances, cannot be exercised at all or only to a limited degree. Health states of individuals or specific effects of a health disorder or injury can adversely affect their performance of self-care operations and the operability of their foundational capabilities and dispositions for action. At particular times, persons can be so adversely conditioned by human and environmental factors that their self-care agency is not operative or only partly operative for some time.

The adequacy of self-care agency is critical in nursing practice situations. Lack of adequacy and the health or health-related reasons for lack of adequacy of self-care agency of persons seeking nursing determine the legitimacy of nursing practice situations. Critical judgments of nurses about the adequacy of patients' self-care agency presume knowledge of patients' calculated therapeutic self-care demands or components of them and the capabilities required for meeting them and making needed adjustments. Nurses must also know the degree of development and operability of persons' developed powers of self-care agency in making final judgments about adequacy and the reasons for the adequacy or the degree of inadequacy of self-care agency of individuals under nursing care.

Self-Care Limitations

Persons who engage in self-care know themselves, their functional states, and the care that they need. They want to know. They appraise, investigate, and make judgments and decisions. They engage in result-achieving courses of action and are able to manage themselves in their environments. Self-care capabilities are expressions of what persons have learned to do and can do in the investigative and decision-making phase of self-care and in its production phase under presenting human and environmental conditions. Self-care limitations are expressions of that which restricts individuals from providing the amount and kind of self-care that they need under existent and changing conditions and circumstances.

Self-care limitations are expressed in terms of restricting influences on the operations of self-care. Three kinds of limitations are identified: restrictions of knowing, restrictions on judgments and decision making, and restrictions on result-achieving actions in either the investigative or production phases of self-care.

Limitations of knowing about one's own functioning, about needed self-care, and about the operations through which self-care is accomplished are associated with individuals' past experiences and with what is being experienced in the present. Some conditions and factors associated with limitations of knowing are identified in three sets.

Set One

- Changed modes of functioning that are new and are not understood; lack of fit between what one has experienced and what one is experiencing
- New unrecognized requirements for self-care associated with changed functional states
- New self-care requisites that are parts of a prescribed regimen of health care that are not understood
- Lack of knowledge essential for performing the operations needed to meet specific self-care requisites, using specified methods and measures of care

Set Two

- Impairments of sensory functioning or perception and memory or attention deficits that interfere with the acquisition of empirical knowledge or recall of knowledge
- Disturbances of human integrated functioning that adversely affect empirical consciousness, cognitive functioning, and rationality associated, for example, with (1) organic conditions that are productive of toxic states, (2) mental and emotional illness, (3) brain disorders, and (4) effects of substances such as prescribed or unprescribed drugs

Set Three

- Dispositions and orientations that result in perceptions, meanings, and appraisals of situations that are not in accord with reality
- Movement away from taking action to acquire new and essential knowledge
- Modes of cognitive functioning that affect mental operations associated with knowing when action is to be taken, adjusting action to existent or emerging conditions, and knowing when to stop action, and with organizing sets of actions into meaningful sequences toward result achievement

The three sets of limitations of knowing differ in kind; therefore, persons with such limitations require different kinds of help with respect to self-care. The first set expresses absence or lack of required knowledge. The second set expresses limitations for knowing environmental conditions and for knowing self and environment. The third set expresses psychic and cognitional limitations for developing insights about situations, for seeking to acquire knowledge, and for the knowing that is basic to doing in result-seeking endeavors.

Limitations for making judgments and decisions about components of a therapeutic self-care demand or about the regulation of the exercise or development of self-care agency are associated with individuals' views of themselves, their habits of investigation and reflection before making decisions about what action to take, their desires to take action that is appropriate and beneficial, and their having requisite knowledge and skills. Eight factors or conditions that set limitations on individuals' judgment and decision making with respect to self-care matters are expressed.

Set One

- Lack of familiarity with a situation and lack of knowledge about appropriate questions for investigation
- Insufficient knowledge or lack of necessary skills for seeking and acquiring appropriate technical knowledge from individuals or reference materials
- Lack of sufficient and valid antecedent and empirical knowledge to reflect and reason within a self-care frame of reference

Set Two

- Interferences with the direction and maintenance of voluntary attention necessary to investigate situations from the perspective of self-care, for example, limitations of consciousness, intense emotional states, sudden or strong likes and dislikes, overriding interests and concerns
- Inability or limited ability to imagine alternative courses of action that could be taken and the consequence of each

Set Three

- Reluctance or refusal of individuals to investigate situations of self-care as a basis for determining what can and should be done
- Reluctance to stop reflection and make a decision once a desirable and suitable course of action is identified and understood

• Refusal to make a decision about a possible course of self-care action or about the exercise or development of self-care agency

Limitations expressed in sets one and two interfere with individuals having or getting an adequate base of information for judgment and decision making. Limitations in set three indicate avoidance of decision making. Such limitations may reflect patterns of behavior typical of individuals, or they may reflect individuals' attachment of meaning to a situation and movement away from involvement in it.

Limitations for engagement in result-achieving courses of action within the investigative and production phases of self-care, including limitations for self-management, are associated with human functional states and with environmental conditions and circumstances. The following examples of limiting factors and conditions are expressed in four sets.

Set One

• Lack of knowledge or developed skills needed to operationalize decisions about self-care
• Lack of resources for self-care

Set Two

• Lack of sufficient energy for sustained action in the investigative and production phases of self-care
• Inability or limited ability to control body movements in the performance of required actions in either or both phases of self-care
• Inability or limited ability of individuals to attend to themselves as self-care agents and to exercise vigilance with respect to existent and changing internal and external conditions

Set Three

• Lack of interest in meeting self-care requisites
• Lack of desire to meet perceived needs for self-care
• Inadequate goal orientations and values placed on self-care that do not sustain engagement in the investigative and production actions essential for knowing and meeting therapeutic self-care demands

Set Four

• Family members' or others' deliberate interference with the performance of the courses of action necessary for individuals to know and meet their therapeutic self-care demands
• Patterns of personal or family living that restrict engagement in self-care operations
• Lack of social support systems needed to sustain individuals when self-care is complex, time-consuming, and stressful
• Crisis situations in the family or household that interfere with self-care
• Disaster situations that interfere with engagement in self-care and with the usual ways for meeting self-care requisites

The first three of the four sets of interferences express absence of conditions necessary for self-care. The fourth set of interferences is associated with individuals' conditions of living.

This approach to the formulation and expression of types of self-care limitations was taken because it fits the conditions found in concrete situations of practice. The presence of evidence of the named types of limitations singly or in various combinations in persons under nursing care provides one basis for nurses to determine the amount and kind of nursing required. It provides a basis for nurses' judgments about valid methods of helping and judgments about interpersonal processes to foster or maintain patients' readiness to receive help through nursing.

SELF-CARE DEFICITS

The term **self-care deficit** refers to the relationship between self-care agency and therapeutic self-care demands of individuals in which capabilities for self-care, because of existent limitations, are not equal to meeting some or all of the components of their therapeutic self-care demands. Self-care deficits are associated with the kinds of components that make up the therapeutic self-care demand and with the number and variety of self-care limitations.

Self-care deficits are identified as complete or partial. A complete self-care deficit means no capability to meet a therapeutic self-care demand.

Partial deficits for self-care may be extensive or may be limited to an incapacity for meeting one or several self-care requisites within a therapeutic self-care demand. Nurses' knowledge of the extent and causes of self-care deficits in individuals in concrete situations of nursing practice is a result of nursing diagnostic activities to determine individuals' self-care abilities and limitations and of identification and particularization of their self-care requisites. However, experienced nurses in their initial contacts with patients habitually make observations to answer one of the initial questions of nursing practice: Is there gross evidence of a self-care deficit that is health-derived or health-related? This question could be phrased differently: Is it reasonable to assume, in light of known conditions, that there is an existent or emerging self-care (or dependent-care) deficit?

Presence of one or some combination of the following named conditions would constitute gross evidence of a self-care deficit:
- Absence of ongoing engagement in self-care or gross inadequacy of what is done to meet self-care requisites
- Limited awareness or loss of awareness of self and environment, excluding losses due to natural sleep
- Inability to recall past experience in the control of conduct
- Limitations for judgment and decision making about self-care associated with lack of knowledge and unfamiliarity with internal and external conditions
- Events indicative of disordered or impaired functioning giving rise to new health-deviation self-care requisites and for adjustments in one or some or all of the universal self-care requisites

• Needs of individuals to incorporate newly prescribed, complex self-care measures into their self-care systems, the performance of which requires specialized knowledge and skills to be acquired through training and experience

In seeking understanding of self-care agency, self-care limitations, and self-care deficits, it is important to recognize two dimensions of self-care. One dimension relates to the deliberate action operations of self-care, involving self-awareness, rational thought, conscious purpose, plan of procedure, and willingness and resolution in proceeding according to an initial or revised plan. This is the personal, purposive dimension of self-care in the full human and psychologic sense. The second dimension of self-care is having knowledge of valid and reliable care measures. Validity relates to the events that occur within individuals and their environments as a result of the joint presence of particular inputs or regulatory factors from performance of care measures and the existent

----

Exercise

Exercise to Aid in Understanding Self-Care Limitations

1. Read and think about the three kinds of self-care limitations described in the section Self-Care Limitations.
2. For nurses to make judgments about the absence or presence of these limitations, nurses must obtain particular kinds and amounts of data, facts about reality conditions and events on which to base their judgments.
3. Think about the question: How would I know if such limitations were or were not present in a particular patient?
4. Then consider the kinds of data and the sources of data that would be necessary to make judgments about the absence or presence of:
   a. Limitations of knowing
   b. Limitations for making judgments and decisions
   c. Limitations for engagement in result-achieving courses of action
5. Select one of the kinds of self-care limitations, *a* or *b* or *c* above, and develop a tool for use in obtaining data about one or more limitations named in a set, for example, limitations of knowing, set one, limitations 3 and 4. In developing the tool, seek answers to these questions for each limitation:
   a. To what do I attend?
   b. What information do I need?
   c. How can I obtain the information?
   d. What will be the form of my data?
   e. How much data will I need?
6. As part of the process of finding answers to these questions, talk informally to *individuals* about their experience of such limitations and to *nurses* about their identification of such limitations in their patients.
7. Refine the tool. Have it reviewed to get answers to this question about each limitation: If I obtain the kinds of data indicated in the tool, will I have an adequate basis for making a judgment about the presence or absence of the limitation?

human or environmental conditions. When particular inputs—for example, some amount and quality of ingested food—correlate directly with human or environmental variables or factors to bring about sought-after and desired conditions, the self-care measures performed have validity.

In individuals' development of self-care agency, both dimensions of self-care must be learned. This includes knowing the kind and amount of data needed to make judgments about internal and external conditions, knowing how to obtain the data, and making judgments on the basis of particular kinds and amounts of data. It also includes knowing what should and should not be done under certain conditions. Thus the development of self-care agency goes beyond learning culturally prescribed self-care practices. Self-care deficits are associated not only with individuals' limitations for performing care measures but also with the lack of validity or effectiveness of the self-care in which they engage.

DEPENDENT-CARE AGENCY

The terms **dependent-care, dependent-care agency,** and **dependent-care agent** were introduced within the frame of self-care deficit nursing theory when the need for them became evident during the 1970s. The terms were introduced in the course of curriculum revision deliberations by nursing faculty of Incarnate Word College, San Antonio, Texas. Since then, the terms have come into wider use. There are increased needs for dependent-care agents with the growth in the aging population; in numbers of persons with chronic illness, debilitating illnesses, and disabling conditions; and in the number and complexity of health-deviation self-care requisites to be met by or for individuals after hospital discharge (Figure 11-5).

The concept dependent-care agency is in the process of formalization. Like self-care agency, its broad conceptual structure is formed by capabilities to perform estimative, transitional, and productive operations in knowing and meeting the therapeutic self-care demand of another (or components thereof). There are enabling power components specific to the operations as operations relate to knowing and meeting components of the other's therapeutic self-care demand. Both of these depend on foundational capabilities and dispositions, with adjustments to focus on meeting another's needs and working with the bodily parts of another person.

Dependent-Care Agency Described

Dependent-care agency is the complex, acquired ability of mature or maturing persons to know and meet some or all of the self-care requisites of adolescent or adult persons who have health-derived or health-associated limitations of self-care agency, which places them in socially dependent relationships for care. With respect to infants and children, dependent-care agency is the complex acquired ability to incorporate knowing and meeting health-deviation self-care requisites of infants and children and needed adjustments in universal and

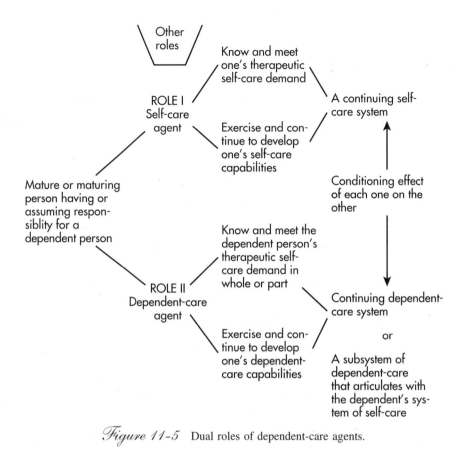

Figure 11-5 Dual roles of dependent-care agents.

developmental self-care requisites into ongoing systems of infant care, child care, and parenting activities.

Dependent-care agents may work in close association with the physician of the persons they help or take care of. They may be contributors to an ongoing nursing system or work with nursing supervision and consultation.

The development of dependent-care agency by individuals is usually a response to needs of family members or friends for help with their continuing self-care. Dependent-care agency is developed to meet known existent and, at times, emerging needs of the persons to be helped or taken care of. More likely than not, the primary focus in development is mastery of production operations of self-care, for example, maintaining cleanliness of wounds, including dressing changes, as well as meeting requisites for maintenance of sufficient intake of water and food. When production operations must be adjusted to specific human and environmental conditions, as in the administration of some prescribed medications, there is need for development of capabilities for performing estimative and transitional operations of self-care. There is always need for development of capabilities to recognize emergency situations and to act promptly and effectively.

Dependent-Care Agents

Nurses are increasingly placed in positions in which they must work with families or individuals to identify and select persons psychologically and physically able and willing to function as dependent-care agents for family members or friends. This is a demand on both nurses in hospitals and home care nursing programs. Nurses recognize the importance of protecting the health and well-being of dependent-care agents. They understand the energy-depleting effects of maintaining systems of dependent-care in the home and the stress associated with it. Therapeutic self-care demands of dependent-care agents must be calculated and means for meeting them established. Figure 11-5 shows the dual care demands on dependent-care agents.

The amount of instruction needed for persons to develop dependent-care agency requisite for situations in which they will function varies with their life experiences, their knowledge, and their developed skills that can be adjusted to the care situation. The relationship of the dependent-care agent to the person to be helped, the willingness of this person to accept help, and the sense of duty on the part of each will affect what can be accomplished. Studies of situations in which dependent-care agents function are ongoing, as well as studies of ways and means to assess the potential of individuals for this function or their developed dependent-care capabilities.

The incidence of chronic illness, the aging population, and the growing need for long-term care brings to the fore the increase in need for dependent-care and its importance. Who will provide it and where it will be provided are the critical questions. Which family member(s) will be the caregiver(s) is a family issue. Whether care will be provided in the home or in a long-term care facility is another question that families must investigate and answer. These are problems of whole societies, not just families. The nursing profession should investigate the kinds of contributions it can make in investigating and finding solutions to the needs for dependent-care in communities.

SUMMARY

The identification of self-care agency as a human capability—a power— associates it with the nature of human beings. This power is represented as one that develops and one that can decline, one that can be exercised or not exercised. The model of the structure of self-care agency provides insights about factors that affect both its development and its exercise. The idea of self-care deficits, their extent, and factors that produce them constitute knowledge that can and should be put to use in nursing practice. The increased need in societies for dependent-care indicates the importance for nurses of understanding dependent-care and their relationships to dependent-care agents.

References

1. Harré R: *The principles of scientific thinking,* Chicago, 1970, University of Chicago Press, pp 269-282.
2. Nursing Development Conference Group, Orem DE, editor: *Concept formalization in nursing: process and product,* ed 2, Boston, 1979, Little, Brown, pp 135-141, 183, 192-193, 195-196, 205.
3. Backscheider JE: Self-care requirements, self-care capabilities and nursing systems in the diabetic nurse management clinic, *Am J Public Health* 64:1138-1146, 1974.
4. Parsons T: *The structure of social action,* New York, 1937, McGraw-Hill, pp 44-45.
5. Pridham KF: Instruction of a school-age child with chronic illness for increased self-care, using diabetes mellitus as an example, *Int Nurs Stud* 8:237-246, 1971.
6. Arnold MB: *Emotion and personality.* vol II, *Neurological and physiological aspects,* New York, 1960, Columbia University Press, pp 54-55.

CHAPTER 12

Nursing Agency: The Nurse Variable

Nursing agency is a theoretic concept that was first formalized in 1971 after a prolonged process of exploration by members of the Nursing Development Conference Group. Members were guided in their discussions and analyses of nursing cases by the simple idea: *under these given conditions and circumstances, nurses will require these capabilities to nurse effectively.* To be guided by this idea it was necessary for group members to take the stance of conceptual theorists and not the stance of nursing practitioners investigating this or that concrete situation of practice. The history of the process of the initial formalization and expression of the nursing agency concept is enlightening (pp. 155-167).[1]

Nursing agency as a conceptual element of self-care deficit nursing theory is identified as the essential element of the theory of nursing system (see Chapter 7). The central idea of this theory expresses the broad purpose of nursing: to compensate for or overcome known or emerging health-derived or health-associated limitations of legitimate patients (or clients) for self-care (or dependent-care). The theory of nursing system attributes to nurses the power of nursing agency, the exercise of which results in produced action sequences toward accomplishment of nursing purposes that are contributary to the life, health, and well-being of nurses' patients.

Nursing agency is understood as a power developed by maturing or mature persons through specialized education, training of self to master the cognitive and practical operations of nursing practice, clinical experiences in nursing practice situations under the guidance of advanced nursing practitioners, and clinical nursing experiences in providing nursing to persons representing some range of types of nursing cases. The power that is named nursing agency is understood as a set of developed and developing capabilities that persons who are nurses exercise in the provision of nursing for individuals or groups. These capabilities are the focus of this chapter.

The first presentation is a summary view of the substantive structure of nursing agency. This is followed by presentations of:

1. An overview of the interlocking operations of nurses in nursing practice situations.
2. An example of a nursing and dependent-care design for the production of regulatory care for a person representative of a type of nursing case.
3. The professional-technologic operations of nursing practice—nursing diagnosis, nursing prescription, nursing regulation or treatment, evaluation and control, and case management; this presentation includes process models.
4. The use of basic conditioning factors in the practice of nursing.

The chapter concludes with an expression of ideas about nurses' maintenance of an overview of each nursing practice situation.

NURSING AGENCY: THE SUBSTANTIVE STRUCTURE

The theoretic concept nursing agency is a formulation of insights about powers of nurses to deliberately interact with persons with legitimate needs for nursing and to produce nursing for them and, when possible, with them. Nursing agency is analogous to self-care agency. They differ in that nursing agency is developed and exercised for the benefit of others and self-care agency is developed and exercised for the sake of one's self. Because the capabilities named nursing agency are exercised for the sake of others, nursing agency encompasses capabilities specific to the social and interpersonal as well as the professional-technologic features of nursing practice situations. Table 12-1 represents the parts of nursing practice situations as person elements, nurses

Table 12-1   Three Dimensions of Nursing Practice

Features	Element		Type of Relationship
	Person in Role	Person in Role	
Social	In position of *nurse* who can legitimately enter into negotiations for providing nursing	In the position of becoming a nurse's patient	Contractual for nursing
Interpersonal	*Active role* as person who is qualified and functioning as nurse	*Active role* to *no instrumental role* as person who is, was, or can be his or her own self-care agent	Professional, helping, nursing
Technologic	*Nurse role set* defined by (1) the work operations of professionals and (2) the presence of a self-care deficit in the patient, including extent and causes	*Patient role set* as defined by (1) the process of diagnosis to determine needs for nursing assistance and (2) the presence and characteristics of an identified and described self-care deficit	Nursing as specified by role sets of patient and nurse

and nurses' patients, and as social, interpersonal, and technologic features and relationships.

Enabling Capabilities of Nursing Agency

Nurses' performance of the operations of nursing practice to know and meet patients' therapeutic self-care demands and to protect and to regulate the exercise or development of patients' self-care agency requires enabling capabilities or power components. These are analogous in kind to the named power components of self-care agency (see Chapter 11). The power components include valid and reliable knowledge of all three areas of nursing operation (social, interpersonal, professional-technologic), intellectual and practical skills specific to the three areas, sustaining motives, willingness to provide nursing, ability to unify different action sequences toward result achievement, consistency in performance of nursing operations, making adjustments in them because of prevailing or emerging conditions, and ability to manage self as the essential professional operative element in nursing practice situations.

The foregoing summary of the enabling power components of nursing agency was developed into a set of desirable nurse characteristics—social, interpersonal, and professional-technologic. These characteristics when present in life situations are viewed as evidence of nurses' capabilities, their power of nursing agency.

Suggested Desirable Nurse Characteristics

Social

- Is well informed about and accepts the general social and legal dimensions of nursing situations; has specialized knowledge of the particular social and legal dimensions of types of nursing situations in his or her practice area
- Has knowledge of cultural differences among groups and among members of groups and understands the significance of persons' cultural orientations in their contacts and communications with others
- Has a repertoire of social skills, including communication skills, sufficient for effecting and maintaining contacts with individuals and multiperson units from a range of social classes and culture groups
- Accepts and respects himself or herself and others as developing persons, recognizing that each person has characteristic ways of conducting himself or herself in interpersonal situations
- Is courteous and considerate of others
- Is responsible in the provision of nursing to individuals or multiperson units within defined types of nursing situations
- Understands nursing with its domain and boundaries as one of the health services provided for by society
- Understands the nature of contractual and professional relationships and is able to perform the operations of nursing practice within limits set by these relationships

Interpersonal*

- Is well informed about the psychosocial dimensions of human functioning
- Has knowledge of factors that facilitate or impede interpersonal functioning
- Has knowledge of conditions necessary for the development of helping relationships
- Is interested in identifying and resolving human problems that interfere with satisfying relationships with others and produce emotional pain or suffering
- Has a repertoire of interpersonal skills that can be adjusted to infants, children, and adults, including those who are ill, disabled, or debilitated, and that enable the nurse to:
  1. Be an active participant in relationships with patients and their significant others
  2. Be a participant observer in interpersonal relationships with patients and their significant others with the goal of identifying personality characteristics (e.g., being controlling or passive) significant in the relationship; the

---

*The identified characteristics pertain to interpersonal operations needed in all types of nursing situations. Some methods or technologic approaches to meeting certain self-care requisites or to regulating self-care agency are purely interpersonal in nature; such interpersonal methods are considered as being within the technologic operations of nursing practice. Mental health nursing specialists caution against the indiscriminate use of regulatory technologies that are valid for use in situations in which patients have grave interpersonal problems.

existence and degree of emotional suffering or emotional pain (anxiety) and physical discomfort and pain (if both are severe, they can interfere with the patient's observation of events, resulting in a lack of knowledge of the interpersonal situation and sometimes in misinterpretation of it)

3. Reduce patients' emotional pain and physical discomfort and pain by effecting conditions that increase patients' comfort and satisfaction within the nurse-patient relationship
4. Increase awareness of the interpersonal situation in terms of the desirable or undesirable factors that affect meeting patients' therapeutic self-care demands and regulating their self-care agency

- Is able to relate to patients and their significant others in a manner that conforms to the conventional form for human interactions (e.g., making eye contact when engaged in conversation, maintaining a conversational tone when seeking information)
- Has a repertoire of communication skills (adjusted to the age and developmental state of individuals, their cultural practices, and communication problems resulting from genetic defects and pathologic processes) sufficient for effecting and maintaining relationships essential in the production of wholly compensatory, partly compensatory, and supportive-educative nursing systems for patients (see Chapter 13)
- Accepts persons who are under nursing care and works with them in accordance with their roles in self-care and dependent care
- Identifies broader social and legal aspects of interpersonal situations (e.g., who is legally responsible for the patient) and is able to represent these in a prudent way to patients or their significant others

Technologic

- Has mastery of valid and reliable techniques for nursing diagnosis and prescription; for meeting the therapeutic self-care demands of individuals with various mixes of universal, developmental, and health-deviation self-care requisites; and for regulating the exercise of the self-care agency of individuals, its protection, and its development
- Is experienced or becoming experienced in using valid and reliable techniques in performing the technologic operations of nursing practice in defined types and subtypes of nursing situations and in producing nursing systems within these situations
- Is able to integrate the use of methods of helping with the technologic operations toward the production and management of effective nursing systems for individuals and multiperson units
- Is alert, at ease, and confident in nursing situations; is relaxed but able to mobilize for immediate and effective action to protect patients' well-being and to regulate the variables of nursing systems and the relationships among them
- Seeks nursing practice experience and supervision as well as specialized education and training to extend or deepen his or her area of nursing practice with respect to nursing populations

- Works toward the formulation and testing of methods and techniques for technologic operations of nursing practice within his or her nursing specialization
- Strives to increase ability to apprehend those factors in nursing situations that condition the values of the patient variables, self-care agency, and therapeutic self-care demand and thus set up requirements that nursing agency be of a particular value
- Identifies the results obtained in specific nursing situations from the use of specific methods in meeting patients' therapeutic self-care demands and in regulating their self-care agency, compiles results over time by types of nursing situations, isolates factors associated with types of results, and compares results in the different types of nursing situations

Art and Prudence

Nurses function in nursing practice situations as persons with developed and developing qualities of personality and character. Nurses work in person-to-person relationships with others as they not only exercise but also continue to develop the capabilities that define their nursing agency at specific times. Closely allied to nurses' capabilities to produce nursing for others are the good habits (or virtues) of art and prudence. Both art and prudence are associated with the human power to engage in goal-oriented deliberate actions, as previously described. Art and prudence are acquired, settled qualities of persons, disposing them to act in particular ways.

The proper interest of prudence is the morality, the goodness of individual human actions in concrete situations of daily living. Prudence is right reason about things to be done. It ranges over consideration of what should be done to judgment about what the individual should choose to do, and it is completed with the decision about what will be done and the command to operationalize the decision. Prudence operates in a world of particularity, of distinctiveness and variety, and is content with what is probable and what is good in concrete situations. Prudence is a virtue of the mind and of the character of individuals.[2]

Art is understood as an intellectual quality of persons that is revealed in what they make, that is, the products of their endeavors. Art is concerned with the practical, with insights about what can be made that does not presently exist. Art is concerned with creating something, moving an idea of what can be to the actuality of existence.

The art of nursing is the intellectual quality of individual nurses that allows them to make creative investigations, analyses, and syntheses of the variables and conditioning factors within nursing situations in order to work toward the goal of the production of effective systems of nursing assistance for individuals or multiperson units. *Nursing prudence* is the quality of nurses that enables them (1) to seek and take counsel in new or difficult nursing situations, (2) to make correct judgments about what to do and what to avoid when particular conditions prevail or suddenly develop in nursing situations, (3) to decide to act in a particular way, and (4) to take action. Both nursing art and nursing prudence aid in and are essential for the production of effective systems of nursing assistance, but in different ways.

Through their art, nurses envision, design, and produce nursing assistance for others, assistance that is in accord with why and how persons can be helped through nursing. Art is concerned with creating systems of nursing assistance or care. Nursing prudence is concerned with doing this or that act at particular moments in light of one's knowledge of the situation. Both the art of nursing and nursing prudence develop with experience and with diligent efforts toward their development. The degree to which and the manner in which they develop in individual nurses are associated with nurses' talents, personality characteristics, developed and preferred modes of thinking, stages of personal moral development, abilities to conceptualize complex situations of action and to analyze and synthesize factual information, and the kinds of life experiences they have had, including nursing experiences. Nursing prudence also demands that nurses continue to advance themselves in the nursing sciences and in foundational disciplines. With the rapid advances in the sciences, it is unrealistic to think that prudence has a single base, practical experience in nursing.

The good habits of art and prudence serve nurses in their performance of the interrelated operations of nursing practice.

OPERATIONS OF NURSING PRACTICE: AN OVERVIEW

The position is taken in this text that nursing students should be introduced to, seek understanding of, and develop bodies of knowledge about, as well as the skills to perform, the essential operation of nursing practice. Operations in this context stand for the processes through which nurses come to know what kind of nursing to produce and actually produce it in concrete life situations.

A comprehensive listing of operations is suggested. The position of an operation in the listing does not necessarily signify the sequence of its performance to completion. It is characteristic of nursing and other human services that in practice situations performance of specific operations is often segmented. Concrete conditions and circumstances may result in one type of operation having performance precedence over another.

Seven operations are identified.

1. Securing demographic data about persons in the role of nurse's patient and information about the nature and boundaries of each patient's health care situation and nursing's jurisdiction within these boundaries
2. The taking of a nursing history to obtain information about persons' perceptions of their therapeutic self-care demands, their development and exercise of self-care agency, and about their conditions and patterns of living (see Appendix A)
3. Establishing and maintaining a legitimate and functional unity of persons for the production of nursing
4. Determining the current values and probable foreseen changes in basic conditioning factors that are affecting or may positively or negatively affect patients' therapeutic self-care demands or their self-care agency

5. Performing the professional-technologic operations of nursing diagnosis, nursing prescription, nursing regulation, or treatment with associated evaluation and control operations and case management
6. Development of designs for the production of regulatory nursing care with attention to continuing nursing diagnosis and prescription
7. Maintaining an overview of the social, interpersonal, and professional-technologic features of each nursing practice situation in the interests of situational management

The first two operations focus on patients and their health and self-care situations. Their performance produces data and information that are used by nurses throughout the duration of nursing practice situations. See design unit A in the nursing case example that follows. The third named operation, along with information from operations 1 and 2, establishes the specific persons who are the person elements of nursing practice situations who should cooperate and function together as a productive unity. See design unit B in the nursing case example.

Operation 4 (basic conditioning factors) and operation 5 (professional-technologic operations), when properly performed and integrated, constitute what is commonly referred to as *nursing process*. It is effective performance of these operations through which nursing requirements and results are identified, nursing is produced, and nursing results attained. See design units D, E, and F in the case example for examples of some results of performance.

Operation 6 identifies the design function of nurses. An adequate nursing design identifies the background information, resources, and role functions that are needed to provide effective nursing. Its purpose is to set forth the reasons for and the results expected from nursing, as well as the person elements, their roles, and their responsibilities. A nursing design is a "blueprint" for production.

Operation 7, maintaining an overview of the social, interpersonal, and technologic features of nursing practice operations, is essentially a control operation. It is directed to the whole of the nursing situation, not just to the professional-technologic features and operations. It is a necessary management operation of nurses in the provision of nursing to individuals and groups.

These operations of nursing practice must be mastered by nursing students and their interrelationships understood. The named operations indicate the complexity of nursing practice and the kinds of responsibilities that nurses are expected to bear and that many nurses do bear. Persons making decisions and setting policy about nursing practice, including nurse qualifications for practice, often do so without understanding the complexities of nursing practice and the responsibilities that nurses bear.

To provide a basis for nursing students' development of insights about the results of and the reasons for performance of the identified operations of nursing practice, a summary description of a nursing design for a nursing case is presented. A nursing design identifies what goes into and is necessary for the production of care to meet identified needs of persons for help in the form of nursing. Nursing designs, like architectural and engineering designs for buildings or bridges, describe in detail what is to be produced or constructed.

AN EXAMPLE OF A NURSING DESIGN

The idea of **nursing design** and the constituent units of design was introduced in the fourth edition of this book. Six design units were specified. Units were identified by the letters A through F. See box below for a concise identification of units that are developed in the presented example of a nursing design.

Throughout this chapter the term **nursing practice situation** is used. This term refers to the entirety of situations when persons are nursed, their person elements and features. The term **nursing case** is introduced in the following example of a nursing design. A nursing case refers to a particular instance of a person with specialized requirements for nursing organized around the person's health-associated self-care deficits. The nursing case illustrated is an instance of group 7 in the classification of nursing situations by health focus in Chapter 9. It is an example of a situation in which "quality of life is gravely and irreversibly affected," because of the effects of two cerebrovascular accidents.

Summary Description of a Nursing Case by Design Units

Information about patients under nursing care because of cerebrovascular accidents was organized as a typical case. The six design units were used in assigning nursing meaning to relevant available information. There is no suggestion that the exposition of the design features of the presented "case" is complete or even adequate. The presentation illustrates the attachment of nursing meaning to information and the relevance of information to nursing

---

Constituent Units of Designs for the Production of Nursing for Individuals

A. Contract for nursing, nursing's area of jurisdiction in contributing to the achievement of health care goals

B. Establishment of a legitimate functional unity of care providers

C. Descriptions of the components of current or prior self-care or dependent-care systems

D. a. Establishment of the components of a person's therapeutic self-care demands and factors that condition these components

D. b. Identification of resources needed to produce nursing to meet the therapeutic self-care demand

E. Establishment of self-care abilities and roles of persons under nursing care

F. Establishment of the design for the production of nursing for the person under care by defining role responsibilities for knowing and meeting the person's therapeutic self-care demand and for regulating the person's development or exercise of self-care agency

design and production. The case is presented by design units A through F. The case material presented is for a time period when health state was relatively stable. The case description by design units should be read with understanding of the grave potential for unfavorable changes in health state that can occur at any time. There is no focus on all possible conditions that appear in cases of this type.

A–Contract For and Jurisdiction of Nursing

Information, judgments, and decisions specific to this design unit are presented under 10 headings.

Person to be Nursed

Mary Doe, a 70-year-old wife of Harry and mother of adult married children, resides in the family home as part of an extended family.

Reason for Seeking Nursing

Mrs. Doe has a complete self-care deficit following a second cerebrovascular accident.

Prior Caregivers

Previous caregivers, in regressive order, are nurses in Hospital X, husband in home, nurses at rehabilitation center, nurses at Hospital X, self before first stroke.

Request for and Projected Requirements for Nursing

Hospital referral to Home Health Care Association after Mr. Doe and family (in collaboration with Mrs. Doe's physician) had made the decision to take care of Mrs. Doe in her home. Proposal: A dependent-care system in the home that would be articulated with a periodic system of nursing produced by association nurses who would be responsible for instruction of family members. Nursing will be provided by association nurses until home care is no longer appropriate for Mrs. Doe. Nurses and assistants will provide direct nursing of Mrs. Doe. Nurses will provide instruction, guidance, and direction that is needed by family members contributing to the dependent-care system. Nursing would include monitoring Mrs. Doe's condition, monitoring results of care, and evaluation of adequacy of the combined systems. Nurses will make referrals about needs for special services or equipment to the association or to other agencies.

Position in Health Care System

Mrs. Doe is under the care of a physician who is a specialist in internal medicine because of diabetes mellitus and two cerebrovascular accidents, the second of which affected the brainstem.

Nurses' Knowledge of Impact on Family

The hospital social worker advised the family to have Mrs. Doe provided with care in a nursing home. Despite stress associated with Mrs. Doe's previous illness, the family said the only acceptable course was to have Mrs. Doe in her own home.

Number and Qualifications of Nurses and Assistants to Nurses

A primary nurse is required, with provision for a replacement nurse. The primary nurse has educational qualifications for entry to professional level practice with 10 years of nursing practice experience. A home health aide, with provision for replacement, is also required. The aide is trained vocationally with 8 years of experience in the association. The primary nurse will provide nursing daily or adjust schedule in accord with Mrs. Doe's nursing requirements. The home health aide will provide care for Mrs. Doe daily.

Contracting Parties

Mr. Doe (in collaboration with Mrs. Doe's physician) and the Home Health Care Association are the contracting parties.

Resources Required and Obtained

Resources include a hospital bed, lift, suction equipment, and other standard equipment.

Method of Financing

Third-party payment is available.

B—Legitimate Functional Unity of Care Providers

Mrs. Doe has no active participatory role and limited awareness, but does react to some events. Legitimate care providers are the association nurses and home health aides, the three family members, and association personnel, such as a physical therapist and speech therapist, who provide for Mrs. Doe's special requirements.

C—Current or Prior Self-Care or Dependent-Care System

Not relevant at this time period.

D—Therapeutic Self-Care Demand

Mrs. Doe's therapeutic self-care demand is conditioned primarily by her health state and by her condition of living, that is, confinement to bed. Her state of health is characterized by impaired neuromuscular functioning resultant from cerebrovascular accidents, including inability to speak, to swallow, or to manage the position of her body and its parts. Her cardiac and respiratory functioning are stabilized, but there have been periods when breathing was in the Cheyne-Stokes pattern. Cough reflex is diminished, with inability to handle her own secretions. There is no bladder or bowel control. Mrs. Doe has a gastrostomy tube that is sutured in place. Mrs. Doe has diabetes mellitus with a care regimen of prescribed morning dose of insulin and prescribed diet, which her family understands and manages. Level of awareness fluctuates during the day and over time periods from alertness to grogginess.

The components of Mrs. Doe's therapeutic self-care demand are universal self-care requisites and health-deviation requisites. Developmental self-care requisites are not considered apart from the universal requisites of prevention of hazards and promotion of normalcy.

The factors that condition each universal and health-deviation self-care requisite are presented along with summary listings of technologies and actions. Technologies and associated care measures are presented as action statements without detailed development of action sequences.

Maintaining a Sufficient Intake of Air

Normal pattern of inspiration and expiration is obstructed at times by the following conditioning factors, each of which may affect sufficiency of air intake: Cheyne-Stokes pattern of breathing; diminished cough reflex with inability to manage secretions; confinement to bed and inability to manage self, to turn, to sit up.

Technologies and actions include the following:
- Position in bed to facilitate breathing; transfer to upright position in chair; change position in bed.
- Observe for open airway.
- Suction to remove secretions.
- Regulate airflow and humidity in room.
- Observe for respiratory distress.

Maintaining a Sufficient Intake of Water

The process of securing and consuming water is affected by inability to speak, move, and swallow. Technologies and actions include the following:
- Know and maintain a standard for fluid intake for Mrs. Doe.
- Adjust fluid intake to fluid loss.
- Give water through gastrostomy tube at intervals throughout the day other than after prescribed feedings.
- Give water after each gastrostomy feeding.
- Observe for signs of dehydration or overhydration.

Maintaining a Sufficient Intake of Food

The process of securing and consumption of food by Mrs. Doe is interfered with or conditioned by her inability to speak, move, or swallow, and by her diabetic condition.

Technologies and actions include the following:
- Have available the medically prescribed, prepared formula for feeding Mrs. Doe, the caloric and protein adequacy of which has been evaluated by the dietitian associated with the Home Health Care Association.
- Prepare the formula and feed Mrs. Doe through her gastrostomy tube four times daily; administer water after feeding.
- Administer prescribed insulin dose each morning.
- Observe for signs of hypoglycemia and hyperglycemia.
- Observe for signs of hunger.
- Observe for signs of inadequate nutrition.

Providing Care Associated with Eliminative Processes and Excrements

The meeting of this universal self-care requisite is affected by absence of bladder and bowel control, inability to move, composition and consistency of tube feedings, and amount and sufficiency of water intake.

Technologies and actions related to urinary output include:

- Urine elimination through Foley catheter involving periodic change of catheter and a routine of catheter care to ensure safety, effectiveness, and prevention of infection.
- Ensure that the standard for intake of water is met.
- Observe urine for color, clearness, and odor; measure urine output and record amount as well as observed features.
- Dispose of urine in a sanitary manner.
- Care for urine drainage bag.

Technologies and actions related to bowel evacuation include the following:

- Develop and maintain a regimen for bowel evacuation. This may require medication to counteract the effects of the composition and consistency of gastrostomy tube feedings on bowel evacuation.
- Stimulate through activity spaced throughout the day such as turning and repositioning.
- Hygienic care of body parts and surfaces after bowel evacuation; maintain clean clothing and bed linen.
- Use sanitary procedure to dispose of feces and to handle soiled linen.
- Observe and record consistency of the stool, its color, and the amount of fluid in the evacuation.
- Record time of evacuations.
- Take appropriate action when diarrhea or constipation occurs.

Technologies and actions related to the excretory activities of the skin include the following:

- Perform regular personal care related to insensible perspiration, including bathing of all body surfaces, keeping clothing and linen clean.
- Know patient's body temperature and the environmental temperature.
- Regulate room temperature; adjust weight and amount of clothing and airflow to maintain a physical environment that supports normal body temperature.
- Observe for sweating and its associated signs and symptoms. Act to ensure that patient is warm and dry. Act to determine the underlying reasons and institute appropriate regulatory action.

Maintaining a Balance Between Activity and Rest and Between Solitude and Social Interaction

Maintaining these balances for Mrs. Doe is affected by her inability to move and speak and by alternating periods of alertness and extremely limited awareness during the course of a day or over a period of days. Mrs. Doe can hear and see and reacts or responds to events by gaze.

Technologies and actions related to maintenance of a balance between activity and rest include the following:
- Support Mrs. Doe's diurnal wake-sleep pattern.
- Provide for periods of stimulation and rest during the day.
- Prepare for sleep at night.
- Select stimulation to which Mrs. Doe responds favorably, such as television or persons whom Mrs. Doe wants to be with her and who relate to her with speech.
- Provide for physical movement: passive exercises of the extremities; move from bed to chair at least once a day.
- Recognize and respond appropriately to signs of fatigue brought about by care activities.

Technologies and actions related to maintenance of a balance between solitude and social interaction include the following:
- Recognize and respond to Mrs. Doe's signals for solitude (wanting to be left alone) with knowledge of what she preferred when well.
- Interact with Mrs. Doe during each caregiving contact. Limit verbalization during care in the interest of preventing fatigue.
- Show interest in and concern for Mrs. Doe, at the same time affording her rightful independence as a person.
- Be "caring" as "taking care of" activities are performed.
- Allow Mrs. Doe to select visitors through the use of the picture communication board to which she responds with a specific gaze.
- Provide for television viewing.

Preventing Hazards

The meeting of this universal self-care requisite is viewed as related to meeting the previously described requisites. It is affected by Mrs. Doe's lack of self-management capabilities, limited awareness, inability to swallow, absence of bladder and bowel control, use of a Foley catheter, gastrostomy tube, and insulin-dependent diabetes mellitus.

Technologies and actions for meeting this requisite include the following:
- Recognize signs of clinical emergency situations and respond appropriately.
- Take action to prevent untoward events associated with Mrs. Doe's confinement to bed for the major portion of every day and in moving from bed to chair to bed.
- Maintain conditions to prevent respiratory distress and respiratory infections.
- Maintain actions to prevent hazards associated with the use and care of the Foley catheter, including infection.
- Maintain actions to prevent hazards associated with use and care of Mrs. Doe's gastrostomy tube and administration of feedings. These include infection, tube displacement, and feeding-associated diarrhea.
- Maintain action to minimize stress and physical exhaustion resultant from performance of care measures by others without ability to participate.

- Know fluid intake and fluid loss (sweat, urine, bowel evacuations) and take action appropriate to maintain fluid balance.
- Maintain observations relative to Mrs. Doe's safety and to the occurrence of emergencies with immediate reporting to physician, the Home Health Care Association, emergency medical services as appropriate.

Being Normal

All the conditioning factors identified in prevention of hazards are relevant to Mrs. Doe's normality. The lack of self-management capabilities and the limitation of awareness are most significant.

The following technologies and actions are important:
- Recognize when Mrs. Doe is aware; approach her and respond to her as a person.
- Maintain features of family living familiar to Mrs. Doe, including Mrs. Doe in accord with her family roles.
- Maintain Mrs. Doe's contacts with friends, church members, and other social contacts that she prefers.
- Contribute to development and to Mrs. Doe's use of a pictorial system of communication.
- Recognize evidence of discomfort and pain and act to relieve these experiences by elimination of causes, soothing care measures, and use of prescribed medication if needed.
- Know Mrs. Doe's religious orientations and practices and assist appropriately in their maintenance.
- Foster Mrs. Doe's maintenance of her sense of self.
- Provide care to maintain Mrs. Doe's integrity to the degree possible with respect to, for example, grooming, body alignment, body temperature, fluid balance.

All of the described universal self-care requisite components of Mrs. Doe's therapeutic self-care demand are adjusted to factors derived from the results and effects of two cerebrovascular accidents, to her condition of insulin-dependent diabetes mellitus, and to health care system factors such as the fixed gastrostomy tube and use of insulin. Other health-deviation self-care requisites to be met continuously are identified.

Health-Deviation Self-Care Requisites

Mrs. Doe's other health-deviation self-care requisites that would constitute components of her therapeutic self-care demand at a minimum include the following:
- Securing appropriate assistance from Mrs. Doe's physician by telephone or visit in the event of occurrence of signs and symptoms of another cardiovascular accident; substantial neurologic change; elevated blood pressure; signs and symptoms of hyperglycemia, hypoglycemia, urinary tract infection, or infection in the area of the gastrostomy tube; respiratory distress; fever; unexplained pain; a fall.

- Effective conduct of the medically prescribed diabetes mellitus management regimen including morning insulin in the prescribed dose, observation of blood glucose levels, calculation of insulin dose within the prescribed range if afternoon insulin is required, administration of prescribed feedings by gastrostomy tube, and observation for signs of hypoglycemia or hyperglycemia.
- Observe for the status of and changes in Mrs. Doe related to specific aspects of her functioning and her known pathologies, including attention to features of and changes in cardiac functioning, respiratory functioning, kidney functioning, circulation, neurologic functioning, the integrity and condition of skin and mucous membranes, and bowel functioning.

E–Self-Care Capabilities and Roles, Dependent-Care Capabilities and Roles

Mrs. Doe has no known operational capabilities to engage in self-care. There is no known potential for restoration of prior capabilities or for development of new capabilities. Mrs. Doe has some ability to convey her reactions through her gaze.

Adult members of Mrs. Doe's family have learned and continue to learn to meet components of Mrs. Doe's therapeutic self-care demand by performing some care measures that must be performed at specific times, as well as ones that may need to be performed any time of the day. They provide care consistently, safely, and effectively. Dependent-care capabilities of family members are not adequate for meeting all components of Mrs. Doe's therapeutic self-care demand or for knowing when and how to make adjustments or major changes.

Some family members experience psychologic and physiologic dependent-care limitations. Other family members recognize when this occurs and are flexible in compensating for what one family member cannot do at a particular time.

All family members are subject to fatigue and what they can endure relative to the dependent-care situation.

F–Design Features of the Nursing System and Dependent-Care System

The nursing system for Mrs. Doe is a periodic system that is in operation each day but not continuously. The nursing system articulates with a dependent-care system for Mrs. Doe that is in continuous production. There is provision for communication of dependent-care agents with the primary nurse or the Home Health Care Association at times when nurses are not present in Mrs. Doe's home.

The nursing system and the dependent-care system were initiated upon Mrs. Doe's return home from the hospital. Both systems have achieved a degree of operational stability but continue to develop as nursing problems are recognized and resolved, and solutions found. The nursing system is produced and managed by the primary nurse with assistance of the home health aide(s). The dependent-care system is produced and managed primarily by three members of Mrs. Doe's family, working collaboratively.

Broad Role Responsibilities of the Primary Nurse

The primary nurse has two broad responsibilities: (1) to govern, produce, and manage the nursing system in accord with its constituent action elements, articulating primary nurse contributions with those of the home health aide and the person and action elements of the dependent-care system, and (2) to determine the elements and the relations among elements of the dependent-care system, to identify signs of its adequacy and effectiveness, and to confer with family members to guide them in their endeavors and in effecting needed adjustments and changes.

Specific Role Responsibilities of the Primary Nurse

The following is a development of these responsibilities:
- Instruct and guide family with respect to meeting components of Mrs. Doe's therapeutic self-care demand.
- Guide and direct the home health aide as changes occur in Mrs. Doe's condition; be accessible to the home health aide for supervision and consultation.
- Assess Mrs. Doe's vital signs. Conduct a physical assessment for Mrs. Doe once a week or more frequently as indicated. Do blood glucose checks to determine effectiveness of care measures for management of diabetes mellitus.
- Obtain information about and judge the nursing or medical relevance of the Cheyne-Stokes pattern of breathing when it occurs.
- Obtain information from home health aide and dependent-care agents about the presence or absence of respiratory distress or airway problems and their management when present.
- Observe for and make judgments about matters that should be referred to Mrs. Doe's physician. Advise family about nurse-perceived needs for contacting physician.
- Make judgments about situations when the nurse should communicate directly with the physician.
- Instruct family about signs of emergency situations and emergency care, including notification of Mrs. Doe's physician or emergency medical services when emergencies arise.
- Manage care related to use of the Foley catheter and its periodic replacement. Observe for signs of urinary tract infection.
- Observe for the integrity of patient's tissues, with concern for the condition of mouth and the skin and with attention to tissues surrounding the permanent gastrostomy tube.
- Know nutritional and fluid intake and make judgments about its adequacy.
- Know urinary and bowel output and assess and judge quality and quantity.
- Observe for hazardous conditions in Mrs. Doe's environment and in care performance and work with home health aide and dependent-care agents to remove them or to institute safety measures.
- Work with home health aide and dependent-care agents to identify new and emerging self-care requisites and to design means for meeting them.

- Work cooperatively with speech therapist in the development and use of picture charts to aid Mrs. Doe to communicate.
- Work cooperatively with the physical therapist with respect to rules of body alignment, passive exercise, protective measures, transfer from bed to chair and return, and use of needed equipment.
- Consult with dietitian associated with Home Health Care Association for reevaluations of Mrs. Doe's diet.
- Document immediately observations and measures of care performed and problems encountered with recommendation for follow-up.
- Work with family members to guide and support them with respect to knowing and meeting components of their therapeutic self-care demands associated with or affected by their dependent-care activities.
- Consult with dependent-care agents about their assessments of the quality and effectiveness of Mrs. Doe's care and problems they are encountering.
- Endeavor to know what Mrs. Doe's family is experiencing and support them in ways that are helpful but not intrusive.
- Assist the family to become an operational unit with the nurses and home health aide in designing and providing care for Mrs. Doe, with understanding of areas of independence and interdependence.
- Be judicious in the use of nursing supplies and equipment and in protecting household furnishings that are used in Mrs. Doe's care.
- Periodically assess personal capabilities and actions in governing, producing, and managing the periodic system of nursing for Mrs. Doe and in cooperative functioning with Mrs. Doe's family. Identify needs for knowledge, new skills, or improvement of skills.
- Seek nursing consultation and supervision from the assigned nurse in the Home Health Care Association.

Role Responsibilities of the Home Health Aide

The following is a development of these responsibilities:
- Communicate with patient as care is provided.
- Bathe patient; provide mouth care; care for hair; exercise concern for Mrs. Doe's privacy.
- Perform range of motion exercises.
- Position Mrs. Doe to facilitate comfort and support unobstructed breathing; protect extremities.
- Inspect skin and report problems of skin integrity to nurse.
- Use clothing and coverings for Mrs. Doe that are appropriate for maintaining normal body temperature under prevailing environmental conditions.
- Provide Foley catheter care according to the specified regimen.
- Empty and care for urinary drainage bag; record urinary output.
- Provide care within the regimen for bowel evacuation and note features of bowel movements, including fluid content of evacuations.
- Provide care in a manner that prevents psychological stress and prevents or minimizes physical exhaustion for Mrs. Doe.
- Cooperate with family members who provide care.

- Be judicious in the use of resources and protect the household furnishings in Mrs. Doe's room.
- Document immediately care provided and report information to the primary nurse and nursing supervisor.
- Seek supervision as needed.
- Assess personal capabilities and contributions to Mrs. Doe's care. Identify need for additional skills and supporting knowledge.

Broad Role Responsibilities of Dependent-Care Agents

These responsibilities include taking care of Mrs. Doe 24 hours of each day safely and effectively and being with her and performing care measures at specified times or when the need for them occurs. Dependent-care agents must be flexible in accepting changing responsibilities for performance of care measures to ensure continuity of care and operational unity in the provision of care. There is the broad responsibility to accept Home Health Care Association nurses into the household and to work with them, not as strangers or intruders, but as professionals to be collaborated with in the care of Mrs. Doe.

Specific Role Responsibilities of Dependent-Care Agents

These responsibilities are developed as follows:
- Give fixed prescribed dose of morning insulin; give afternoon dose if needed according to the prescribed sliding scale.
- Prepare and give prescribed feedings by gastrostomy tube four times a day; give water after and between feedings.
- Empty urinary drainage bag; measure and record amount of urine; observe characteristics of urine, noting changes in color or clarity.
- Change Mrs. Doe's position in bed; position to facilitate inspiration and expiration.
- Keep Mrs. Doe clean and dry after bowel evacuation; note color and consistency of stool and the amount of fluid in the evacuation; record.
- Maintain weight of Mrs. Doe's clothing and covering in accord with environmental conditions to prevent chilling and sweating.
- Manage environmental conditions and Mrs. Doe's position in bed or chair to provide some balance between activity and rest.
- Manage social conditions to provide for a balance between solitude and social interaction.
- Act to prevent development of hazardous conditions and to ensure Mrs. Doe's safety if they occur. This includes maintenance of a clear airway.
- Maintain environmental conditions to assure Mrs. Doe that she is at home with her family.
- Work with nurses and home health aide to ensure that Mrs. Doe's self-care requisites are known and met.
- Seek guidance and direction from primary nurse when courses of care action are unclear or instruction is needed.

- Notify the primary nurse or the Home Health Care Association when nursing help is needed.
- Communicate with Mrs. Doe's physician as requested by the physician; convey information to the physician that the primary nurses identify as important for the family to report.
- Know the indications of emergency situations; observe for such evidence; report and seek help from Mrs. Doe's physician or from emergency medical services.
- Perform family-related role responsibilities including (1) supporting one another in providing care to minimize stress and prevent fatigue, (2) ensuring that each family member's therapeutic self-care demand is calculated and met, (3) observing family members for signs of stress and fatigue and act to provide relief, (4) observing effects of providing home care for Mrs. Doe on individual family members and the family as a structural and functional unity, and (5) taking action to prevent family dysfunction or to restore family stability.
- Maintain a care record.

Basic Conditioning Factors Summarized

The foregoing example of design unit information for a type of nursing case reveals the social, interpersonal, and technologic features of the case. It also highlights the active conditioning effects of patients' self-management abilities, self-care agency, and therapeutic self-care demand of patients on requirements for care. The contractual and interpersonal features of the case were conditioned by the patient's complete self-care deficit and by loss of self-management capabilities associated with the results and effects of two cerebrovascular accidents (health state factors). The contract for nursing was not with the patient but with the patient's husband, who would be legally responsible for her. Interactions of nurses with the patient were one-sided, with patient reactions as the only contributions to the process. Nurses interacted with family members in the initiation, development, and maintenance of interlocking nursing and dependent-care systems.

The factor actively conditioning the patient properties of self-care agency and therapeutic self-care demand was health state with age and development state, affecting therapeutic self-care demand to a minimal degree. Age in this case was not actively related to developmental state as it would be with infants and children because maturation had been achieved. If or how psychologic or personal development could proceed in cases of this type is unclear. Health state factors expressed as the results and effects of two cerebrovascular accidents imposed on the patient a style of living that did not permit movement from one place to another unless moved or transported physically by other persons. It also required the patient to remain in a health care system, including nursing and dependent-care, for the duration of life.

Family system factors, sociocultural factors, socioeconomic factors, and available resources were relevant to family decisions. They would be condition-ers of the willingness and the developing ability of the family and of the availability of time, labor, and resources to provide a continuous system of dependent care in the home and to articulate it with a periodic system of nursing. This case can be summarized as well as typed according to its health care focus, the causes and the extent of the self-care deficit, the components of the therapeutic self-care demand, the complexity and stability of the therapeutic self-care demand, and the type of nursing system that would be the product of the work of nurses expressed in terms of the compensatory or educational features of the action system and its continuous or periodic production.

PROFESSIONAL OPERATIONS IN HEALTH SERVICES

Professional practice within the health service professions varies in accord with the proper object of each health service, the state of development of each service's practical and applied sciences, and the kind of preprofessional and professional, including advanced professional, education of its practitioners. Operations that are specifically professional-technologic are identified as (1) diagnostic, (2) prescriptive, (3) treatment or regulatory, and (4) case management. These operations are directed to and performed for the sake of persons receiving the specific health services singly or in groups. Each of the named operations has a general meaning that becomes specific within the individual health service.

Diagnostic operations involve a process of careful and directed investigation, with an examination and analysis of data descriptive of a particular person and the person's conditions and circumstances of living in an attempt to understand or explain the nature of existent or changing condition(s) for which health service is sought. What health service professionals diagnose and the diagnoses they make are specific to each service. Diagnostic operations precede prescriptive operations, which precede treatment or regulatory operations. Diagnostic operations result in answers to the questions: What is? What are the distinguishing characteristics of what is? What is its nature and meaning? Why is it as it is? Diagnostic operations incorporate investigative operations to accumulate data that is relevant to the problems for which people seek care from specific health services.

Prescriptive operations are practical judgments followed by decisions about courses of action to be followed if particular diagnosed conditions exist. Prescriptive processes answer the questions: What can be done, given the known present and projected state of affairs and the means available? What should be done in light of the total situation of the person and the conditions and circumstances of living, not just this or that single aspect of the situation?

Treatment or regulatory operations are the practical activities through which what is prescribed is executed and through which the diagnosed condition or problem is treated in order to remove it, control it, or keep it within boundaries compatible with human life, health, and well-being.

Case management operations are concerned with controlling, directing, and checking each of the diagnostic, prescriptive and treatment, or regulatory operations. Controlling includes evaluation. Case management is concerned with the integration of technologic operations to form a dynamic system of health service that is effective and judicious in the use of resources and that minimizes both psychological and physical stress for persons seeking and receiving the health service.

The technologic operations of professional practice are particularized for each health service. Particularization occurs when professional providers of a service recognize and accept that they must know the conditions of members of society that render them to be in need of that service. This is another way of saying that providers of a service must know the proper object or focus of the service and its boundaries. The focus of each service (the human condition[s] that renders persons to be in need of it) undergoes development as professionals conceptualize and theorize about it.

The professional operations described here have not had widespread acceptance in nursing, for a number of historically based reasons. However, professionally prepared nurses should know and accept the reasons for nursing's existence and continued acceptance in society, be able to theorize about what nursing is and what nursing should be, and accept and engage in fulfilling their responsibilities to develop the nursing sciences. The professional-technologic operations of the health services are the bases for the development of practice models and rules of practice. (See Figure 8-3 on stages of understanding nursing.)

PROFESSIONAL-TECHNOLOGIC OPERATIONS OF NURSING

Nursing process is a term nurses use to refer to nurses' performance of the professional-technologic operations of nursing practice. These operations are conceptualized and named by nurses in a variety of ways. *Process* is used in the sense of a continuous and regular sequence of goal-achieving, deliberately performed actions of particular kinds carried out in a definite manner.

In this text nursing process is understood to be constituted from nurses' performance of diagnostic, prescriptive, and regulatory or treatment operations, with associated control operations including evaluation. Nurses perform these operations within the context of their enabling interpersonal relationships with patients and their contractual agreement to provide nursing. The operations are performed in sequence. For example, nursing diagnosis precedes nursing prescription but the nursing diagnostic operation is not necessarily complete before prescriptions are made and regulatory care provided. This is illustrated in a case study developed by Susan G. Taylor in consultation with Jeanne Saathoff (pp. 59-68).[3] A 34-year-old man was hospitalized with diabetes mellitus out of control, a submandibular abscess, high fever, and a leg ulcer that resulted from a tick bite. An immediate decision was made for medical and nursing staff to take over the "regulation and production of self-care." All care measures to meet known components of the patient's therapeutic self-care demand, "including routine hygiene, were performed or initiated by the nursing staff." The health focus of care of nurses and physicians was (1) treating the infection and (2) regaining some control of the diabetes mellitus. With improvement in the patient's condition, the medical focus shifted to "evaluating his general condition," including the use of intrusive medical diagnostic measures. "The nursing focus during this period was on support" because of the patient's anxiety about "procedure and outcomes." The nursing focus shifted "to one of evaluating and improving" the patient's "self-care system when he was able to attend to this" (p. 61).[3] This focus moved nurses back to nursing diagnostic operations related to the patient's self-care agency—his capabilities and limitations for self-care. The nursing diagnoses are expressed in a paragraph that is explanatory of the patient's self-care limitations and his past failures to know and meet components of his therapeutic self-care demand (p. 64).[3]

The initial decision that nurses would be the producers of continuing care to meet components of the patient's therapeutic self-care demand was based on the unexpressed nursing diagnosis that the patient was not able to engage in self-care because of the urgency for meeting his health-deviation self-care requisites, and because his acute infection and hyperglycemia limited his ability to attend and his available energy. Health state, including acuity of illness, was the major dynamic variable in this first phase of nursing, affecting both the patient's self-care agency and the components of his therapeutic self-care demand.

The preceding example demonstrates the necessity for nurses to avoid conceptualizing the provision of nursing as a linear process moving from a complete, definitive nursing diagnosis to nursing regulation and evaluation. This experience may occur on occasion but is far from what should be expected.

The technologic orientations and operations of nurses in practice situations are summarized in the box on p. 311. The orientations are to the powers of persons to engage in self-care and to the knowing, continuous, and effective meeting of persons' therapeutic self-care demands. The operations are expressed according to these two orientations.

Nursing's professional-technologic operations are described in subsequent sections.

Nursing Diagnosis and Prescription

Nursing diagnosis necessitates investigation and the accumulation of data about patients' self-care agency and their therapeutic self-care demand and the existent or projected relationships between them. Nurses in practice understand or should understand that investigation should not go beyond what is needed for nurses to make valid judgments about existent conditions. Experienced nurses can quickly apprehend many facets of each practice situation and know the kind and amount of information they need as they proceed to nurse patients. In nursing, diagnosis is focused on persons who are accepted as having therapeutic self-care demands, the components of which are based in their particularized self-care requisites and have self-care agency, which may be in various stages of development and may

Technologic Orientations and Operations of Nursing Practice

1. The power of others to engage in self-care
   a. Diagnose the values of the constituent elements of self-care agency of the other in terms of:
      (1) Degree of development
      (2) Degree of operability
      (3) Adequacy as related to the operations required for meeting an existing or a projected self-care demand (2f below)
   b. Determining the presence or absence of a deficit relationship between existing powers of self-care agency and the action demands on it (2f below)
   c. Prescribe how self-care agency should be regulated
   d. Represent to the other need for and the rationale for and assist the other with:
      (1) The immediate exercise of self-care agency
      (2) The withholding of the exercise of self-care agency in a prescribed manner
      (3) The adjustment or development of one or more of the constituent elements of self-care agency in a prescribed manner in order to meet existing or projected self-care requisites
2. The continuous and effective meeting of the self-care requisites of others in accordance with 1a, 1b, and 1c
   a. Diagnose existing or projected self-care requisites
   b. Particularize the value(s) of each self-care requisite by determining the active conditioning effects of such factors as age, gender, developmental state, health state, sociocultural orientation, and available resources
   c. Determine the method(s) through which each existng or projected self-care requisite can be met
   d. Select the method(s) for meeting each self-care requisite that is both safe and effective in view of the age, developmental state, and health state
   e. Set forth the courses or systems of action required to use the selected method in meeting each particularized self-care requisite
   f. Calculate, in light of the foregoing, the totality of the courses of action required to meet existing and projected self-care requisites, using selected methods (the therapeutic self-care demand), and then design the total action system
   g. Prescribe the role that the other can safely and effectively take in self-care in light of 1a
   h. Prescribe the role that the nurse (or a nonnurse) can and should take in meeting the therapeutic self-care demand of the other, including selecting and presenting valid and reliable ways of helping
   i. Perform and manage role operations to meet each self-care requisite of the other according to the selected or adjusted method(s), the determined action system, and the prescribed roles (2g and 2h)

or may not be operable in whole or in part. Nurses also require facts to make judgments that self-care agency, if it is developed and operable in individuals, will be exercised by them and adequate for meeting their therapeutic self-care demands.

In nurses' development of the process operations of nursing practice, the term *nursing assessment* has been in common use to identify the initial step of the process of nursing, the operation referred to here as *nursing diagnosis*. Assessment in its extended use (use beyond placing monetary values on things) implies a process of determining or estimating the exact value, extent, or character of a thing before making judgments about it or using the assessment as a ground for decision making. In the following description and explanation of nursing diagnosis, *assessment* is *one type of action* within the process of nursing diagnosis, but it is not the whole of the process. Additionally, assessment is a feature of all the other operations of nursing practice, namely, prescriptive and regulatory or treatment operations with associated control operations, including evaluations.

Nursing diagnosis is a process of carefully collecting, examining, and analyzing data, with assessment of its validity and completeness for making nursing judgments about persons, their properties, their movements, or changes in properties to explain (1) relationships between basic conditioning factors and existent self-care requisites and means for meeting them; (2) the patient's repertoire of self-care practices as related to known components of the therapeutic self-care demand; (3) limitation for deliberate actions that interfere with estimative (investigative) judgment and decision making, and the production phases of self-care; (4) adequacy of knowledge, skills, willingness, and other power components to perform self-care operations to meet each component of the therapeutic self-care demand; and (5) potential for the future exercise or for the development of self-care agency.

Diagnostic statements can be expressed in various ways with respect to the five types of explanations. However, it should be remembered that technically an explanation expresses a relationship between entities. In the nursing case design described in this chapter, where information was sorted by design units, diagnostic statements to describe the five explanations named in the preceding paragraph could be expressed appropriately as follows:

1a. All universal self-care requisites and means for meeting them are conditioned by the results and effects of the two cerebrovascular accidents (health state factors).

1b. There is a set of health-deviation self-care requisites associated with the condition of insulin-dependent diabetes mellitus with the continuing possibility to probability for the emergence of additional requisites of this type.

1c. There are health-deviation self-care requisites of a monitoring (watching or checking) nature related to the emergence of evidence of changes in vital functions.

1d. Developmental self-care requisites are for protection of human integrity and maintenance of a sense of self.

2, 3, 4. There is a complete deficit for engagement in estimative judgment and decision making, and production of self-care operations in knowing and meeting the therapeutic self-care demand. This deficit is associated with the absence of self-management capabilities and limited cognitional functioning resultant from the effects of two cerebrovascular accidents.

5. There is no known potential for the future exercise or development of self-care agency because of the results and effects of the cerebrovascular accidents.*

Prescriptive operations specify (1) the means to be used to meet particularized self-care requisites, and the courses of actions, care measures, to be performed in using the means to meet the requisite; (2) the totality of care measures to be performed to meet all components of the therapeutic self-care demand, including a good organization of the care measures from the various components; (3) the roles of nurse's (nurses') patient and dependent-care agent(s) in meeting the therapeutic self-care demand; and (4) roles of nurses, patient, and dependent-care agents in regulating the exercise or development of self-care agency.

Diagnostic and prescriptive self-care operations that relate to patients' therapeutic self-care demands and self-care agency are summarized in Tables 12-2 and Table 12-3, respectively. These operations are expressed within the context of interpersonal and contractual operations of nursing practice.

In nursing diagnostic and prescriptive operations, as well as in regulatory or treatment operations, patients' and families' abilities and willingness to collaborate with nurses affect what nurses can do. Patients, members of their families, and others who are acting for patients may or may not be interested in the need or psychologically able to accept the need to collaborate with nurses or to become active participants in their own self-care or the care of their dependents. Thus it is important for nurses to make initial observations about patients and their families to provide themselves with information they can use to guide their interactions and communications with patients.

From this perspective, nurses should concern themselves with (1) identifying overt evidence of personality characteristics of patients and others related to them that will significantly affect the nursing situation (e.g., passivity-activity) and (2) identifying and exploring patients' concerns that may block their active collaboration with nurses and their participation in health care. To obtain this information, nurses must make observations about and elicit subjective information from patients. Nurses should also be alert to situations in which patients never question what nurses say and do. It is important for nurses to know whether patients are understanding and accepting, uninvolved, always accepting

---

*A contrasting case in terms of potential for development of self-care agency is reported by Smith MC: An application of Orem's theory in nursing practice, *Nurs Sci Q* 2:159-161, 1989.

Table 12-2 Operations Related to Determining Patients' Therapeutic Self-Care Demands

Interpersonal and Contractual Operations	Professional-Technologic Operations	Type of Operation
Enter into and maintain effective relationships with patient, family, or significant others		
Reach an agreement (implicit or explicit) with the patient or family to seek answers to the questions: What is the patient's therapeutic self-care demand at this time? In the future?		
Collaborate with the patient or family	Determine the existing and projected self-care requisites, their particular values, and expected changes in their values:	*Diagnostic* of self-care requisites
Review with patient or family	*Existing requisites* / *Current values* / *Projected requisites* / *Projected values* Universal — Universal / Developmental — Developmental / Health-deviation — Health-deviation	
Collaborate with patient or family	Determine the methods through which each existing or projected self-care requisite can be met, i.e., methods that are valid and reliable in relation to the patient's age, developmental state, health state, and other conditioning factors	Preliminary—*prescriptive*
Review with patient or family	Select the methods that will be used for meeting each particularized self-care requisite, with knowledge of the safety and degree of effectiveness of each method	*Prescriptive* of methods

Review with patient or family	Lay out the procedures or care measures required for using the selected method(s) for meeting each of the requisites	*Prescriptive* of measures
Review with patient or family	Calculate the ideal therapeutic self-care demand and identify self-care requisites with high priorities:	*Prescriptive* of the ideal therapeutic self-care demand for some duration
	Self-care requisites *Values* *Methods* *Measures for meeting* Universal Developmental Health-deviation	
Reach agreements with patient or family about the constituent parts of the therapeutic self-care demand, and give the final prescription of the therapeutic self-care demand to the patient or family	Make adjustments as required in the therapeutic self-care demand to bring it into accord with what is possible (and necessary) to accomplish	*Final—prescriptive* of the therapeutic self-care demand
Specify nurse, patient, or family roles in making adjustments	Identify factors that will require changes in the values of self-care requisites. Indicate how to calculate value changes and to make adjustments in methods or procedures as needed	Specification of rules for making changes in the therapeutic self-care demand

Table 12-3 Operations Related to Self-Care Agency and its Regulation		
Interpersonal and Contractual Operations	Professional-Technologic Operations	Type of Operation
Enter into and maintain effective relationships with patient, family, or significant others		
Reach an agreement (implicit or explicit) to seek answers to the questions: To what degree can the patient engage in required self-care at this time? At a future time?		
Collaborate with patient or family	Identify and describe the patient's repertoire of self-care practices and the usual components of the patient's self-care system	*Diagnostic of self-care agency* Specific existent abilities
Collaborate with patient or family	Identify and describe limitations for deliberate action that interfere with the decision-making and productive phases of self-care, including medically prescribed restriction of activity	Specific existent limitations
Review conclusions with patient or family	Make inferences about the general abilities and limitations of the patient for engagement in the decision-making and productive phases of self-care; formulate and express as judgments	Specific existent abilities and limitations by phases of self-care
Collaborate with patient or family	Validate inferences through continued observation of what the patient does and does not do	Confirmed self-care abilities and limitations

Table 12-3   Operations Related to Self-Care Agency
and its Regulation—cont'd

Interpersonal and Contractual Operations	Professional-Technologic Operations	Type of Operation
Collaborate and reach agreements with patient or family	Determine the adequacy of the patient's knowledge, skills, and willingness to meet each self-care requisite, using particular methods and measures of care	Adequacy of self-care abilities in relation to components of the therapeutic self-care demand
Inform patient or family of the judgment about the presence or absence of a self-care deficit	Make and express judgments about what the patient is able to do, not able to do, and should not do in meeting the prescribed therapeutic self-care demand at this time or at a future time	*Diagnostic of* the presence or absence of a self-care deficit—existing; projected
Reach agreements about prescribed roles with patient or family, nurses, or dependent-care agents	In light of the presence and nature of a self-care deficit, determine what the patient should do, should not do, and is willing to do in the immediate meeting of the prescribed therapeutic self-care demand	*Prescriptive of* patient role and nurse role (or dependent-care agent role) in meeting the therapeutic self-care demand
Reach agreements with patient about prescribed patient role and related nurse role	In the event of an existing or a potential self-care deficit, determine the potential for the future exercise of or the continued development of self-care agency	*Prescriptive of* patient role and related nurse role in regulating the exercise or development of self-care agency

of what persons in position of authority say, or fearful or unknowing. Such information should be limited to what is essential to know in order to work with patients and families. Patients' interests in and concern for their integrated functioning, their acceptance of the reality of their states of functioning, and their appraisal of their need for particular care measures affect what patients will and will not do. Meeting the universal self-care requisite for promotion of integrated functioning and normalcy can be a first step toward patients' collaboration with nurses and their participation in self-care.

Regulation or Treatment Operations

These operations are performed for the attainment of nursing results for individuals. Nursing results are expressed as the continuous meeting of the patient's therapeutic self-care demand, the regulation of the exercise or development of the patient's powers of self-care agency, and protection of the patient's developed self-care capabilities or potential for further development. Regulation or treatment operations are periodic or continuous and may be performed by nurses in conjunction with patients or dependent-care agents.

As nursing diagnosis and prescription proceed, nurses have degrees of knowledge about components of patients' therapeutic self-care demands and the presence, extent of, and reasons for the existence of a self-care deficit. They have a basis for allocation of roles for performing regulatory or treatment operations.

Designs for Performance of Regulatory Operations

Nurses have knowledge from nursing diagnosis about the instrumental role that the patient can fill in the production and management of self-care (no role, some role). Nursing designs for regulatory care should (1) set forth relationships among the components of the therapeutic self-care demand that will result in good regulation of the health and developmental state of the patient, (2) specify the timing and the amount of nurse-patient contact and the reasons for it, and (3) identify the contributions of nurse, patient, and others to meeting the therapeutic self-care demand, to making adjustments in it, and to regulating the exercise or development of self-care agency.

Nurses should keep in mind certain matters as they design regulatory care for patients. For example, some self-care actions, particularly those involving choice, decision, and will, cannot be performed for a patient by anyone else. The provision of appropriate support and environmental conditions may help the patient to gradually acquire competence in these matters. In relation to a patient's requirements for sleep, rest, and activity, nurses may be able to or help others to establish and maintain environmental conditions that are conducive to rest, sleep, or activity, including control of demands placed on the patient. Nurses should also keep in mind that patients may want to do more than they are physically or psychologically able to do. Provisions to help patients set limits on what they are to do in self-care should be included in the nursing systems design. Some patients may not desire or be willing to engage in self-care, even when they are able by objective standards. Here again, nurses may need to foresee the desirability of providing environmental conditions that will encourage or induce patients to assume self-care responsibility.

Patients who want to perform beyond their capacities may test themselves and learn from experience that they cannot do what they had judged themselves able to do. In the same way, reluctant or unwilling patients, when confronted by nurses who want to and know how to assist them to become self-directing, can often move quickly to engage in decision-making and planning activities relating to self-care and to perform selected self-care tasks. In both instances, nurses and patients do not agree as to who shall do what. They are not cooperating in an agreed-upon manner (positive cooperation); they are engaged in a struggle (negative cooperation) (pp. 62-64).[4] This type of cooperation is valid only if nurses' judgments about patients' abilities are sound and if they are motivated by a sincere desire to conserve patients' energies or to help them assume their self-care responsibility. Nurses must be certain, however, that the basis for action is valid so that the situation will not dissolve into a battle of wills. In designing a regulatory nursing system, evidence that indicates that positive or negative cooperation will prevail should be taken into consideration. An important element in designing a regulatory nursing system for a patient and in planning for the complement of nurses required is the identification of the extent and intensity of nurse-patient interaction that is required to meet nursing requirements. The psychological effects on nurses of nursing in various types of health care situations should be thoroughly studied as one of the principal elements for determining more effective and efficient nursing system designs.

Designing effective and efficient regulatory nursing involves selecting valid ways of assisting a patient. The immediacy of patients' needs for self-care, as well as the nature of their self-care limitations, may affect nurses' choices about ways to assist patients. The nurse uses two types of knowledge. One type of knowledge is factual and is derived from or related to the patient. It describes the patient from a nursing perspective and includes detailed descriptions of his or her abilities and limitations for self-care. The other type of knowledge is general and relates to accumulated information about types of therapeutic self-care demands and how the ways of helping can compensate for or overcome limitations for therapeutic self-care. It takes into account the health-related causes of these conditions and factors that affect the effective use of the ways of helping.

When decisions are made about ways of assisting, a pattern or design of a system emerges (see Figure 13-2). The design of a regulatory nursing system for a specific patient becomes more detailed when the roles of nurse and patient are described in relation to (1) self-care tasks to be performed in coordinated patterns and in particular time sequences, (2) making adjustments in the therapeutic self-care demands, (3) regulating the exercise of self-care agency, (4) protecting developed powers of self-care agency, and (5) bringing about new development in self-care agency (e.g., acquiring knowledge, developing specific skills).

In making decisions about valid methods of helping and how to help patients effectively extend their self-care capabilities, it is necessary for a nurse to have for recall a body of knowledge about self-care as deliberate action. Understanding based on previously presented information about the conditions essential for deliberate action, including self-care (Chapter 3), may be extended by further considering that some self-care behaviors are internally oriented, whereas others are externally oriented. See Figure 11-4, which indicates the directional flow of some of these behaviors.

The internally oriented behaviors required for self-care are:
- Learning activities related to the development of self-care knowledge, attitudes, and skills
- Use of knowledge in initiating, performing, and controlling self-care activities
- Self-care action to control behavior, such as controlling an emotional reaction, facing the reality of one's state of health or disability, or restricting one's activities in order to rest or keep a part of the body immobilized
- Action to monitor one's condition or responses

The externally oriented behaviors required for self-care are:
- Knowledge-seeking activity directed to printed material or to persons who possess knowledge about health, disease, and effective self-care practices
- Resource-seeking activity related to securing equipment, materials, facilities, and services necessary in self-care
- Resource-utilizing activities related to using supplies or equipment in performing self-care
- Action to control factors in the external environment, for example, controlling the movement of air, the number of social contacts, or biological elements in the environment
- Action to seek assistance to accomplish a self-care goal within an interpersonal situation, for example, requesting help in performing a self-care task, seeking validation of a judgment, or asking not to be left alone
- Expressive interpersonal activity, such as when a patient expresses feelings about health or self-care verbally or nonverbally but without a direct request for help
- Action to become aware of one's location in an environment or of environmental conditions

The internally oriented behaviors necessary in self-care depend on awareness of self and environment, developed knowledge and skills, as well as motivation and interest. The internally oriented self-care behaviors of a patient at any particular time always depend in part on acquired knowledge about the goals and practices of self-care. This knowledge may have been acquired in the family setting, in school, in social contacts with friends and associates, or through previous contacts with physicians and other health workers. Limitations in awareness, in valid knowledge about the nature and meaning of self-care, in self-care skills, and in initiating, directing, and controlling behavior to accomplish defined goals of self-care affect a patient's internally oriented self-care behavior.

The externally oriented self-care behaviors are need-fulfilling behaviors with an external environmental orientation. Factors in the patient or in the environment may be instrumental in prompting a person to behave in one of these ways. Ability to engage in specific goal-seeking activities is a prerequisite for the externally oriented self-care behaviors listed earlier. In a nursing situation, the kinds of externally oriented behaviors in which a patient will seek to engage, or should be helped to engage, are related to the patient's self-care habits, perceived needs for care, objective requirements for care, and need to express feelings or impart or secure information. Environmental conditions, as well as the person's capabilities for various forms of deliberate action and existent self-care limitations, are relevant to these behaviors.

In summary, an effective nursing system provides ways to relate behaviors of both nurse and patient to the accomplishment of nursing goals appropriate to the situation. Adjustment of nurse and patient behaviors to immediate conditions and to projected future conditions is accomplished through the selection of helping methods and definition of roles. The nature of the patient's specific limitations for self-care and the patient's degree of deficit for self-care are important and continuing considerations, as is the health care focus.

When a nurse selects a system of assistance for the immediate care of a patient, she or he may not have sufficient knowledge for making projections about how the selected forms of assistance should change with anticipated changes in the patient's condition. Nurses should systematically collect information about their patients to enable them to project requirements for changes in the initially selected system. Designing systems of nursing assistance for individual patients is not a commonly recognized activity of nurses in health care agencies. Designing is an essential professional nursing activity because a nursing plan has as its central focus the delivery of some selected system of nursing assistance.

Planning for Regulatory Operations

Planning as an aspect of the technologic nursing process is the movement from designs for nursing systems or for portions of such systems to ways and means for their production. A plan sets forth the organization and timing of essential tasks to be performed in accordance with role responsibilities. If a design is partial, the plan for using the design to guide nursing actions will also be partial. *Partial* is used in the sense of not complete, related to the duration of time that a person will be under nursing care. At times, nurses may not separate design and planning operations from diagnostic and prescriptive operations. In such instances, plans are short-term and integrated with nurses' judgments and decisions about the specific task performance roles of nurses and patients.

Planning adds to the proposed nursing system design specifications of the time, place, environmental conditions, and equipment and supplies required for the production of the system. Planning also produces specifications for and selects the number of qualified nurses or others necessary to produce a designed nursing system or a portion thereof, to evaluate effects, and to make needed adjustments. When planning is for the immediate performance of a selected self-care task, it may amount to a judgment by a nurse that, under prevailing conditions, "The patient can and should do this. I will remain here to support the patient. Betty will get the supplies needed." In scheduling the performance of self-care measures, nurses should take into consideration (1) the relationships among the components of a patient's therapeutic self-care demands, for example, arranging the performance of measures of self-care to enable patients to have periods of uninterrupted rest and sleep, and (2) the provision for assistance when patients need it, for example, in helping patients with elimination.

Production of Regulatory Care

Regulatory nursing systems are produced when nurses interact with patients and take consistent action to meet their prescribed therapeutic self-care demands and to regulate the exercise or development of their capabilities for self-care. A valid design for one or a series of nursing systems to be instituted for a patient can be used as a guide in the production and management of regulatory care. The planning for implementation of the design and related procurement activities will determine when nurses should be with patients and when essential materials and equipment will be available and ready for use. In this, the third step of the technologic nursing process, nurses act to help patients meet their therapeutic self-care demands and regulate the exercise or development of their abilities to engage in self-care.

Systems of nursing oriented to regulation or treatment should be produced and managed for patients as long as the self-care or dependent-care deficits exist. Systems for regulatory nursing at times are replaced by systems of assistance provided by persons other than the nurse who are prepared to perform some measures of self-care for others. In such instances, nursing consultation and supervision should be available to both the person with the care deficit and the persons providing care. In all such situations, a professional nurse should participate in the development of the regulatory care system design whenever patients and families cannot.

Regulatory nursing systems are produced through the actions of nurses and their patients during nurse-patient encounters. Nurses during these encounters will take action to:

1. Perform and regulate the performance of self-care tasks for patients or assist patients with their performance of self-care tasks
2. Coordinate self-care task performance so that a unified system of care is produced and coordinated with other components of health care
3. Help patients, their families, and others bring about systems of daily living for patients that support the accomplishment of self-care and are, at the same time, satisfying in relation to patients' interest, talents, and goals
4. Guide, direct, and support patients in their exercise of, or in withholding the exercise of, their self-care agency
5. Stimulate patients' interest in self-care by raising questions and promoting discussions of care problems and issues when conditions permit; be available to patients at times when questions are likely to arise

6. Support and guide patients in learning activities and provide cues for learning as well as instructional sessions
7. Support and guide patients as they experience illness or disability and the effects of medical care measures and as they experience the need to engage in new measures of self-care or change their ways of meeting ongoing self-care requisites
8. Monitor patients and assist patients to monitor themselves to determine if self-care measures were effectively performed and to determine the effects of self-care, the results of efforts to regulate the exercise or development of self-care agency, and the sufficiency and efficiency of nursing action directed to these ends
9. Make characterizing judgments about the sufficiency and efficiency of self-care, the regulation of the exercise or development of self-care agency, and nursing assistance
10. Make judgments about the meaning of the results derived from nurses' performance of the preceding two operations for the well-being of patients and make or recommend adjustments in the nursing care system through changes in nurse and patient roles

The first seven operations constitute direct nursing care, that is, the action system that makes up the treatment or the regulatory phase of nursing. These operations are performed by nurses at moments when patients can benefit from these seven operations. They are selected and performed by nurses in accordance with the presenting needs and conditions of patients. The last three operations are for the purpose of deciding if direct nursing care should be continued in the present form or if it should be changed. Nurses' performance of the first seven operations and facts about patients' presenting needs and conditions are recorded in *patients' charts to document nurses' day-to-day direct care actions.* The results and recommendations resulting from nurses' performance of the last three operations are recorded as *progress notations.* Such notations document the basis for nurses' judgments about the effects of patients' current self-care regimens, their self-care agency, and the sufficiency and efficiency of nursing.

The direct nursing care actions of nurses may be started during nurses' first encounters with patients during the period of initial nursing diagnosis. Assisting patients with self-care or performing direct care operations cannot be deferred until nursing diagnosis is complete or until there is a formalized design for a regulatory nursing system. Diagnostic, prescriptive, and design and planning operations may be sequentially performed with the interposition of direct care actions whenever needed by the patient.

To understand the production of regulatory nursing care, it is necessary to visualize the distribution and duration of nurse-patient encounters, the kinds of operations nurses engage in during these encounters, the nursing focus maintained by nurses in relation to known health care focuses, and the helping methods nurses select in relation to the presenting needs and conditions of the patient and existing environmental conditions. The need for the performance of some self-care tasks at particular times can be anticipated. The degree to which tasks to meet patients' therapeutic self-care demands and to regulate self-care agency can be programmed by time and place varies with the stability of patients' health states and their health care regimens. The number of nurses required to produce a system of nursing for a patient varies with the intermittent or continuous nature of patients' self-care requisites, degrees of physical helplessness and dependency on others, states of development, the degree of stability of health states, the familiarity or strangeness of the environments in which health care is received, and, of course, what individual nurses can and should do within a particular time period. The frequency and duration of contact between nurse and patient must be sufficient for the intermittent or continuous performance of some or all of the 10 operations required for the production of effective regulatory nursing care.

Nursing practice situations in which patients require nursing over the 24 hours of the day range from those in which a professionally qualified nurse is unable or just able to provide continuous nursing for one patient without assistance, to those in which one nurse can effectively provide care to a number of patients during the same time period with or without assistance. In ambulatory care, nurses may carry large case loads of patients, the number of patients being related to the frequency of required nurse-patient contacts and the length of visits. When nursing is provided through home visits by the nurse, the number of patients in a nurse's case load is affected by the frequency of visits, the kind and amount of care provided, and travel time. When more than one nurse is contributing to the production of nursing, there are requirements for coordinating nursing operations, clarifying the goals being sought through nursing, and socializing patients to a number of nurses. In a situation of this type, patients without guidance and direction may be unaware of their own roles and the roles of nurses with whom they have contact.

Control Operations

Control operations include observation and appraisal to determine (1) if regulatory or treatment operations are performed periodically or continuously according to the design for the system of nursing under production for a patient; (2) if the operations performed are in accord with the conditions of the patient or the patient's environment for the regulation of which they have been prescribed, or if the prescription is no longer valid; and (3) if regulation of patient's functioning is being achieved through performance of care measures to meet the patient's therapeutic self-care demand, if the exercise of patient's self-care agency is properly regulated, if developmental change is in process and is adequate, or if the patient is adjusting to declining powers to engage in self-care.

Control operations answer certain questions. The first control operation asks the question: Is this person receiving regulatory nursing treatment? The second asks the question: Are regulatory and treatment operations valid in relation to prior conditions and/or current conditions? The third control operation asks the question: Are nursing results being achieved and to what degree? All questions demand investigation, including observation of what is currently existent or in process, and all demand a standard against which appraisals are made.

The standard for the first question is the role responsibility of nurses, patients, and others and the use of methods of helping implicit in the statements of role responsibilities for (1) performance of self-care measures or (2) the regulation of the exercise or development of self-care agency. There are two standards for the second operation. The first is the continued existence of the human or environmental conditions they were prescribed to regulate. The second is the presence of new, not previously existent conditions or the absence of prior conditions. The third operation has as its standard the therapeutic self-care demand prescribed and its potential for bringing about functional stability or desired functional change in the patient. It also has as its standard the patient's prescribed roles in self-care and the patient's potential for developmental or regressive change.

Control operations are professional-technologic operations of nursing practice that can be performed concurrently with regulatory or treatment operations of nursing practice. They can also be performed in separation from them at intervals during the period when the patient is being nursed and before discharge from nursing or transfer to another nursing service. The second volume of the report of the Horn and Swain study of criterion measures of nursing care[5] provides nursing students and nurses with finely developed examples of measures for appraisal of nursing care. The process for developing these criterion measures of nursing care is described in a 1977 article by the nurses who formulated them (pp. 41-45).[6]

BASIC CONDITIONING FACTORS AND NURSING OPERATIONS

The self-care deficit theory of nursing presents conceptualizations of two patient variables—therapeutic self-care demand and self-care agency. Nurses direct the exercise of their powers of nursing agency toward identification of the features of these variables and toward their regulation. Development of the theory revealed 10 **basic conditioning factors** (Chapter 8) that can affect not only individuals' self-care requisites and valid methods for meeting them but also their development and exercise of self-care agency. The 10 factors are shown in Figure 12-1.

Nurses' use of the factors in performing the operations of nursing practice is evident in design units A, B, D, and E and in the background information of the nursing case design in this chapter. Basic conditioning factors that are obstacles to meeting the universal self-care requisites are presented in Appendix C. Many of the identified obstacles are physical or psychic health state factors; other types of factors are included in the listing.

To further clarify the use of the factors in nursing practice, an example of use by clinical nursing specialists in one hospital is presented. This is followed by a description of the practical value of the basic conditioning factors.

Pattern of living
of
THIS INDIVIDUAL
MAN, WOMAN, CHILD
of this

Age   Gender

in this

Development state   Health state

affected by
Health care systems factors

Family system factors   Sociocultural factors

Availability of resources
and
Environmental factors

Figure 12-1   Types of factors that condition the values of or means for meeting or regulating the patient variables therapeutic self-care demand and self-care agency.

Nurses' Use of Basic Conditioning Factors, an Example

Basic conditioning factors can be used and grouped in a number of ways. One organization of factors was revealed by an analysis of material descriptive of nursing cases reported by clinical nursing specialists in a hospital serving a population, the members of which had many characterizing features in common.[7]

In analysis of described cases it was found that information about basic conditioning factors was used and organized in four sets in the process of describing nursing cases. The first set of factors described the person who was nursed. The factors in the set included the following:

- The age and gender of the patient and age by dates of admission for health care in the specific hospital
- The residence of the patient and its environmental features (an environmental factor)
- Family system factors including patient's position in the family and information about other family members, with relevant details about residence and relationship with the patient
- Sociocultural factors including education, occupation, occupational experiences, or life experiences
- Socioeconomic factors including resources currently available or potentially available

These factors describe the person who is in the position of nurses' patient and provide one empirical knowledge base that nurses use in nursing patients.

The second set has only one factor, that is, the pattern of living of the patient. Information sought included usual and repetitively performed daily activities, including self-care measures performed daily; activities performed at other intervals of time, including recreational activities and self-care measures; amount of time spent alone and with others; adjustments in pattern of living imposed by health state or health care system factors; and responsibilities for other persons, a household, pets, a garden, or a business or farm.

The third set of factors included the factors of health state and health care system factors. Health state was conceptualized as having anatomic, physiologic, and psychologic features. Attention was given to the following:

- Documented conditions of health before and during current care period and on discharge: (1) physician's medical diagnosis and named documented conditions and (2) nurse-determined, -named, and -documented conditions
- Health state features identified and described by (1) patient or (2) patient's family members
- Health care system features described by discipline (nursing, medicine, others by name) and by form of care (active, supervisory, consultative) before admission for care or during current care period

The fourth set included the factors of developmental state (adult oriented) in its relation to the existence and the meeting of developmental self-care requisites under known environmental conditions. The focus of the set was on:

- Nurse-observed and patient-described current and future self-management capabilities in relation to current and projected conditions of living within specified physical and social environments and under conditions imposed by health state features
- Patient- and nurse-identified factors necessary for self-management or factors that adversely affect self-management
- Personal developmental potential evidenced by (1) patients' views of the future and goals held and (2) objective appraisals

Practical Value of Basic Conditioning Factors

Basic conditioning factors as understood and worked with by members of the Nursing Development Conference Group "increased the ability of members to deal with the complexity of concrete complementary elements in concrete situations of practice" (p. 170).[1] For example, a person under nursing care is a concrete element in a nursing practice situation, but to know the person as a concrete element the nurse must know the person's health state because of its conditioning effects, that is, the way the person is affected. As "insights about the functions of basic conditioning factors increased so did Group members' understanding of how to sort out and relate patient data in nursing practice situations as well as their understanding of points of articulation of the subject matter of nursing with the subject matter descriptive and explanatory of the . . . factors" (pp. 170-171).[1]

The selection and use of named basic conditioning factors are based on the premise that persons who seek and receive nursing are individuals who at the same time are members of families—families that are units of larger sociocultural groups living in some place or places during the period of each individual's existence in the world.

The basic conditioning factors group themselves into three categories: (1) factors descriptive of individuals who are nurses' patients singly or in groups, (2) factors that relate these individuals to their families of origin or families of marriage, and (3) factors that locate these individuals in their worlds and relate them to conditions and circumstances of living.

Factors descriptive of individuals include age, gender, and developmental state. Factors that locate persons within family constellations and sociocultural groups are broadly expressed as sociocultural orientations and family system factors. The factors that describe individuals in their worlds of existence include health state, health care system factors, patterns of living, environmental factors, and resource availability and adequacy.

Information that describes basic conditioning factors in each nursing case must be obtained by nurses initially and on a continuing basis as necessary throughout the duration of the provision of nursing. Some factors will remain stable; others will fluctuate or change. Relationships among factors must be understood. With infants and children, age is actively related to developmental state and health state to both age and developmental state. With mature adults both age and developmental state have achieved their own stability, and health state may be the most active conditioning factor. With persons in advanced age, the condition of aging and health state factors will be seen as related factors.

In nursing practice situations nurses obtain information about basic conditioning factors in a variety of ways. Information is obtained from patient records, including medical history and the medical diagnosis and medical prescriptions, by direct questioning of patients or members of their families, by observing what patients and family members say and do, and more formally by taking a nursing history and by health state assessment. Nurses obtain such information to have it available for making nursing judgments and decisions and for guiding the practical endeavors of nurses.

Nurses' use of information about basic conditioning factors relative to the societal, interpersonal, and interactional aspects of nursing has been described in some detail. The use of such information, as it affects the patient properties of self-care agency and therapeutic self-care demand, has been developed. To further understand this, the relationships of basic conditioning factors to the substantive structure of self-care agency and therapeutic self-care demand should be made explicit.

Information about each of the 10 basic conditioning factors may be necessary for use in calculating patients' therapeutic self-care demand. The information is necessary for (1) particularizing universal self-care requisites and (2) identifying obstacles to be overcome if universal self-care requisites are to be met, as well as factors that condition the selection and use of particular technologies or methods for meeting requisites (see Appendix C). Information about health state, health care system factors, pattern of living, and environmental factors is relevant to the identification and description of the health deviation components of patients' therapeutic self-care demands. Information about age and gender, developmental state, and sociocultural factors may be relevant in formulation of the therapeutic self-care demand. It is always relevant to the interpersonal dimensions of nursing and to insights about self-care agency. The identification and description of developmental self-care requisites require information about the age and gender of individuals, family system factors, patterns of living, health state and health care system factors, and relevant environmental factors. Sociocultural factors may be of special relevance.

Information about basic conditioning factors to identify self-care capabilities and limitations of patients should be related to the substantive components of self-care agency, with a primary focus on use of information about health state and health care system factors. This process of relating basic conditioning factors to the substantive components of self-care agency can begin with the self-care operations (estimative, transitional, productive) or the power components of self-care agency or with the various sets of capabilities and dispositions foundational for engagement in self-care (see Chapter 11). For example, if there is health state information that a person is comatose, that person can engage in no self-care operations because the person cannot exert and maintain voluntary attention, is not perceptive of his or her life situation, and cannot manage self and act deliberately. Persons who have not developed and incorporated a concept of self as self-care agent into their self-concepts may not be motivated and maintain willingness to consistently perform measures to meet components of their therapeutic self-care demand.

The conditioning factors of age, health state, and health care system factors are considered in some detail with respect to nursing situations and nursing cases in Chapter 13.

OBTAINING AND MAINTAINING AN OVERVIEW OF EACH NURSING PRACTICE SITUATION

Nurses maintain overviews of nursing practice situations for which they bear responsibility in order to manage their own nursing actions as part of their management of nursing cases. Experienced nurses are able to maintain overviews of nursing situations as part of their ongoing nursing activities. Nursing students and nurses not familiar with overviews must learn to recognize the situational elements and features that they should be aware of within the context of the wholeness of situations of nursing practice. The situational elements are persons in different roles with stable or changing social, interpersonal, and professional-technologic orientations and relationships.

Social Features and Relationships

Features and relationships of nursing practice situations that relate such situations to legal and regulatory features of the society include (1) the legitimacy of persons seeking or under nursing care identified in terms of the presence of health-derived or health-associated self-care or dependent-care deficits, (2) the legitimacy of nurses expressed in terms of their competency as responsible persons and the adequacy of their powers of nursing agency in relation to nursing requirements of patients derived from the nature and extent of patients' health-associated self-care deficits, and (3) the contractual relationship of nurses and patients. Patients or their significant others seek help in the form of nursing within the frame of community provisions for health services; nurses (or their employing institution) agree that nursing will be provided. This part of the agreement in many instances is quite vague (see Chapter 4). Nurses usually must clarify with patients and persons responsible for them the role responsibilities of nurses in health care situations and determine what patients expect from nurses.

Social features of nursing practice situations change. Patients' requirements for nursing may increase or decrease in number or kind. Nurses specialized for practice in specific areas of nursing practice may be needed. The number of nurses required to provide nursing during time periods may increase or decrease. Adult patients may move from states of inability to make judgments and decisions about themselves to states of competence or the reverse. Patients' next of kin or legal guardians can move in and out of the status of being decision makers for patients. Nurses in practice situations may make the judgment that their nursing capabilities are no longer adequate as conditions of patients change.

These are only some of the changes that occur in the societal aspect of nursing practice situations. Both nurses and patients (or persons responsible for patients) must initially establish and take action to maintain the legitimacy of the social features and the contractual relationships within the legal and regulatory requirements of the society and the nursing profession.

Interpersonal Features and Relationships

The interpersonal features of nursing practice situations encompass the person elements of each situation and the relationships between or among them. Person elements in nursing situations, as previously indicated, include nurses, nurses' patients, and patients' guardians or next of kin when patients are incapable of decision making about themselves and their affairs. Each legitimate person in a nursing situation must be accepted as a person with role responsibilities and worked with in terms of his or her personality, style of communication, and ways of relating to other persons in face-to-face situations. Individuals may differ in their understanding of their own roles and the roles of others.

Role-determining relationships may need to be clarified initially and throughout the duration of nursing. Nurse relationships to patients within a contractual frame of reference are specified as (1) professional, (2) helping, and (3) nursing. Patient roles within this contractual frame are as partner to an agreement to receive professional service in the form of nursing and as person in need of help in the form of nursing (see Figure 13-1).

Maintaining an overview of the interpersonal features of nursing practice situations includes determining if person elements are present or absent and if persons are interacting, communicating, and cooperating in fulfillment of role responsibilities. It also demands awareness of need for patient role changes and changes in the nature or causes of patients' self-care deficits. This in turn may call for changes in nurses to ensure that nursing agency of nurses is operative and is adequate for the achievement of nursing results for patients. Maintaining an overview also requires recognition of incompatibility and destructive or obstructive behavior on the part of nurses or patients (or persons responsible for them).

Technologic Features and Relationships

Professional-technologic features of nursing practice are determined by nursing identification of the nature, causes, and extent of self-care deficits of patients and their overriding reasons for being under health care. Emerging features include definitions of nurse roles and patient roles (1) in knowing and meeting patients' calculated therapeutic self-care demands in time and over time and (2) in the regulation of the exercise or development of patients' self-care agency (dependent-care agency). Role definition may be followed by role performance by nurses to introduce patients to their roles and by guidance of patients in needed role learning and role performance. When patients can have no role in their care, the nurse(s) bears the entire responsibility. The technologic features of nursing practice situations are produced within a developing or developed interpersonal relationship. These features, too, should conform to the contractual features of the nurse-patient relationship.

Maintaining an overview of a nursing practice situation requires time-specific information about whether self-care requisites have been determined and therapeutic self-care demands have been calculated and self-care limitations diagnosed. It also requires determining if there is continuing action to meet the component parts of patients' therapeutic self-care and if results achieved are positive or negative; if self-care limitations are being overcome, are stable, or are worsening; and determining the nature, degree, and frequency of change in components of the therapeutic self-care demands of patients.

SUMMARY

The content of this chapter is oriented to features and aspects of nursing practice that represent developments of self-care deficit nursing theory within the stages of development of nursing represented in Figure 8-3.

The treatment of nursing agency is a substantive development of the concept introduced in the theory of nursing system, a stage I development. The proposition that *nursing agency varies over a range* is qualified by the specification that the range is *partially determined* by the broad health care focus (groups 1 to 7) of nursing situations and by the types of cases within the groups. This is a beginning of stage II development of the nurse variable nursing agency.

The described nursing practice operations define the developed power that is nursing agency. They promote formulation of developing models and rules of nursing practice, stages IV and V developments. The example of nursing case design represents the results of performance of some of the operations in provision of nursing for a type of nursing case (complete self-care deficit associated with cardiovascular accident) within the more general focus of health care in situations where "quality of life is gravely and irreversibly affected (group 7)." This provides a partial model for compiling information about nursing cases, stage III developments.

The content of the chapter provides some foundation for understanding the complexity of nursing. Nursing education has tended to avoid dealing with nursing's complexity. Teaching nursing as task performance—and this includes the tasks of nursing process—without a general orienting nursing frame of reference is a disservice to nursing students and to society.

References

1. Nursing Development Conference Group, Orem DE, editor: *Concept formalization in nursing: process and product,* ed 2, Boston, 1979, Little, Brown, pp 155-167, 170-171.
2. Gilby T: Introduction and appendix 2, 3, 4: In St. Thomas Aquinas: *Summa theologiae,* vol. 36, Prudence, New York, 1974, McGraw-Hill, pp xiv-xvii, 176-184.
3. Orem DE, Taylor SG: Orem's general theory of nursing. In Winstead-Fry P, editor: *Case studies in nursing theory,* New York, 1986, National League for Nursing.
4. Kotarbinski T: *Praxiology: an introduction to the science of efficient action* (translated by Wojtasiewicz O) New York, 1965, Pergamon, pp 62-64.
5. Horn B, Swain M: *Development of criterion measures of nursing care.* Vol II, *Manual for instrument of health status measures,* University of Michigan-Ann Arbor, 1977, US Department of Commerce, National Technical Information Service PB-267 005.
6. Clinton JI et al: Developing criterion measures of nursing care: case study of a process, *J Nurs Adm,* 7:41-45, 1977.
7. Nursing cases of clinical nursing specialists, The Harry S. Truman Memorial Veterans Hospital, Columbia, Mo., presented at The School of Nursing, University of Missouri, Columbia, Summer Institute on Self-care Deficit Nursing Theory, June 12, 1986.

PART IV

The Practice of Nursing

CHAPTER 13

The Practice of Nursing: The Individual as the Unit of Service

To practice nursing means to be regularly engaged in and responsible for the nursing of one or more persons (singly or in groups) in their time-place locations. Nurses' engagement in the practice of nursing may be continuous; persons for whom nursing is provided change. To practice nursing means to enter into the life situations of others (usually strangers) to function as nurse with social and nursing legitimacy.

335

Persons provided with nursing during the same time duration measured in hours, days, weeks, or months constitute the **case load** of a nurse. The amount of time necessary to provide the kind and amount of nursing required continuously or periodically by nurses' patients affects the number of persons or numbers of groups of persons constituting nurses' case loads. The extensity and intensity of nursing requirements of individuals affect the time requirements for providing nursing and, therefore, the number of patients that nurses can nurse effectively.

Nursing persons in health care situations classed in groups 5 and 6 (Chapter 9) at times may require the continuous presence of more than one nurse at the same time and over the 24 hours of each day. At the other extreme, nurses who practice in nurse-managed clinics and work primarily with ambulatory patients with therapeutic self-care demand components associated with pathologies or with the results and effects of medical treatments that must be met continuously (a subgroup of group 5, Chapter 9) may have very large case loads. Patient clinic visits are scheduled periodically according to need or on request, and visits of individuals do not consume the major portion of a nurse's day.

This chapter further develops the practice features of nursing when nursing is provided for individuals who have health-related self-care deficits. Chapter 14 focuses on practice variations for the provision of nursing to multiperson units of service, including families. The professional-technologic operations of nursing are relevant to the production of nursing for individuals as well as for multiperson units with adjustments for types of units.

The practice features of nursing that are addressed include the following:
1. Stages of nursing and rules of nursing practice
2. Types of **nursing systems**
3. The design function in nursing practice
4. The production of nursing
5. Major factors affecting nursing practice for individuals

These practice features of nursing, when carefully examined, provide a basis for developing insights about the time requirements for the provision of nursing to individuals and also about the extent and complexity of educational preparation required by nurses for the safe and effective practice of nursing. Too many health service organizations that offer *nursing* have no interest in or even an awareness of their need to study the populations they seek to serve from the point of view of their members' requirements for nursing and about the qualification of nurses able to meet a diverse population's requirement for nursing. This chapter and the classification of nursing situations by health care focus repeated from Chapter 9 (see box) provide foundations for the study of nursing requirements of populations and the preparation of nurses that will enable them to care for persons with nursing requirements specific to some range of types of nursing situations.

Nursing Situations by Health Focus

1. Life cycle oriented
2. Recovery oriented
3. Illness or disorder of undetermined origin
4. Defects of a genetic or developmental nature or the biologic state of the premature or low-birth-weight infant
5. Regulation through active treatment of a disease, disorder, or injury of determined origin
6. Restriction, stabilization, or regulation of human integrated functioning
7. Regulation of the effects of processes that have disrupted human integrated functioning, with quality of life gravely affected

STAGES OF NURSING AND RULES OF PRACTICE

Nursing care for individuals is produced in time and over time. The production of nursing by nurses for and with patients or clients is the actual concrete distribution of the health service nursing. Nursing, as previously represented, has the nature of a product, that is, something made. No product in its entirety, including human services, can be made instantaneously. The stage of production described here should not be equated with nurses' instantaneous recognition of a person's need for performance of an emergency care measure and nurses' immediate carrying out of the measure. Stages of production should be recognized in nursing as well as in the manufacture of concrete products. The **stages of production** of nursing, as well as variations within the stages, can be identified in concrete nursing practice situations. Definitive nursing research could be directed to investigation of stages of production of nursing in relation to studies of **nursing cases.**

Three stages in the production of nursing can be recognized in nursing practice situations.
1. The stage of initial contact of nurse(s) and persons requiring nursing care
2. The stage of continuing contacts of nurses and persons who are nurses' patients over some time duration for the production of nursing care
3. The stage of preparation of nurses' patients for discharge from nursing as it is presently being produced for them; discharge from a currently produced system of nursing may be a return to self-care or to dependent-care with or without nursing consultation and supervision or discharge to another arrangement for the provision of nursing

Each of the stages may vary in duration and in the sequence of operations performed by nurses. Each stage places demands on nurses to conduct themselves in ways that recognize and support their patients and are conducive to achievement of nursing goals in relation to broader goals of health and well-being for patients.

The three stages for the production of nursing are further developed in terms of the orientations and operations of nursing practice and rules that should guide nurses' behaviors and functioning in practice situations. **Rule** is used to mean a principle that governs the conduct of nurses in practice situations by specifying proper ways of thinking or acting to achieve nursing results for patients. Rule is not used in the sense of regulation but in the sense of instructive and prudential rules (pp. 93-136).[1] The rules presented are general rules, applicable in all situations of nursing practice by stage or by the identified orientation. It should be understood that rules do not hold under all conditions and circumstances. The content of the chapter may appear to be repetitious. It is the context within which content is presented that is important to student learning.

The stages of production of nursing provide the format for nurses' documentation of their own actions, their observations of patients, patients' statements about themselves, and patients' requests. Stages also provide the format for making statements about nurses' judgments concerning the progress of patients (nursing progress notes) with respect to knowing and meeting their therapeutic self-care demands (including cooperation with others) and in the use or development of their self-care capabilities.

The Initial Period of Contact

Nurses in the initial period of contact with patients reveal to themselves and to others their acceptance of themselves as responsible nurses, their degree of socialization to nursing practice and to particular types of nursing situations and nursing cases. One general goal of nurses in initial periods of contact is to convey to the other (the patient) personal acceptance and recognition of the individuality of the other, for example, by addressing the patient and by forms of address used. The right of the other to seek nursing is recognized. The need to determine if and what kind of nursing is required, if the need is not overt, is expressed. Nurses with recognition that self-care requisites must be met continuously but periodically in time will take action to ensure that immediately required self-care measures are performed.

The duration of initial periods of contact and the goals sought and action taken by nurses during this period vary with the "health focus" of the broad health care situation of the patient (groups 1 to 7 health care situations, Chapter 9 and box on p. 333). Duration also varies with the self-management capabilities of patients, their developed and operative powers of self-care agency, and the urgency of meeting presenting or emerging self-care requisites. Ten rules to guide nurses in their initial periods of contact with patients are offered. Types of variations in the presenting condition of patients would determine need for nurses' adjustment of rules. Rules to guide nurses in the initial period of contact include:

1. Enter nursing situation in accordance with held credentials for nursing practice and occupational-professional status.
2. Initiate contacts with potential or actual patients in accordance with social norms, with receptiveness, and in a manner that is adjusted to patients' overtly perceptible states of health and well-being.

3. Convey in initial contacts with patients and their families what knowledge you have about reasons for patients being under health care for confirmation or the raising of questions that will provide historical or current information about patients' health care situations.

4. Determine in initial contacts with patients the presence or absence of gross evidence of a self-care deficit (see Chapter 11) and whether immediate regulatory nursing care to meet one or a number of self-care requisites takes precedence over engagement in detailed nursing diagnostic procedures.

5. Accept each patient as having continuing requirements for self-care and from some capacity to no capacity for its provision.

6. Determine in initial contacts with patients or with persons acting for them who has been the continuous provider of care to meet patients' therapeutic self-care demands and then come to an agreement about who will be the care agent(s) during the processes of nursing diagnosis and nursing prescription. Possibilities include the following:

   a. Patients will continue to meet the usual components of their therapeutic self-care demands. Patients will have appropriate guidance and directions from nurses if there are needs for adjustments.

   b. Patients will continue under a system of dependent-care. Dependent-care agents will have appropriate guidance and direction from nurses if there are needs for adjustments.

   c. Patients and nurses together will maintain the continuing system of care to meet the usual components of patients' therapeutic self-care demands, making adjustments as needed.

   d. Nurses become the agents who maintain patients' continuing systems of self-care.

7. Know the parties to, the conditions of, and the place of self as nurse in the agreements under which nursing is provided to patients for some specified or unspecified duration of time.

8. Confirm one's relationship as nurse to patients. Express the bases for the relationship, role responsibilities as nurse, and manner and procedure of working with patients and patients' families.

9. Elicit patient or family expectations of the nurse(s) and their insights about their immediate roles in the nursing situation as a basis for confirming that roles are understood or for negotiating roles.

10. Assess one's legitimacy as nurse in the situation and one's willingness and fitness to proceed with the provision of nursing.

Variations in Practice in the Initial Period of Contact

The practice endeavors of nurses in the initial period of contact vary with the physical and psychic states of patients and their immediate requirements for care. Three variations and the bases for them are identified: variation 1, with overt evidence that patients' powers of self-direction and self-management are operational; variation 2, with overt evidence of extensive limitations for engagement in self-care and presenting needs for the immediate performance of care measures; variation 3, with overt evidence of physical and psychic distress, acuity of illness, debilitation, or disordered vital processes. What nurses should do in initial contacts with patients varies with the named presenting conditions of patients.

Variation 1. Nurses who initially encounter persons who evidence capabilities in self-management, are self-directing, and can follow directions (variation 1) proceed according to the presented rules of practice. Information sought and action taken follow nursing design units A, B, and C (see box and subsequent section of this chapter). In general, nurses seek to:

1. Establish the legitimacy of the nursing practice situation.
2. Determine the health care situation of the patient and presenting evidences of overt or predictable requirements for nursing.
3. Begin socialization of self and patient to the new developing nursing practice situation.
4. Identify by conversing with patient his or her awareness of self-care requisites to be met by the immediate performance of care measures; if there are, assist by helping the patient perform the measures or by performing them (to the degree possible) for the patient.
5. Identify with or for the patient the care measures within the patients' ongoing system of self-care or dependent-care; add new medically prescribed care measures and nursing prescribed measures.
6. Reach agreement with patient about nurse, patient, or dependent-care agent roles in the continuous provision of self-care during the ensuing process of nursing diagnosis and establishment of a regulatory regimen of self-care and nursing. See rule 6a, b, c, and d for possible role allocations.

Nurse and patient should then be ready to move to the second stage.

Variation 2. Nurses who initially encounter persons who have extensive self-care limitations and immediate need for care move in accord with the overt condition of the patient. Nurses proceed immediately to diagnose and meet

---

Units for Designing Nursing Systems

A. Delineation of the contract for and jurisdiction of nursing
B. Establishment of a socially legitimate and functional unity of persons within nursing practice situations
C. Identification of current or prior components of patients' self-care or dependent-care systems
D. a. Establishment of the components of patients' therapeutic self-care demands
   b. Establishment of resources required to meet the components of patients' therapeutic self-care demands
E. Establishment of self-care capabilities and roles of patients
F. Establishment of the design for the production of nursing, with definitions of and differentiations of roles, statements of nursing results sought, and identified factors that would indicate a need for change in the design

patients' self-care requisites and to ensure the safety, the peace of mind, and the comfort and well-being of the patient. Nurses may then proceed as in variation 1 situations, following the rules of practice for initial period of contact and adjusting them to existent conditions and circumstances. Design units D and E are begun.

Variation 3. In initial encounters of nurses with patients who are in distress, acutely ill, or with disordered vital processes, nurses act to protect patients and to relieve distress. Nurses act in concert with physicians and other care providers to regulate life processes. Nurses ensure that universal self-care requisites are met, using means that overcome identified obstacles to meeting them. The nurse acts for the patient and supports and guides the patient until a degree of stabilization is achieved. In such situations nurses conform to the rules of practice but make adjustments to fit existent conditions and circumstances. Nurses act to formulate design units D and F to ensure continuous adequate and effective nursing in subsequent periods.

Period of Continuing Contacts

The stage of continuing contacts of nurses and patients in nursing practice situations often divides itself into phases. Phases are the function of the initial health care focus of a patient's situation (groups 1 to 7) and health state changes that occur. For example, in a variation 3 initial contact situation the health care focus for the patient is a group 6 focus *stabilization of integrated functioning.* With *stabilization* of functioning the situation changes to a *regulation* focus, group 5, and may proceed to *recovery* with or without permanent dysfunction, group 2 focus.

The duration of this stage varies with the health state of the patient and the features of the total health care situation. The period of continuing contacts of nurses and patients involves nurses in continued nursing diagnoses and prescription and the design, operationalization, and production of systems of nursing regulation or treatment.

Adjustments in the care system are made in accord with changes in patients' health states, changes in medical diagnoses and treatment, changes in patients' self-care capabilities or limitations, and progress of patients in knowing and meeting their therapeutic self-care demands.

A critical nursing feature in the stage of continuing contacts is the provision of a developmental environment, as well as nurses' use of support and other appropriate methods of helping. Six general rules of nursing practice for the stage of continuing contacts and 11 rules to guide the production of nursing for patients are suggested.

The 6 general rules to guide nurses in their contacts with patients and families of patients include the following:

1. Initiate and maintain the amount and kind of interpersonal contact and communication with patients that is essential for achieving nursing results with respect to knowing and meeting patients' therapeutic self-care demand and regulating the exercise or development of their self-care agency.

2. Keep the number and timing of contacts with patients adjusted to patients' capabilities for self-protection, self-management, and the attainment of nursing results.

3. Initiate and maintain contact and communication with family members of patients or with persons legally responsible for patients to help them understand the nursing aspects of patients' health care situations now and in the future.

4. Accept patient-initiated contacts with you as nurse as requests for nursing and respond to them with social and nursing appropriateness.

5. Assist patients to become able to initiate contacts with you or designated nurses whenever specific conditions are perceived or whenever patients or their dependent-care agents are unknowing about how to proceed with matters related to patients' therapeutic self-care demands.

6. If you need to be replaced temporarily or permanently, make sure that the nurse is as competent as you.

The 11 suggested rules of practice to guide nurses in their production of nursing are as follows:

1. Engage in nursing diagnosis initially and on a continuing basis to obtain and organize data in order to assess and make and verify judgments about patients' self-care abilities and self-care limitations, self-management abilities within their environmental situations, and the number and characteristics of existent and emerging self-care requisites as a basis for calculating patients' therapeutic self-care demands.

2. Calculate and prescribe patients' therapeutic self-care demands or components thereof.

3. Express and document nursing judgments about the presence, reason for, and extent of patients' self-care deficits.

4. Determine patients' potential for the initial or continuing development of self-care agency or its redevelopment when necessary.

5. Prescribe means for the regulation of exercise or development of self-care agency.

6. Recognize, express, and document the value of effective nursing for the life, well-being, and health of patients with the understanding that, at times, nursing may be essential for life and for maintaining human integrated function or for preventing deterioration of functioning, that nursing may be helpful in maintaining or promoting states of health and well-being of patients, or that nursing should be a limited adjunct to patients' ongoing system of self-care or dependent-care.

7. Design, operationalize, and manage systems of nursing for patients, keeping nurse and patient roles and methods of helping adjusted to changes in patients' self-care agency and in their therapeutic self-care demands.

8. Manage self-as-nurse and features of the environmental setting toward maximizing high-level coordination with patients and their families and toward economy in use of time, energy, and resources.

9. Seek nursing consultation for self and patients with respect to matters of nursing diagnosis, prescription, and regulation whenever you as nurse or patients and their families are unsure about what should be done to attain nursing results or the progress being made in attaining them.
10. Maintain a professional level of documentation of nursing operations performed and results attained.
11. Begin, when patients' condition permits, instructional systems for the preservation and development of their existent self-care or dependent-care capabilities and the preservation of their sense of self.

The Stage of Preparation for Discharge

This third stage of practice in nursing situations is concerned with helping patients and their families to become ready to move from a currently provided system of nursing to another care system. This stage of nursing practice for individuals necessitates that nurses consider the matter of discharge of patients from nursing care as separate from the process of discharge from active medical care or discharge from care facilities such as hospitals. There are failures of nurses and care providers at all levels to adequately attend to this matter of discharge from nursing or to admit that it is or should be a matter of concern for health care providers at the agency or community level.

The number and complexity of components of patients' therapeutic self-care demands and patients' mastery of these components, including observation of factors that require making adjustments to them, are one consideration in making decisions about nursing discharge. Another consideration is patients' operational capabilities and continued limitations (if any) for knowing and meeting the care demand. A third consideration is patients' capabilities for self-direction and management of self and personal affairs. A fourth consideration is the question of whether existent self-care limitations are being or can be gradually overcome or whether they are permanent limitations. To make correct judgments and decisions, nurses must have valid data about the considerations named and the insight and creativeness to know what should be done under existent conditions and circumstances. Nurses must also have knowledge about resources available to patients and their families.

The time period for the stage of preparation for nursing discharge naturally overlaps with and may be a natural part of the prior stage of regulatory nursing care. Regulatory nursing is concerned with the continuous knowing and meeting of patients' therapeutic self-care demands and with the protection of patients' powers of self-care agency and the regulation of its exercise and development toward patients' ability to know, meet, and make adjustments in their own therapeutic self-care demands. Patients' achievements in care in relation to instructional experiences begun in the prior stage should be assessed and decisions made about needs for continued learning, valid instructional methods, and continued contact with nurses.

Nurses' judgments about readiness for discharge are conveyed to patients, their physicians, and patients' families or responsible others. Final decisions of patients and their responsible others include:

1. Return to a system of self-care or dependent-care with or without access to nursing consultation or supervision
2. Return to a system of self-care with an adjunct dependent-care system with or without provision for nursing consultation or supervision
3. Assumption of the responsibility for self-care including the selection, direction, and supervision of assistants or helpers who do the required manipulation and ambulatory work required for performance of self-care measures
4. An articulation of a self-care system or a dependent-care system with a periodic nursing system
5. Movement to residence in a care facility with or without provision for design and development of a professional-level nursing care system

Nurses understand that decisions made by patients and families affect what they should do or can do in the discharge stage of a nursing situation.

Several rules of practice are suggested as guides for nurses in this third stage of provision of nursing.

1. Initiate conversation with patients or their responsible others to recount with them the components of the patients' therapeutic self-care demands, a good order for performing the care measures, resources required, and sources for resources, components, and care measures that require adjustment with change in health state and other factors, and the procedures for making adjustments.
2. Elicit from patients or dependent-care agents their judgments about their capabilities in producing and maintaining an adequate self-care system and their judgments about the amount and kinds of help needed.
3. Provide patients or their dependent-care agents with written prescriptions for the therapeutic self-care demand to be followed and guides for the exercise or development of self-care agency.
4. Initiate and conduct or participate in referrals of patients and families to agencies providing the kinds of nursing or household assistance required.
5. Develop and transmit nursing care summaries and nursing prescriptions as appropriate when patients are transferring to another agency for the provision of nursing.

Common Features of Stages of Nursing

Each stage of nursing involves nurses in interpersonal relationships with patients and with other nurses and care providers. Nurses' interpersonal relationships with patients develop for good or ill as the stages of nursing progress. Incompatibility of nurse and patient is not an uncommon occurrence. From the perspective of both nurses and patients, frequent changes in nurses are not conducive to the production of effective care.

When nursing is provided throughout the 24 hours of a day, more than one nurse will be engaged in providing nursing to a patient. Patients must become acquainted with and interact with a number of nurses. The continuity of nursing may be disrupted, and the demands on patients may produce stress. Without adequate design, planning, and coordination of effort, multinurse situations and frequent change of nurses are stressful for nurses. The number of health professionals providing service to a nurse's patient places both interactive and coordinating demands on patients and nurses.

Rules to guide nurses in interpersonal situations and relationships with other nurses and care providers are suggested.

Rules for interpersonal functioning include:

1. Relate and attend to patients in ways that will protect, preserve, or promote their integrity as human beings, promote well-being, and foster continuing movement toward maturity.
2. Recognize patients' degrees of socialization to their roles in the health care situation.
3. Approach and work with patients as persons who are at specific stages of growth and development, including cognitive development, from particular families, with orientation to self and family, with likes and dislikes, and with values, habits, and lifestyles, and who may or may not view or value themselves as self-care agents or have positive orientations to health.
4. Relate and attend to patients with knowledge of their self-management capabilities based on evidence of their (a) levels of awareness of self and environment, (b) degrees of physical strength and vigor, (c) control of movements, (d) affective state, (e) long- and short-term memory, and (f) cognitive functioning.
5. Become insightful about the expressed perceptions, the overriding interests and concerns, and the fears of patients that interfere with fulfilling their role functions with respect to self-care or to the exercise or development of their self-care agency.
6. Work with patients and members of their families to help patients become active participants in their own care whenever and to the degree that self-care is possible and at the same time compatible with the health results being sought.

Rules to guide relationships with other nurses and other care providers include:

1. Know and communicate with other nurses who participate in the production of nursing for one's designated complement or caseload of patients.
2. Ensure that nursing consultation is available as needed, and keep abreast of rules and procedures for obtaining specialty nursing consults.
3. Maintain and use open channels of communication with the attending physicians of patients under nursing care as needed for nursing purposes and for the achievement of health results for patients.
4. View and accept medical orders written by physicians for their patients as prescribed medical diagnostic or treatment measures that are within the

domain of medical care but may need to be incorporated into these persons' therapeutic self-care demands and their systems of self-care or, when under nursing care, into a nursing system.

5. Maintain and use open channels of communication with other health workers participating in the care of persons under nursing care as needed for nursing purposes and to attain health results by patients.

The rules are general and useful as guides in all types of nursing situations. They provide nursing students with structures for organizing knowledge. They also provide bases for developing more detailed specifications for practice by nurses in various practice settings or specialty areas of nursing who work consistently with particular nursing populations.

NURSING SYSTEMS IN CONCRETE PRACTICE SITUATIONS

In a general sense all the actions of nurses performed in their relationships with specific patients constitute an action system. Nurses' actions with social, interpersonal, and professional-technologic orientations for purposes of analysis could be separated out and considered as subsystems (Fig. 13-1). The theory of nursing system (see Chapter 7) conceptualizes the professional-technologic orientations and operations of nurses, stipulating their occurrence within existent and developing interpersonal frames of reference with contractual features.

This section is a further development of the concept of nursing system with a focus on the *regulatory-productive operations* of both self-care and nursing. Self-care has been described as a regulatory function of mature human beings (Chapter 3). Self-care agency has been identified as the power to engage in the estimative, decision-making, and production operations of self-care (Chapter 11). Nursing has been described from a technologic perspective in terms of nurses' performance of the essential operations of nursing diagnosis, nursing prescription, and nursing regulation or treatment. The ensuing description of nursing systems assumes nurses' prior and continuing performance of diagnostic operations. It assumes nursing diagnosis of the nature and causes of patients' self-care deficits, the calculation of patients' therapeutic self-care demands (see Chapter 10), and valid identifications of patients' self-care capabilities and action limitations (see Chapter 11).

The classification of nursing systems offered in this section represents nursing prescriptions for nurse and patient role allocations and subsequent agreements about roles. Roles specify responsibilities for (1) knowing and meeting patients' therapeutic self-care demands in order to regulate the patients' physical and psychic functioning and development and (2) regulating patients' exercise or development of their powers of self-care agency.

In summary, the concrete elements of nursing systems are the persons who occupy the status of nurse and the status of nurse's patient and the events that transpire between them. These persons are conceptualized as having attributes and powers that legitimate their occupancy of the status of nurse and the status of nurse's patient. Legitimate patients have (1) a therapeutic self-care demand to

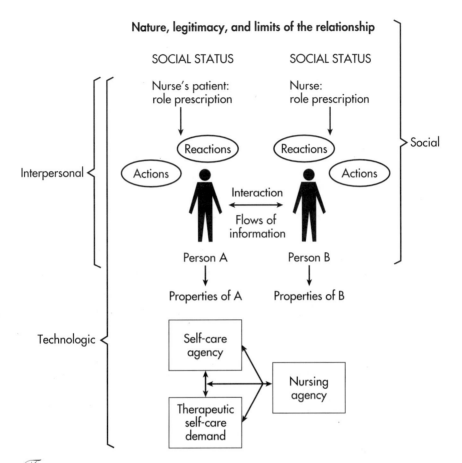

Figure 13-1 Social, interpersonal, and technologic elements of nursing systems.

be met, (2) self-care agency in some state of development and operability, and (3) a deficit relationship between (1) and (2); that is, self-care agency is not adequate in quality or operability for meeting the existing or projected therapeutic self-care demand because of health or health-related factors. Nurses have the power of nursing agency and are willing to exercise their nursing abilities for the benefit of others with health-derived or health-related self-care deficits. These attributes and powers of patients and nurses are viewed as the variables of the technologic (the clinical) component of nursing systems. The relationships between and among the variables in concrete nursing situations are indexes of the nature and purposes of nursing systems.

Nursing systems exist as systems of concrete action produced from the deliberate, discrete actions of nurses and patients in nursing situations. Nursing system projections that nurses (or nurses and patients) make about future actions in regulating patients' self-care agency and in meeting their therapeutic self-care demands are care system designs. Projected nursing systems exist as prescriptions, that is, statements of the type(s) of nursing system that has been judged both effective and reliable in light of the nature of and the factors associated with existing or projected patient self-care deficits. Nursing systems come into existence when nurses and patients operate according to their role prescriptions.

Ideally, nurses see how patients should be immediately helped and foresee how they can and should be helped over some time period. The actual design of a concrete nursing system emerges as nurses and patients interact and take action to calculate and meet patient's therapeutic self-care demands, to compensate for or overcome the identified action limitations of patients, and to regulate the development and exercise of patients' self-care abilities.

Projected designs for nursing systems can be developed when nurses have the necessary knowledge, foresight, imagination, and creative abilities to make a structural design for nurse and patient actions for some projected time period. Nurses who function at the professional level should be skilled in making and projecting designs for nursing systems; all nurses must have some skills in designing or making adjustments in the design of nursing systems. As previously indicated, projected designs for nursing systems for patients are analogous to an architectural blueprint. Projected and emerging designs of nursing systems make clear (1) the scope of the nursing responsibility in health care situations; (2) the general and specific roles of nurses, patients, and others; (3) reasons for nurses' relationships with patients; and (4) the kinds of actions to be performed and the performance patterns and nurses' and patients' actions in regulating patients' self-care agency and in meeting their therapeutic self-care demand. See the design for nursing Mrs. Doe in Chapter 12.

Nursing Systems as Helping Systems

The basic design of a nursing system is that of a helping system (see Chapter 3). Nurses' review and selection of valid ways of helping individual patients follow (1) partial to complete diagnosis of patients' self-care deficits, (2) knowledge of movements that patients should not perform for health reasons, and (3) knowledge about the therapeutic range for energy expenditure by patients. Implicit in selection of valid ways of helping are decisions about nurse and patient role allocations. Roles specified by methods of helping are described in Table 13-1. The table indicates that patients' and nurses' roles vary with each helping method. When nurses use a combination of helping methods in the care of individuals, both nurses and patients must move from one role to another. That which is constant is the social status of both nurse and nurse's patient.

In understanding and classifying nursing systems as helping systems, it is necessary to address two questions: (1) Who can and should perform the actions through which components of patients' therapeutic self-care demands are met according to current prescriptions for them? (2) Who can and should regulate patients' exercise or development of their powers of self-care agency? When

Table 13-1   Nurse and Patient Roles in Nursing Situations as Specified by Methods of Helping

Method of Helping	Nurse Role	Patient Role
Doing for or acting for another	A person who acts in place of and for the patient	Recipient of care to meet the therapeutic self-care demand and to compensate for self-care limitations Recipient of services relevant to environmental control and resources
Guiding and directing another	Provider of factual or techno-logic information relevant to the regulation of self-care agency or the meeting of self-care requisites	Receiver, processor, and user of information as self-care agent or as regulator of self-care agency
Providing physical support	A partner, cooperating in per-forming self-care actions to regulate the exercise of or the value of self-care agency by patient	Performer of actions to meet self-care requisites or regu-lator of the exercise of or the value of self-care agency in cooperation with a nurse
Providing psychologic support	An "understanding presence";* a listener, a person who can institute the use of other meth-ods of helping if necessary	A person confronting, resolv-ing, and solving difficult problems or living through difficult situations
Providing an environment that supports development	Supplier and regulator of essen-tial environmental conditions and a significant other in a patient's environment	A person who is confronted with living and caring for himself or herself in a way and in an environment that supports and promotes personal development

Teaching	Teacher of:
	  Knowledge describing and explaining self-care requi-sites and the therapeutic self-care demand
	  Methods and courses of action to meet self-care requisites
	  Methods of calculating the therapeutic self-care demand
	  Methods of overcoming or compensating for self-care action limitations
	  Methods of managing self-care
		Learner engaged in the devel-opment of knowledge and skills requisite for continu-ous and effective self-care

*Van Kaam A: The art of existential counseling, Wilkes-Barre, Pa, 1966, Dimension Books.

these critical questions are answered, the basis for the structure of a nursing system emerges. Because nurses may use all the helping methods in the process of nursing an individual, the basic structure for a nursing system requires identification.

Types of Nursing Systems

Three basic variations in nursing systems are recognized: (1) *wholly compensatory* nursing systems, (2) *partly compensatory* nursing systems, and (3) *supportive-educative* (developmental) nursing systems.* This typology of nursing systems is associated with the question: Who can or should perform those self-care operations that require movement in space and controlled manipulation? If the answer is the nurse, the system of nursing is wholly compensatory because a nurse should be compensating for a patient's total inability for (or proscriptions against) engaging in self-care activities that require controlled ambulation and manipulative movements. If the answer is that the patient can perform some but not all self-care actions requiring controlled ambulation and manipulative movements, then the nursing system should be considered partly compensatory. If the answer is that the patient can and should perform all self-care actions requiring controlled ambulation and manipulative movements while engaged in self-care agency development, the nursing system should be of the supportive-educative (developmental) type. Figure 13-2 provides an overview of the basic nursing systems.

These nursing systems describe what would be a good organization of the actions of nurses and patients whenever there are conditions such as (1) the patient has physiologic or psychologic limitations for controlled movement in the accomplishment of required self-care, (2) the patient has a self-care requisite to limit energy expenditures because of health state, and (3) the patient lacks knowledge or skill or is not psychologically ready to perform self-care actions requiring controlled movements that must be performed only once or performed continuously for some time but are technically complex and require informed judgments and decisions at each step of execution. The types are paradigms of nursing systems that vary over a range. Max Black's description of range words and range definitions is a useful guide for understanding the process for identifying the three types of nursing systems as well as in identifying possible subtypes (p. 29).[2]

These systems are derived from and relevant to individual nursing situations. When multiperson units such as families are served by nurses, the resulting nursing systems are usually combinations of the features of partly compensatory

---

*It should not be assumed that there is a direct correlation between these types of nursing systems and hospital patient service units referred to as critical or intensive care, intermediate care, and self-care units. In some self-care units nursing may not be provided; at most there may be some general surveillance from nurses. In intermediate care units, wholly compensatory as well as partly compensatory nursing systems may be required by patients. The same may be true in intensive care units. These patient service units are organized according to the principle of acuteness of illness and rapidity of expected change in the condition of patients and to patients' ambulatory states.

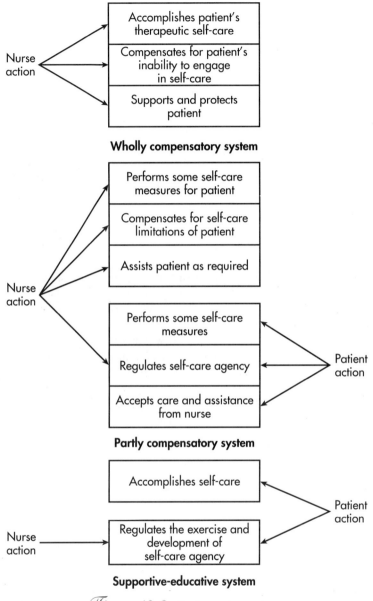

Nurse
action

> Accomplishes patient's
> therapeutic self-care
>
> Compensates for patient's
> inability to engage
> in self-care
>
> Supports and protects
> patient

Wholly compensatory system

Nurse
action

> Performs some self-care
> measures for patient
>
> Compensates for self-care
> limitations of patient
>
> Assists patient as required

> Performs some self-care
> measures
>
> Regulates self-care agency
>
> Accepts care and assistance
> from nurse

Patient
action

Partly compensatory system

Nurse
action

> Accomplishes self-care
>
> Regulates the exercise and
> development of
> self-care agency

Patient
action

Supportive-educative system

Figure 13-2 Basic nursing systems.

and supportive-educative nursing systems. It is within the realm of possibility that families or residence groups would need wholly compensatory nursing systems under some circumstances, but it is advisable at this stage of the development of nursing knowledge to confine the use of the three nursing systems to situations in which individuals are the units of care or service.

Wholly Compensatory Systems

The patient factor that is the criterion measure for identifying the need for a **wholly compensatory nursing system** is inability to engage in those self-care actions requiring self-directed and controlled ambulation and manipulative movement or the medical prescription to refrain from such activity (a health-deviation self-care requisite). Three subtypes of wholly compensatory nursing systems are recognized. Each subtype is based on a complex of limitations for deliberate action that interferes with controlled movements necessary for deliberate actions, including self-care. Persons with these limitations are socially dependent on others for their continued existence and well-being. The subtypes are:

- Nursing systems for persons unable to engage in any form of deliberate action, for example, persons in coma
- Nursing systems for persons who are aware and who may be able to make observations, judgments, and decisions about self-care and other matters but cannot or should not perform actions requiring ambulation and manipulative movements
- Nursing systems for persons unable to attend to themselves and make reasoned judgments and decisions about self-care and other matters but who can be ambulatory and may be able to perform some measures of self-care with continuous guidance and supervision

Persons who fit the first subtype of wholly compensatory nursing are (1) unable to control their position and movement in space, (2) unresponsive to stimuli or responsive to internal and external stimuli through hearing and feeling, or (3) unable to monitor the environment and convey information to others because of loss of motor ability. These persons will be confined to one location in space, unless they are moved by others. They must be protected and cared for. The valid helping method is that of doing and acting for. Nurses and others should speak to these persons with a conversational tone, handle them gently, maintain continuous or frequent contact, and maintain environmental conditions that protect and support normal functioning.

Persons whose action limitations fit the second subtype differ from persons in the first subtype by being (1) aware of themselves and their immediate environment and able to communicate with others (communication powers may be normal or greatly restricted); (2) unable to move about and perform manipulative movements because of pathologic processes or the effects or results of injury, immobilizing measures of medical treatment, or extreme weakness or debility; or (3) under medical orders to restrict movement. These persons may be mentally competent and capable of making accurate observations. They may be involved in making judgments and decisions about self-care and perform self-care actions that do not require movement. They must exercise self-control and develop a style of living that promotes normalcy of outlook and continued personal development and must maintain their willingness to be cared for by others regardless of their reluctance to do so. Nurses use a number of methods to help patients in the second subtype, with emphasis on maintaining a developmental environment and doing and acting for the patient. Patients with these limitations will suffer when neglected by nurses and others and when their interests and concerns are not solicited or are ignored. Psychological support, guidance and direction, and teaching are therefore valid methods also. Prevention of hazards and promotion of normalcy must be given special attention because of the possible deleterious effects of inactivity, restricted environments, and awareness of one's helplessness.

Persons in the third category differ from those in the first two subtypes in that (1) they are conscious but are unable to focus attention on themselves or others for purposes of self-care or care of others, (2) they are not consistent in making rational judgments and decisions about their own care and daily living without guidance, or (3) they can ambulate and perform some measures of self-care with continuous guidance and supervision. Persons characterized by such limitations may bring about hazardous conditions for themselves and, at times, for others. They should be taken care of and protected, and others may need to be protected from them. The helping methods associated with this set of limitations include providing and maintaining a developmental environment, guiding and directing, providing support, and doing or acting for the other.

Wholly compensatory nursing systems have social, interpersonal, and technologic dimensions that must be understood by nurses. These dimensions are related to the extremely restricted ability or inability of persons to manage themselves and to control environmental conditions. From the nursing viewpoint, nurses are not only major providers and managers of patients' self-care but also the makers of judgments and decisions about the self-care requisites of their patients and the designers of nursing care. Nurses have the responsibility to meet all three types of self-care requisites—universal, developmental, and health-deviation—for persons with the types of limitations described here. Nurses must be in close contact and communication with family members, know who is responsible for the patient's affairs, and be able to sort out the nursing responsibility for the patient from family members' rights and responsibilities. The social, interpersonal, and technologic dimensions of these nursing situations require that nurses be the major, and in some instances the sole, contributors to action systems produced to meet the self-care requisites of patients and protect patients' powers of self-care agency and their personal integrity.

Because of the labor involved in providing continuous care to persons with the action limitations identified here, persons other than nurses are frequently placed in positions of responsibility for patients requiring wholly compensatory nursing systems. Nurses have a social responsibility as members of the nursing profession to act to ensure safe and effective care to persons with extensive limitations of self-care agency. This responsibility can be fulfilled when nurses are free enough as professionals to accept the responsibility and are creative and knowledgeable enough to design, put into operation, and manage effective care systems for these persons. They should also be knowledgeable enough to set the specifications for and guide and supervise others who can contribute to the operation of wholly compensatory care systems.

Partly Compensatory Systems

The second system is for situations in which both nurse and patient perform care measures or other actions involving manipulative tasks or ambulation. The distribution of responsibility to nurse or patient for performance of care measures varies with (1) the patient's actual or medically prescribed limitations for ambulation and manipulative activities, (2) the scientific and technical knowledge and the skills required, or (3) the patient's psychologic readiness to perform or learn to perform specific activities. The patient or the nurse may have the major role in the performance of care measures. A **partly compensatory nursing system** may take a number of forms. In one form, patients perform universal measures of self-care, and nurses perform medically prescribed measures and some universal self-care measures. A second form is for these situations in which patients are learning to perform some new care measures. In partly compensatory situations all five helping methods may be in use at the same time.

Supportive-Educative Systems

The third system is for situations in which the patient is able to perform or can and should learn to perform required measures of externally or internally oriented therapeutic self-care but cannot do so without assistance. Valid helping techniques in these situations include combinations of support, guidance, provision of a developmental environment, and teaching. This is a **supportive-educative system.** It is the only system in which a patient's requirements for help are confined to decision making, behavior control, and acquiring knowledge and skills. There are a number of variations of this system. In the first, a patient can perform care measures but needs guidance and support. Teaching is required in the second variation. In the third, providing a developmental environment is the preferred method of helping. The fourth variation is in situations in which the patient is competent in self-care but requires periodic guidance that he or she is able to seek; in this variation, the nurse's role is primarily consultative.

Nursing Practice Implications

The production of each of the three types of nursing systems in concrete situations of nursing practice requires facilitating interpersonal conditions and nurse-patient interactions. The defining of role responsibilities clarifies nurses' responsibilities for their own actions, including their responsibilities for protection of patients, for providing guidance and support, for establishing and maintaining conditions that support development, and for the production of instructional systems. This defining of nurses' role responsibilities has legal as well as professional-ethical connotations.

One or more of the three types of nursing systems may be produced for a single patient over the duration of a period of nursing. For example, patients who are receiving nursing because of surgical treatment involving anesthesia and organ removal may progress from a supportive-educative system to a partly compensatory system to a wholly compensatory system, then back to a partly compensatory system and, finally, to a supportive-educative system before being discharged from nursing. Other patients, especially those in ambulatory care services, may take part in supportive-educative nursing systems, shifting at times to partly compensatory nursing systems. Nurses should select the type of nursing system or sequential combination of nursing systems that will have the optimum effect in achieving the desired regulation of patients' self-care agency and the meeting of their self-care requisites.

Through nursing, patients with extensive action limitations may develop the capabilities needed to design and manage their own self-care and to guide and direct a helper in the provision of care. With nursing consultation and medical supervision, other patients may become able to identify their self-care requisites and to design, provide, and manage their own self-care toward the regulation of the effects of pathology (pp. 422-427).[3,4] The descriptions of the three types of nursing systems and the criterion measures for determining the kind(s) of system(s) needed should be used in examining information about patients' self-care abilities and limitations before prescribing nurse and patient roles. They can also be used to determine whether nurse and patient roles in active nursing situations are in accord with patients' self-care abilities and limitations. This further development of the conceptual structure of the theory of nursing systems articulated in Chapter 7 provides nurses with knowledge that can guide their decision-making and evaluative actions in situations of nursing practice.

The utility of the basic design of nursing systems has been pointed out in relation to the specification of nurse and patient roles and the assisting techniques that the nurse would need to use. Thus, the three nursing systems suggested for the purposes of this text could serve as a guide in the development of a typology of nursing situations for use within health care agencies or communities. Each patient presents specific requirements for assistance that describe his or her need for one or a combination of the three nursing systems. Professional nurses are responsible for accumulating information about patients that describes commonalities and differences in their nursing requirements, including both requirements for assistance with self-care and overcoming obstacles of self-care. The commonalities among specific types of patients, or nursing cases, if identified in terms of factors that specify roles and requirements for specific assisting techniques, would indicate the health agency or community requirement for particular systems of nursing assistance. This information is important in planning for the number and kinds of nurses and nurses' assistants needed to provide a nursing service that will be adequate for a particular population. It is also important for nursing education.

Nursing Systems and Dependent-Care Systems

Changing health care systems brought expectations that persons with major health deviation self-care requisites, major adjustments in the particularization of universal self-care requisites, and the need for specialized technologies in meeting them can be cared for in their homes. Situations range from very young infants born prematurely to children and adults with catastrophic illness and terminal and chronic illness to debilitated elderly persons. Some hospitals, nurses, physicians, or whole communities do not attend to or make provision for ensuring the availability of nursing to individual families with these tremendous care responsibilities. On the other hand, there are outstanding examples of movement to provide not only nursing in the home but also other support services for those needing health care and their families.

Family members in positions of responsibility for ensuring the continuing self-care of others in their homes often strive to develop the knowledge, skills, and interpersonal capabilities and to maintain their willingness for providing continuing dependent-care of others. These persons continue to bear responsibility for their own health and well-being as persons who are self-care agents. Some nurses in hospitals see themselves as responsible for preparing not only patients but also their family members or friends who will bear dependent-care responsibilities for the return home. Nurses have come to see more and more clearly the need to make appraisals, not just of dependent-care capabilities, but also of the health states of persons who are taking on dependent-care responsibilities, including the probable effects of the burden of care on them. This problem is addressed by Taylor and Robinson-Purdy in a reported study "to describe the development of self-care, dependent-care, and professional nursing care systems for hospitalized, about to be discharged patients with physical illness or injury" (pp. 4-16).[5] This paper, an important approach to descriptive studies, identifies, for example, significant limitations of nurses, failures of nurses to assess prospective caregivers, the importance of patients and caregivers coming together to talk about and plan for care at home, and factors that result in dependent-care agents' unrealistic estimates about their capacities to provide dependent-care. The study introduces approaches for continued exploration of this nursing and family problem.

Nurses' contributions to the design of dependent-care systems and planning for their operation and maintenance should be an important consideration in endeavors to develop nursing services that meet needs of communities. The articulation of nursing systems with dependent-care systems is an important consideration whenever there is a need for periodic nursing that is conjoined with a wholly compensatory system of dependent-care (see Chapter 12, example) or with combined systems of self-care and dependent-care.

THE DESIGN FUNCTION IN NURSING PRACTICE

Nurses are admonished to develop plans for nursing care in concrete practice situations, but over the years scant attention has been given to comprehensive design as a function of the professionally educated nurse engaged in nursing practice. Design is recognized in professional fields as prior to and as an essential basis for development of detailed plans for using product and production designs to achieve goals. Design (p. 622),[6] like plan, denotes a proposed way of making or doing something. Design, however, sets forth the disposition of individual elements and details of elements through careful ordering and calculation and suggests a definite pattern for the work to be done. Design implies reference to the achievement of order and the elimination of friction or lack of harmony among the distinct parts or elements of a complex whole. Design also designates attention to integrity of the parts as well as the order, harmony, and integrity of the whole that is to be produced.

The elements of the self-care deficit theory of nursing and their designated relationships identifies or points to concrete conditions and factors that become entities or parts to be dealt with in the production of nursing. Through working with these parts and understanding them and the relationships among them in concrete nursing situations, nurses and nursing students become able to design and produce nursing. Nursing is not a naturally existent entity. It is something constructed and produced by nurses. It is made in time and over time in some place(s) by one or more persons for another person or persons. Simon[7] refers to structured validated knowledge about what is constructed or made as "sciences of the artificial."

Nurses provide help or care in the form of nursing for persons of different ages, in different stages of development, in different health states, and in different time-place localizations. Those who can be helped through nursing become the center of any design for nursing. Men, women, and children who are patients of nurses are unitary beings with singular ways of living and singular life histories. Their behaviors may be disorderly or abberant, spontaneous and unpredictable, or they may behave with accountability and responsibility. All are subject to conditions and conditioning, but it is the individual man, woman, or child who provides that which can be affected (conditioned) (p. 50).[8]

The self-care deficit theory of nursing, with its focus on the realities of men, women, and children, their properties and powers that are nursing-relevant, and the motion or change that occurs in nursing practice situations, points to elements and features of concrete situations of nursing practice with which nurses must deal. These elements and features must be known in detail by nurses, known in their relations to the essential work of producing systems of nursing care for individuals or units composed of individuals. Designing systems of nursing rests on nurses' knowledge (1) of the work to be done and (2) the realities to be dealt with in doing the work. Effective nursing rests on creative design but design that conforms to what is needed and what can be done in practice situations at this time(s), in this place.

Direct personal health services such as nursing are directed to the health and well-being of individuals singly or in groups. Systems of nursing care or systems of medical care are constituted from action sequences, series of events over time to which persons who are nurses' or physicians' patients contribute according to their capabilities. Results of direct personal health care are understood in terms of changes in human or environmental features. Results of health care do not take on existence apart from persons in environments. Nor can the work of designing nursing for a particular individual or group occur in a time period that differs from the time period when nursing care is needed and is being produced. In fields such as architecture and engineering, design is complete, as are plans and specifications, before construction is begun. In both fields, however, professionals must know the work to be done and the concrete realities to be dealt with in designing and doing the work.

A Design Model

Any exercise in explicating the design function in nursing practice demands recognition that through performance of this function nurses form **units of design,** which, when ordered to one another and finally arranged in a creative, orderly, harmonious fashion, constitute patterns for the production of nursing systems toward attainment of nursing results. Design activity begins before production and before planning for production, although there may be the appearance of simultaneity. Understanding the design function in nursing requires acceptance that units must be designed one by one and that the nature of the work of designing of one unit differs from the work of designing other units. Nurses must know the realities to be dealt with in designing each unit; they must also know that different units of design may deal with the same concrete entities and use the same data.

When formed, units of design may exist only within nurses as images of selected elements and features of nursing practice situations in relationship one to another and together constituting a unitary structure. Units of design may be recorded in writing, or they can be communicated verbally. Units of design represent *results* of performance of nursing operations that precede or are concurrent with knowing and meeting components of patients' therapeutic self-care demands and regulating their self-care agency. The design model described here in detail was used in developing the design for the nursing case presented in Chapter 12.

The six design units in the model are based on assumptions that:
1. Nursing has social, interpersonal, and technologic aspects.
2. The self-care deficit theory of nursing, through the substantive structure of its conceptual elements, points to the realities that nurses deal with in nursing practice situations.
3. Nursing design is accomplished through analysis and synthesis of concrete elements of nursing practice situations, bringing them into an orderly relationship to form structural units, the elements of which can be creatively brought together to constitute a pattern to guide the production of systems of regulatory nursing toward attainment of nursing goals.

The units that constitute the model are summarized before presentation of the elements of each unit (Figure 13-3).
A. Delineation within the contract or agreement to receive nursing, nursing's area of jurisdiction in the health care of persons for whom nursing is sought, and an outlining of the health care goals to which nursing will contribute.
B. Establishment of the main features and relationships of a socially legitimate and functional unit of individuals who are person elements of nursing practice situations.
C. Identification of the usual or current components of self-care or dependent-care systems being produced by or for persons who are nurses' patients

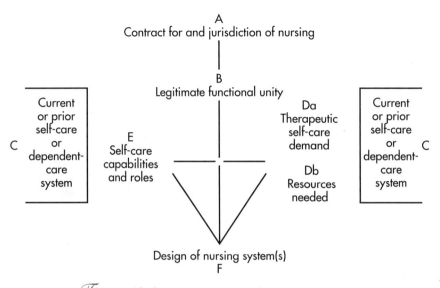

A
Contract for and jurisdiction of nursing

B
Legitimate functional unity

| Current or prior self-care or dependent-care system | E Self-care capabilities and roles | Da Therapeutic self-care demand | Current or prior self-care or dependent-care system |

C   C

Db
Resources needed

Design of nursing system(s)
F

Figure 13-3 Design units, nursing practice situations.

whenever this information is nursing relevant as a base for judging adequacy of care and approaches to change when change is required.

D.a. Establishment of the components of therapeutic self-care demands of persons under nursing care necessary for continuing regulation of their functioning and development, keeping the components in conformity with (1) changes in the number and kinds of self-care requisites and changes in the values at which each should be met and (2) factors that condition the means that can be validly and reliably used to meet self-care requisites, and

D.b. Establishment of the resources needed to meet the components of patients' therapeutic self-care demands.

E. Establishment of the degree to which persons who as nurses' patients (1) can responsibly exercise their developed and operational self-care capabilities without harm to self and (2) continue to develop, improve, or increase their self-care capabilities. Degree would be established in relation to components of the therapeutic self-care demand and the frequency of meeting components.

F. Establishment of the design(s) for the production of a system(s) of regulatory nursing with definitions of and differentiation of nurse roles, patient roles, and roles of participating others, with specification of methods of assistance to be used, the nursing results to be sought, and factors the presence of which would indicate the need for change in the design of the nursing system or a transfer from a nursing system to a self-care or a dependent-care system. Roles are expressed in terms of actions to be performed in order to continue to know and meet patients' therapeutic self-care demands and to protect or to regulate the exercise or development of self-care capabilities or dependent-care capabilities.

Through the work of development of the six design units, nurses establish the patterns, boundaries, and specifications within which they proceed through nursing to overcome or compensate for the action limitations of their patients for knowing and meeting their therapeutic self-care demands and for protecting and regulating patients' exercise or development of their capabilities to engage in self-care within the framework of their self-management capabilities.

Design units serve different purposes. Design unit A sets limits on what nurses do; for example, nursing's area of jurisdiction in a health care situation may range from nurses providing help in knowing and meeting certain identified components of a person's therapeutic self-care demand to nurses' continuous care of persons in comatose states. Design unit B describes the person elements of the operational unit involved in the provision of nursing. Design unit C provides information about the qualitative and quantitative features of current or past self-care or dependent-care systems as one basis of measuring adequacy and determining the need for and possibilities for bringing about change. Design unit D develops the characteristics of and the details for the work of meeting the self-care requisites of patients and the resources needed. Design unit E sets limits for what patients can and probably should do in knowing and meeting their own therapeutic self-care demands and in their regulation of the exercise or development of self-care capabilities. Design unit F provides the pattern for the production of a system of regulatory nursing through establishment of role responsibilities and relationships. See the nursing case design, Chapter 12.

As previously indicated, the development of design units proceeds along with the production of help and care. Nursing design units with their elements enable nurses to seek understanding of their need, not only for conceptualizations of elements but also for images of the details, features, and relationships of all the elements that give form and pattern to the work of nursing. Nurses who accept the foregoing suggestions about the function of nursing design must work through the fit of this function into their already formulated conceptualizations of nursing process. Nursing students who learn how to develop nursing design units and also learn the process operations of nursing practice (investigative and diagnostic, prescriptive, and productive) will be less confused and will understand how design units relate to nursing process.

To the degree that values of their elements remain stable, design units provide the standards and rules nurses need to meet and follow to overcome or compensate for self-care limitations of patients in knowing and meeting their own therapeutic self-care demands and in regulating the exercise or development of their self-care capabilities (or dependent-care capabilities). The process operations of nursing as they relate to design units are identified in Chapter 12.

Design Units

Nursing design in the concreteness of nursing practice situations has its foundation in the contract or the agreement between parties to provide and receive nursing. The first suggested unit of design is concerned with laying out nursing's area of jurisdiction within the context of the health care and the family or broader social situation of persons seeking nursing. The parts of this and other design units are presented in outline form. The parts of units are expressed as types of information required and the kinds of judgments to be made and statements about how nurses use the resulting information and judgments.

Design Unit A: Contract for and Jurisdiction of Nursing

The development of design unit A establishes for nurses who is to be nursed and the person's position(s) in the structure of a family or a residence group and in the health care system, the names of the contracting parties, the general framework for cooperation and coordination of action and functions of communication, and the fit of nursing into the broader systems of health care of persons seeking nursing. It ensures the legality of the nursing situation. If nurses are to have this kind of foundational framework for their nursing endeavors, the following elements of investigation and judgment are suggested:

A.1 Person(s) to be nursed by name, age, gender, position in family, residence, and marital status; if single, name and residence of next of kin; if married, name and residence of spouse

A.2 Reasons for seeking nursing at this time

A.3 Prior caregivers: self, dependent-care agent, nurse

A.4 Time of request for nursing

A.5a Projected character of requirements for nursing in terms of extent and whether periodic or continuous

A.5b Projected time duration of requirements for nursing

A.6 Location(s) for receiving nursing

A.7 Parties to the agreement or contract for nursing:
   a. Adult person(s) who require nursing or next of kin or spouse by name or adult legally responsible for a dependent person, adult or child, who requires nursing by name
   b. Health care agency by name or nurse in private or group practice of nursing by name(s)

A.8 Position in the health care system:
   Under active medical care from physician(s) by name
   Under medical supervision from physician(s) by name
   Under care of other health professionals by name and field

A.9 Reason(s) for being in the health care system

A.10 Health care goals being sought; nursing's fit as contributory to goal achievement

A.11 Impact of reasons for person(s) being in the health care system on their families or friends; obvious requirement for concern for, attention to, or provision of guidance and counseling for families and friends

A.12 Establishment of the authority and responsibility of nurses in accord with nursing's area of jurisdiction

A.13 Number and qualifications of nurses needed and the kinds of resources required

A.14 Method of financing nursing

Design unit A requires for its development information generally obtained when persons are admitted to residence health care agencies or institutions or placed on patient rosters of home health care agencies or clinics. However, nurses must obtain some information from patients, from relatives, or from their physicians. The elements of design unit A established in each concrete situation of nursing practice must be held in mind by nurses throughout the nursing period.

Design Unit B: A Legitimate and Functional Unity

Identifying the persons and the relationship among them, with respect to their functioning, in the nursing practice situation is done initially and thereafter as frequently as necessary. This design unit establishes the persons to be associated with one another; establishes general requirements for communication, coordination of action, and cooperation; fosters persons acting with an operative, dynamic sense of duty; and establishes the characterizing developmental and functional features of the person(s) to be nursed. It ensures the nursing legitimacy of the situation of nursing practice. The following are the suggested elements established and ordered in relationship to one another.

B.1a Capabilities of persons who are nurses' patients for self-management in a customary or a changed environment

B.1b Self-management limitations associated with age and developmental stage, health state factors, health care system factors, environmental features

B.2a Degree to which persons who are nurses' patients have been providing their own self-care, or have been provided care within a dependent-care system, degree to which assistance with self-care has been provided and by whom

B.2b Existent limitation for engagement in self-care by type of self-care operation—estimative, decision making, productive

B.3 Projections about probable emergence of types of self-care limitations or worsening of existent ones or overcoming existent ones

B.4 Degree to which members of families or friends will be involved with the nurses' patients and their needs for association and communication with nurses

B.5 Existent and required capabilities and areas of nursing responsibility of nurses who are operational participants in the nursing situation during specified time periods with specification of areas of independence and interdependence and modes of communication

B.6 Needs and provisions for nursing consultation and supervision

B.7 Interpersonal features of the nursing situations according to the general characteristics of the agreement or contract for nursing with general role specifications

B.8 Modes of communication and documentation relative to the kinds of events that demand immediate communication, for example, patient to nurse,

nurse to patient, nurse to nurse, patient and nurse to physician, patient to family, nurse to family, family to nurse

B.9 Communication channels for nurses' patients who need assistance with respect to personal affairs and interests outside the domain of nursing

B.10 Modes for fostering an active, operative, dynamic sense of duty in all participants

Design unit B identifies the operational participants in the nursing situation, recognizes areas of independence and interdependence of functioning, designates modes and channels of communication, and identifies general areas of responsibility of participants.

Design Unit C: Self-Care or Dependent-Care System Components

Given nursing's area of jurisdiction in a health care situation, it may be necessary initially or at other times to know the components of patients' self-care or dependent-care systems. This information is necessary if nurses must know the completeness and adequacy of some or all components or if new components must be introduced.

C.1 Establish what the patient or dependent-care agents customarily do (care practices engaged in) to meet universal self-care requisites and the frequency of use of named care practices.

C.2 Establish the developmental self-care requisites that are understood and the care measures used to meet them.

C.3 Know obstacles that interfere with the methods of care that are regularly used to meet universal and developmental self-care requisites.

C.4 Establish the presence or absence of types of care system components to meet health-deviation self-care requisites, including regulation of symptoms the patient experiences and discernible effects and results of particular medical components.

C.5 Establish how self-care or dependent-care system components articulate with patients' and dependent-care agents' patterns of daily living.

Design unit C is formed through recounting by a patient, family member, or dependent-care agent of what is being or has been done to meet patients' self-care requisites with some degree of stability or what has been recently introduced. Nurses also observe what patients and dependent-care agents do.

Design Unit D: Therapeutic Self-Care Demand

Design unit D establishes the amount and kind of essential to desirable action to control factors (keep them within norms compatible with human life, health, development, and well-being) that contribute to the regulation of human functioning and development. For example, meeting the universal self-care requisite "maintain a sufficient intake of food" provides for an intake of food (the factor being controlled) that is in accord with established norms for quality and quantity of food required according to (1) age and developmental stage and state of an individual; (2) conditions and circumstances under which the person lives, for example, an active or sedentary life, hot or cold climates; and (3) health states characterized by certain disorders.

Design unit D is developed through investigation, data analysis, synthesis of data, and judgments about qualitative and quantitative values at which self-care requisites should be met, along with specifications about frequency and timing. Values of requisites are particularized for individuals, means are selected for meeting requisites, and work of meeting each particularized self-care requisite is outlined in the form of sets of care measures to be performed and resources required.

Details about self-care, self-care requisites, and therapeutic self-care demands are given in Chapter 10. Here only elements of the design unit are set forth.

D.1a Establish from authoritative sources values at which each universal self-care requisite should be met for individuals of the patients' age and gender, developmental stage and state, and environmental conditions under which they live.

Know the values at which universal self-care requisites have been or are being met for the patient.

Know existent or predicted conditions and circumstances that indicate need for change from recommended norms or from values at which universal requisites have been or are being met.

Calculate the qualitative and quantitative values at which each universal self-care requisite should be met.

D.1b Establish from authoritative sources and from experiential knowledge valid and reliable means for meeting each requisite, for example, means for food intake for a 3-month-old infant with a cleft palate.

Know existent conditions and circumstances that interfere with use of the usual valid and reliable means for meeting each requisite, for example, the inability of a patient to swallow as related to maintaining an adequate intake of food.

Know conditions internal to patients as well as external conditions and circumstances that constitute obstacles to or interferences with meeting each requisite, the nature of the interference, tested ways, including medically prescribed ways, for surmounting the interference, and estimating if, how, and to what degree the effects of the obstacle can be controlled, for example, the effects of emphysema on maintaining an adequate intake of air.

Establish for each universal self-care requisite the required process and the means that will be used to meet each universal self-care requisite at values particularized for patients and establish the sets of care measures, which, if effectively performed, should attain these goals of meeting each requisite.

Identify for each universal self-care requisite the resources needed to meet each requisite, using the selected means and identifying resources in relation to each set of care measures.

D.2 Establish the developmental type of self-care requisites that nurses' patients have been, are, or should be meeting.

Know developments that are in process in patients and the environmental conditions that will promote physical, psychological, cognitive, and social developments; know developments that should be brought about because of existent or emerging conditions and circumstances, for example, need for rehabilitation of the patient's self-concept because of the presence of disabling conditions.

Know existent conditions and circumstances that interfere with or are obstacles to development and the degree to which they are controllable through use of valid and reliable means.

Identify developmental self-care requisites associated with patients' age, gender, stage of development, and health state; establish the environmental conditions and other means through which they can be met and the resources required.

D.3 Establish the health-deviation self-care requisite associated with patients' states of health and their system of medical care that patients have been or are meeting.

Identify specific features of the health states of patients and the diagnostic and treatment modalities used in their medical care with knowledge as to how they are being experienced by patients and the impact on patients. Express existent and emerging health-deviation self-care requisites, including the qualitative and quantitative values at which they should be met, including changes in values of universal self-care requisites.

Identify the sets of care measures to be performed, given particular health-deviation self-care requisites, required processes, selected means for meeting them, and the resources required.

D.4 Establish the order that should exist between and among the sets of care measures through which universal, developmental, and health-deviation self-care requisites are to be met.

Structure sets of care measures in relation to time and place of performance, energy demands of performance, economy of use of resources, and other factors such as duration of time required for performance.

Identify essentiality and contributions of sets of care measures to the continuing regulation of patients' functioning and development.

Design unit D, the calculation of patients' therapeutic self-care demands, establishes one of the patient variables identified in the self-care deficit theory of nursing. It specifies the self-care to be produced by or for patients.

Design Unit E: Patients' Self-Care Roles

The outcome of design unit E is the establishment of what patients can do, should do, or should not do in the interest of their own health and well-being while under nursing care to meet specific particularized self-care requisites, to protect their power of self-care agency, and to continue to develop capabilities to know and meet their own therapeutic self-care demands.

E.1 Know the components of patients' therapeutic self-care demands that they (a) have been or are meeting and can continue to meet without assistance and (b) have been or are meeting and can continue to meet with guidance and support.

   Know emerging internal or external conditions and factors that will interfere with one or both of the foregoing and their probable time of occurrence.

E.2 Know the components of patients' therapeutic self-care demands that they cannot or should not meet (for reasons of health and well-being) at this time and for some projected time duration.

E.3 Know the changes that patients should make in their customary systems of self-care with respect to identified and evaluated components in order to bring them in accord with their current, calculated therapeutic self-care demands, including the fit of new or changed self-care components into their patterns of daily living.

E.4 Know the new or adjusted self-care operations (estimative, critical judgment and decision making, and production) that patients or their dependent-care agents must learn to perform and the facilitating powers to be developed if required changes in self-care or dependent-care systems are to be brought about.

E.5 Know patients' or dependent-care agents' capacities for learning and for making required adjustments.

E.6 Know the psychological and physiologic limitations of dependent-care agents.

   Design unit E furthers the establishment of the goals to be sought for and by patients and establishes the foundations for design unit F.

Design Unit F: Design of the Regulatory Nursing System(s)

This unit involves nurses in the creation of designs for unifying nurse action, patient action, and action of participating others to achieve results and goals expressed in terms of (a) knowing and meeting patients' therapeutic self-care demands continuously in time, (b) protecting developed and developing powers of patients to manage themselves and to engage in self-care, and (c) regulating patients' exercise or development of self-care capabilities. The following elements of design are identified.

F.1 Initial and continuing establishment by nurses of their roles in the immediate and subsequent meeting of the therapeutic self-care demands of patients and their use of methods of assistance that conform to patients' self-management capabilities, their stages of development, their levels of available energy, their needs for safety and protection, their overt limitations for engagement in self-care, and their fears and concerns.

Provide for communication of information about and coordination of role responsibilities of nurses who contribute to the immediate achievement of nursing results during the 24 hours of the day or whenever one nurse is replaced by another.

F.2 Nurses' initial and continuing establishment and adjustment of patient roles and roles of participating others in meeting of patients' therapeutic self-care demands in accord with patients' developed and developing and operational capabilities for engagement in self-care, the exercise of which is unrestricted by health state features or health care system factors.

F.3 Nurses' and patients' or participating others' designation of areas of functioning requiring coordination of action and cooperation and use of designated methods of communication if the productive work of meeting patients' therapeutic self-care demands is to be accomplished effectively and economically.

F.4 Nurses' and patients' or participating others' initial and continuing establishment of their respective role functions in protecting the self-management and self-care capabilities of patients and in regulating the exercise or development of patients' self-care capabilities.

F.5 Nurses' continuing establishment of their own professional responsibility for conduct of the provision of nursing with recognition of interdependence of patients and participating others, as well as the independence of each as a legitimate participant in the nursing situation.

F.6 Establishment of conditions that should foster effective functioning and bring about order and a dynamic sense of duty on the part of all—nurses, patients, participating others.

Design unit F sets the specifications for who will do what toward achievement of nursing goals.

Variations in Nursing Systems Design

Variance in nursing system design is described first in relation to nursing's area of jurisdiction in health care situations where nursing is being sought or provided. Then variance is related to role responsibility differences for nurses, patients, and participating others in nursing practice situations.

Variance in Areas of Jurisdiction

Nurses' governing or leadership role in nursing practice situations is determined by nursing's area of jurisdiction in specific health care situations. This role is established by the contract or agreement to provide nursing and to be nursed. This formalizes the reason for seeking nursing and defines the authority of and the responsibilities to be fulfilled by nurses. If an agreement is unfulfilled or improperly fulfilled through failure of health care agencies to ensure the presence of nurses who know what nursing is needed, who design systems to ensure the production of nursing, and who produce it, then agencies may be suspected of contract nonfulfillment. If nurses in situations do not exercise their nursing authority and fulfill their nursing responsibility, they are suspected of malpractice.

Areas of nursing jurisdiction should be expressed in terms of nursing with designation of the following:

- Total to limited responsibility of nurses for the safety and protection of nurses' patients according to their stable or changing self-management capabilities and their self-care limitations in their situations of daily living
- Total to limited responsibility for continuous knowing and meeting of patients' therapeutic self-care demands by overcoming or compensating for patients' self-care limitations
- Areas of responsibility for assisting nurses' patients to protect their developed self-care capabilities and their self-management capabilities
- Areas of responsibility to assist patients to regulate (1) exercise of developed and operational capabilities to engage in self-care and (2) development of new capabilities for self-care or making adjustments in existent ones
- Areas of responsibility for the design of dependent-care systems and the development for role fulfillment of dependent-care agents

Design units A and B are concerned with identifying and laying out the details of nursing's area of jurisdiction and the governing role of nurses in defining and attaining nursing goals within nursing's area of jurisdiction in health care situations.

Establishing nursing's area of jurisdiction sets forth nursing's situational boundaries and should identify points and areas of articulation with medical and other health care systems, as well as self-care and dependent-care systems, that are operational and will continue to be operational as patients are nursed. It also establishes the matters to be communicated and lines of communication.

Role Variance

As identified in the preceding section, the extent of the governing or leadership role of nurses in practice situations is defined by nursing's area of jurisdiction in health care situations. The governing role of nurses extends to all facets of developing nursing situations. It includes the design function as developed in preceding sections. It includes continuous efforts to bring about and maintain association, integration, and interaction among participants in the nursing situation. The governing role also extends to ensuring production of nursing and attainment of nursing goals for patients. The governing role of nurses includes the actual production of continuous nursing whenever the health states of patients are in continuous flux, the therapeutic self-care demand is complex and in continuous change, and the life or integrity of patients is in jeopardy.

Nurses' decisions within the design function about their own roles in the continuing production of systems of nursing are made in relation to decisions about patient roles and roles of participating others in their designs for nursing systems. Nursing system design (design unit F) involves making judgments and decisions about methods of helping that are valid in relation to patients' limitations for engaging in self-care and reasons for or causes of these limitations. Each method of helping described in Chapter 3 casts helpers and those helped into distinct roles (see Table 13-1). Self-care limitations of patients and their developed and operational self-care abilities provide one basis for nurses' decision about methods of helping that are valid for use in the situation and in so doing cast patients in specific roles in relation to the production of care that they need.

Five general roles of adolescent or adult patients appropriate in the designs of systems of nursing are identified. Roles as expressed reflect the operations to be performed.

• No active role as observer or operator whenever there is absence of sensory consciousness in patients

• Active role as participant observer and contributor of nursing-relevant information about self and environmental features

• Active role as a participant operator in meeting components of his or her existent or emerging therapeutic self-care demand

• Active role as a participant investigator in calculating components of his or her therapeutic self-care demand

• Active role as learner in understanding self-care requisites and mastering specific means to meet them.

These roles, except for the first, can be combined. For example, the second and fourth roles can be fulfilled by persons with limitations of movement. Roles two, three, four, and five may be combined according to capabilities of patients and the need for role performance at particular times throughout the period of nursing.

When nurses' patients are infants or children, they should first be considered in terms of their needs to be taken care of and to be cared for in their uniqueness as individuals. Infants and children should be accepted as experiencing, as seeking to know what is around them, and as able to tolerate certain approaches to them but not others. Infants and children should be considered as active participants and be helped to participate in accord with their developmental states in systems of nursing designed for them.

The number of nurses brought into the design of nursing systems in addition to nurses with the governing and leadership role should vary according to (1) the degree of complexity and stability of patients' therapeutic self-care demands, (2) the stability of health states of patients with resultant effects on their therapeutic self-care demands and their self-management and self-care capabilities and limitations, and (3) the essential contribution of nursing to the health and well-being of persons to be nursed. Nurses with vocational or broad, technical-type preparation for nursing are valuable in stable nursing situations. Nurses with deep technical-type preparation and experience are valuable in the production of nursing if intricate technologies are needed to meet self-care requisites of patients. The relationship of these nurses to nurses in the governing or leadership role must be well developed and maintained, and their contributions to the production of nursing for patients over time should be well defined. In some settings, vocationally trained attendants or aides provide care. In settings where attendants and aides are used, nurses may or may not fill governing or leadership roles. In situations where there are no nurses, attendant service, not nursing, takes place.

Other participants in nursing practice situations whose roles should be identified in nursing system designs include members of patients' families or friends who contribute to meeting selected components of patients' therapeutic self-care demands whenever their roles are consistent over time. Also members of families or friends of patients or paid helpers may fill the "sitter" role. Sitters stay with patients to ensure their protection if they are not capable of self-management in their environments, secure help for them when care is needed, and assure patients that they are not alone.

Validity of Nursing Systems Designs

Nursing systems designs are valid whenever the design for what is to be produced conforms with what is and what should be. Validity demands the identification of what is to be produced and for what reasons, the goals to be attained through its production, and the numbers and qualifications of persons by time periods who can produce the designed nursing system. Validity also demands that any designed system meet criteria for effectiveness and economy of time and resources. Specialists in nursing system design (1) know in detail the self-care capabilities and limitations and the therapeutic self-care demands of persons with special health and developmental problems and (2) have participated in developing effective systems for producing nursing that attain nursing goals and results.

Designs for nursing systems are valid only for that period during which elements of design units A, B, D, and E maintain the values initially used by nurses in governing and leadership roles to create the design of a nursing system(s) for particular patients. The initial product of design unit F may be for a series of nursing systems designs to be followed sequentially whenever nurses can predict changes in elements of design units A, B, D, and E in some time frame.

Articulations of Nursing Systems

Known predictable areas of articulations of nursing systems with other systems of care must be incorporated into designs for them. Sometimes this can be accomplished before the actual production of care; at other times, articulations must be designed during production. If there are self-care or dependent-care systems in operation at the time nursing is to be provided, nurses must make judgments and decide which is to be viewed as the major system and which is to be considered the subsystem of care. For example, if a person living at home has help from nurses relative to designated components of a therapeutic self-care demand, the meeting of which are beyond the person's functional competencies, then it is realistic to consider the major system to be the person's ongoing self-care system. The same consideration would hold when nurses contribute a subsystem of nursing to an ongoing dependent-care system for adults or children. On the other hand, nursing is the major system when patients or participating others have defined but limited roles in the production of continuous care of the patient.

Designing and developing articulation of subsystems of action with main systems of action demand timing of performance of care measures with the same goal orientations by persons in different roles. They also demand current information about the effects of performance of care activities to attain one set of goals on care activities directed to attain another set of goals. For example, a person at home may be responsible for all aspects of self-care, including those related to continuous control of a condition of diabetes mellitus and impaired cardiac functioning with help from nurses whose area of jurisdiction is defined in terms of meeting self-care requisites associated with or arising from a leg ulcer and vascular surgery on the same lower extremity. The nurse within this area of jurisdiction must not only know the components of the person's self-care system as related to diabetes and cardiac functioning but also obtain information to judge adequacy of control because of the interrelations of the health disorders and their treatment. The nurse within this defined area of nursing jurisdiction must coordinate nursing efforts with those of the patient's vascular surgeon. However, the nurse's responsibility also extends to advising and counseling the patient about other self-care requisites that are inadequately met. This may include advising the patient to contact the internist or cardiologist.

Nursing systems design can become very complex and require frequent redesign. Nurses must develop habits of mental imagery, allowing them to see whole systems of nursing in terms of parts, function of parts, and articulations among them. Timing and designing articulations with other health services are of great importance when nurses' patients are undergoing extensive medical diagnosis or specialized therapies that place them in contact with a variety of health care workers and often require them to move from one place to another. Under these conditions, control of fatigue and special protection from hazards should be built into patients' therapeutic self-care demands.

MAJOR FACTORS AFFECTING NURSING PRACTICE AND NURSING SYSTEMS DESIGN FOR INDIVIDUALS

The age and related developmental states of patients, their health states, and features of their total health care systems are identified as factors that condition the components of patients' therapeutic self-care demands and their powers of self-care agency (see Figure 11-1). The influence of the named factors, however, extends beyond their conditioning effects on the patient variables therapeutic self-care demand and self-care. For this reason, the three factors are considered in some detail in relation to how they affect persons who are patients and influence nurses and the nursing care they produce.

Age as a Factor in Nursing

A patient's age is an index of both the health care focus and the helping focus of nursing. Personal maturation and organic, psychic, and intellectual functioning vary with the periods of the human life cycle. Basic self-care in meeting universal and developmental self-care requisites varies with periods of the human life cycle; however, the types of universal and developmental self-care requisites to be met remain the same. The variations are in the values at which the requisites should be met (e.g., the kind and amount of rest distributed by these time periods), in how they can be met, and in who will meet them.

Age is one index of the amount and kind of help persons need from nurses or others. This results from the association of chronologic age and developmental state. Capabilities for management of self in one's environment, psychic habits and dispositions, the attachment of meaning to what is perceived, and powers of understanding, reflection, and judgment vary by stages of development.

Both a basic health care focus and valid modes of helping can be inferred from information about a patient's age. Individual differences including developmental differences are recognized and taken into account by nurses. When individuals are in good to excellent states of health, age-relevant care and helping methods suffice other than in periods when special self-care is required, for example, because of an injury or a change in environmental conditions. Care of newborn infants is an example of the need to adjust care to age, to health state of infants, and to the process of infants' adjustments to new environmental conditions. As indicated previously, the basic conditioning factors of age, gender, developmental state, health state, and conditions of living in combination influence both the therapeutic self-care demands and the abilities and limitations of individuals for self-care.

Individuals who can benefit from nursing may be of any age and any state of development and health. When multiperson units such as families become the subject of care and service from nurses, the constituent members of the unit may be of similar or dissimilar ages and states of development and health. Nurses' descriptions of persons who are seeking or under nursing care must consider age, developmental state, and health state. If these three factors are not investigated and characterizing data are not obtained, nurses will not have an adequate basis for understanding the helping and health aspects of nursing because they influence both aspects of nursing. Age as a factor in the production of variety in nursing situations will be discussed. The influences of age and other factors on the production of variations in the therapeutic self-care demands and the self-care agency of patients will then be addressed.

Age of the patient is an important factor in every nursing situation. It normally is closely related to the characteristics of a person's behavior, and it has meaning in relationship to the self-care behavior of the patient and the nursing behavior of the nurse. Age also has a number of meanings in a given society, and these meanings influence the lives of the members of that society. Nurses must be aware of these meanings and their influences because such knowledge is related to the consideration of age in every nursing situation.

The Meaning of Age

Age is most frequently thought of in terms of chronologic age, the period of time between birth and succeeding time periods. Chronologic age is measured in seconds, minutes, hours, days, weeks, months, and years. Nurses may care for infants whose age can be measured in seconds as well as for persons whose age can be measured in decades. In prenatal life, chronologic age is measured in time intervals within the 9-month gestation period (the first, second, and third trimesters).

A person at any age may show failure to grow and develop along organic, psychic, or intellectual dimensions. Every individual should be provided with a type of environment that promotes development not only toward physical maturation but also toward emotional and intellectual maturity. Evidence of particular kinds of retardation of development should be considered as perhaps limiting but not as completely restricting personal achievement and fulfillment. Restraining persons with particular kinds of retardation from involvement in the human scene—for example, keeping them confined without education for self-care and other aspects of personal and community living—is a societally imposed hazard on their development, health, and well-being.

Developmental age refers to the combinations of qualities, powers, and capacities that develop naturally in each person in light of hereditary factors and environmental conditions. The developmental age of an individual is determined by identifying physical and behavioral developments and comparing them with chronologic age-group norms. Characteristic growth and developmental pictures of individuals by chronologic age periods are valuable guides to nurses in understanding health care requirements (including care to promote normal growth and development) and limitations for deliberate action. Each nurse must be constantly alert to advances in the knowledge of human growth and development and in technologies that foster normal growth, development, and health by age-group.

Growth in physical size is readily observable and measurable. Because individuals grow at different rates, children of the same chronologic age may vary in physical size. Persons who are small or large because of hereditary factors or whose natural growth has been retarded in some way, such as through malnutrition, may have problems in accepting themselves and in being accepted by others. Problems may also arise from a child's degree of development or maturity, which determines what a child can do at a particular age. If development is slow, help may be needed in allaying the child's fears that he or she will not be normal or be able to do what other children of the same age can do. If the rate of maturing is rapid, the child may need guidance in accepting himself or herself and relating to other children.

Some societies establish the chronologic age at which individuals, according to law, are capable of making certain decisions, of entering into contracts, and of being held legally responsible for their acts. In the United States, this age is part of either the common law of the country or the civil law of the states. According to common law, for example, the *age of majority,* or adulthood, is 21 years for both men and women. In some states, however, it is 18 years for women. Before a person reaches the legal age of adulthood, the law recognizes other ages, such as the age of discretion, the age of consent, and military age. The *age of discretion* means that a minor at the age of 14 years is recognized as possessing sufficient knowledge to be responsible for certain acts and to exercise certain powers. A minor under 7 years of age is conclusively presumed incapable of criminal intent, and a minor between the ages of 7 and 14 years is considered incapable of criminal intent unless there is proof to the contrary. The *age of consent,* which varies by state, is the age at which a person is recognized as legally competent to consent to marriage and to other acts.

Laws also protect persons who have not reached adult status. These laws hold natural and adoptive parents legally responsible for the support of a child. Support includes the provision of food, clothing, shelter, education, and health care. Legally, parents are responsible for the protection of the health and well-being of their child, including development of personal and social values and movement toward personal maturity.

A person's chronologic age and sex relate to status within a family, for example, the status and roles of husband and wife, mother and father, son and daughter, and brother and sister. Status and role define the duties and responsibilities of the individual toward other members of his or her family.

Age as it is discussed here is a relatively important factor in cultural practices related to infant and child care and supervision, instruction of children in self-care and sex attitudes, education toward independence, teaching skills and beliefs, formal education, care of the aged, marriage, and the family. The respect and care given to the young, to the elderly, and to women during pregnancy and the assistance given to individuals in the transitional period from youth to adulthood all reflect how a society views the importance of these age-related events. A patient's attitude or the attitude of family members and the attitude of the nurse in these areas are important influences in each nursing situation.

Influence of Age on Nursing

The chronologic and developmental ages of a patient affect the health and helping dimensions of the nursing situation in a number of ways. They influence (1) the social relations of nurse and patient, (2) techniques for assisting, communicating, and socializing to roles, (3) appropriate nurse responses to a patient's behavior, (4) frequency and duration of the contacts between nurse and patient, (5) the scope of the nurse's responsibility for protecting the patient as a person, (6) the nurse's relationship to members of the patient's family, and (7) the health and self-care needs of the patient. Understanding these influences requires knowledge of human growth and development, social networks, cultural practices, legal responsibilities of care agents, and communication and social interaction theories and technologies. This knowledge must be applied in collecting descriptive information about patients, interpreting the information, and using it in designing and providing nursing assistance for adults and children.

Nurses and nursing students may be in the adolescent stage of the life cycle, which is preparatory for access to specialized work in the society. They may also be adults preparing for or engaging in specialized work. Their patients may be of any age. Ideally, the nurse's behavior should convey acceptance and respect toward all patients. This is, of course, mature behavior and requires that the nurse recognize each patient as a person, as a member of a family, and as one who has a unique heredity and life history. Mature behavior in interpersonal situations also demands from the nurse an awareness of the need for adjusting his or her behavior to practices in the patient's culture that regulate social relations by age and position in the family or community.

Providing nursing to a child differs in several ways from providing nursing to an adult. The age status of a patient as an adult, a neonate, an infant, a child, or a youth has important implications for nursing, regardless of the patient's state of health and disease. The adult's right and responsibility to make decisions is recognized by society, as is the child's inability to do this. The developed and developing powers of the child must be identified and fostered within the nursing situation. Nurses should be acutely aware of the limits for realistic behavioral expectations for children according to age. Nurses should also provide for differences in environmental needs and be alert to signals of health problems by age-groups. Evidence of failure to grow and develop, as well as evidence of regressive changes and dysfunction by age-group, must be understood by nurses.

Nurses should understand the quality of trust, including its importance in effective interpersonal relations and in human growth and development. The trust a patient has in a nurse, the nurse's acceptance of it, and the nurse's respect for the patient are interacting forces that aid in the maintenance of the nurse-patient relationship. The nurse at times will be required to set limits for the behavior of children, youth, and sometimes adults as it relates to the patient's or the nurse's well-being. When trust, acceptance, and respect prevail, limit setting is more likely to be viewed as help given and not as restraint or coercion.

Age-Specific Factors in Nursing Children

In nursing situations involving infants, children, and youth, the patient continues in his or her role of a *dependent who must be cared for or guided by a responsible adult*. Nursing of young patients is a mix of care measures, which each patient needs because of his or her (1) chronologic and developmental age, (2) genetic heritage, (3) unique personality, (4) physical and social environment, and (5) health state and related health care needs. Nursing in situations in which the patient is young may involve direct care of the patient by the nurse and assistance to parents or guardians in learning to give the continuous care needed by the child or to cooperate with health workers. The nurse's dual relationship to child and to parents makes the nurse role complex and requires that techniques of assisting be adapted to the needs of the child and the needs of the parents, who may be adolescents or adults.

In the direct nursing care of a young patient, the nurse selects ways of assisting that are in accord with the patient's age and stage of growth and development. *Caring for, acting or doing for,* and *providing an environment that promotes development* are valid ways of nursing infants and young children. *Guiding* and *supporting* the child in self-care action are appropriate methods of nursing older children to the degree permitted by their health state and their personal maturity. Older children and adolescents can learn and want to be responsible for their personal health-related care. They will also want and need guidance and supervision from a responsible adult, though at times they will resist these efforts. Sustained interest of the nurse in the health care efforts of the young patient can make a great contribution toward the patient's becoming an effective self-care agent. Nurses should endeavor to help adolescents develop beneficial self-care practices. When nurses know that adult family members have incorporated practices harmful to health into their daily living, guidance of youth toward physical and mental health should be an important nursing concern.

When children have some continuing therapeutic self-care needs that the parents are incapable of meeting, care responsibilities for the child may be distributed between the nurse and the parents. The distribution should be based on an objective consideration of the parents' limitations for giving the needed therapeutic care. When infants and sick children are placed in hospitals or other health care institutions, parents should be permitted to be with the child and fulfill some of the care responsibilities for the child whenever possible and prudent.

When parents cannot be with their child, the child should have a person to whom he or she can relate during various periods of the day. In an institutional situation, this role may be assigned to a person trained in child care rather than in nursing. This practice is appropriate when most of the care needs of the infant or child are not of the specialized type of care required as a result of disease, injury, or defect. Nurses should be able to give both aspects of care to children, but they also should be able to work cooperatively with both parents and with persons trained for child care. In long-term care institutions or when children are ill at home for prolonged periods, their formal education should be continued under the direction of qualified teachers.

The nature of the interpersonal relationship between a nurse and an infant, child, or adolescent patient is of paramount importance. It should communicate trust. Young patients should be able to feel that the nurse is a responsible adult who is interested in them and to whom they can turn for help. The nurse fosters the child's growth and development and at the same time contributes to the achievement of other specific health results. It is thus essential that the nurse know about the present developmental state of the child and how children develop cognitively and use knowledge at various ages.

The relationships between the nurse and the mother, father, or guardian of a child also may be affected by the age of the nurse or of the parents, as well as by cultural factors. In cases in which parents have differing opinions about the care needs of the child, the nurse may find it necessary to work with both parents for the child's well-being. This situation is complex. Some nurses may not be sufficiently competent to cope with it.

A nursing situation in which the patient is an infant, child, or youth continues as long as the patient requires specialized therapeutic care or until the parents or guardians have overcome their limitations for giving the needed care or assistance. Nurses should select methods that will benefit both the child and the parents. For example, if an infant or child has to be fed via a technique adapted for a cleft lip or palate, it may be appropriate for the nurse to involve the parents early in learning to feed the infant. Parents may need periodic guidance and supervision from a nurse when they are giving and managing the continuous therapeutic care required by a sick or disabled child or when they are giving therapeutic care to a well child.

When a child's integrated functioning is seriously disturbed or the health care technologies are complex and interrelated and when the child's suffering is intense, nurses should not involve the parents in the technical (clinical) aspects of the child's health care. If parents must become technically able to participate in or completely provide the continuous health care for their child at home, nurses must carefully determine how the parents can be assisted without harm to them or to the child. If children have birth defects or an illness that places parents in an adverse light with or without reason, or if children are unwanted and rejected, parents may need health care for their own sake as well as for that of the child.

In infant, child, or adolescent nursing situations, there should be an open line of communication between nurse(s) and parents and nurse(s) and physician(s). This is necessary because of the legal status of the patient as a minor and the patient's limitations in understanding and decision making. Because children are immature, they cannot be expected to be responsible agents in their own health care or in coordination of the various parts of care. The role of the adolescent in self-care, including its coordination with other aspects of health care, may be extended with guidance and supervision. The nurse must be aware of prescribed roles, rights, and responsibilities. Parents sometimes may not be in contact with adolescent sons or daughters or assume responsibility for their care or support. Guidance and support from interested and accepting adults are essential to meet developmental needs of young people who have taken on or are about to take on the duties of adult members of a society.

In caring for a minor, physicians must be in direct communication with the child's parents and nurses. The physician has an ethical and legal responsibility to keep parents informed of the child's health state. Some physicians also accept responsibility for guiding parents in fostering the growth and development of the child. A failure in communication between a child's parents and the physician may have adverse effects on the total health care situation, including the nursing component.

In some child nursing situations, it is essential that the child's nurse talk with nurses in another agency in coordinating the care of a child. A nurse giving care to a child at home, for example, may want to discuss nursing information with a nurse in an outpatient clinic or in a hospital before a clinic visit or hospitalization. Nurses, too, may find it necessary to contact the child's teachers and school nurses or assist the child's parents in doing this whenever the child's daily health care needs must be given attention at school. When two or more health care agencies are involved in providing health services, coordination of their activities is important for the effective health care of both children and adults. Channels of communication should be provided and kept open to facilitate interagency coordination of health care for individual patients.

Age-Specific Factors in Nursing Adults

From the viewpoint of the patient's age, adult nursing situations differ from child nursing situations in that adults have the right to decide about the kinds of health care they will accept and the responsibility to act for themselves in matters of self-care and health. Adults may be emotionally or socially dependent on other people as a result of inadequate physical, psychologic, or cognitive development or because of the effects of disease, injury, or disability. However, they are not dependent in the way children are because of their age.

In child nursing situations, the child's age is a signal to the nurse of how to care for and communicate with the child, of growth and developmental needs, and of effects of illness or environmental factors on development. The adult patient's age is a signal to the nurse that the patient is responsible for himself or herself and his or her dependents (unless the patient is incompetent from developmental or health state factors). A patient's age tells the nurse that the patient is able to communicate as an adult but at a level that is influenced by habits of perceiving and thinking and that needs for help in self-care arise from health state or health care requirements. Adult age also may point to needs for assistance in accepting and living in a state of social dependency resulting from illness or treatment, in becoming self-directing about matters of self-care, and in learning to seek and use nursing services, including guidance and consultation in self-care.

In adult nursing situations, a nurse-family relationship may or may not exist. When an adult patient is not physically or mentally competent to manage his or her own affairs to make decisions about health care, nurses may have frequent contacts with a responsible member of the patient's family. When family members in a home provide the continuous care needed by a patient, nurses may instruct, supervise, and consult with family members.

Sometimes adult patients who are incompetent have legally appointed guardians. Adult patients who may be seriously ill or aged may give another responsible adult the power of attorney to transact business for them in accordance with regulations established by law. If adults are unable to decide or act for themselves, a family member, preferably the closest relative, should act for them. Adults often care for their aged parents or for a seriously ill spouse. When an adult has a legally appointed guardian, the guardian occupies much the same position as the natural parents of a child.

Other age-related considerations are of great importance in nursing situations. Adult patients who are aware of their experiences and of the events that occur in the health care situation serve as information and communication centers in the health care situation. They interact with health workers, other persons who provide services, and family members and friends. The frequency and duration of contacts, the variety of social contacts, the content of communications, and a patient's interpretation of and reactions to his or her experiences are influencing factors on health care and nursing. Health workers place demands on patients to make observations, to reveal information, and, at times, to give messages to other health workers and to manage their own care. It is important that adult patients be helped to become responsible agents in their own health care. It is also important that nurses, physicians, and other health workers not burden a patient with their own coordinating duties.

The nursing situation may also be affected by an adult's social responsibilities. The adult patient's health and health care may interfere with family life, work, and other aspects of adult living. The adult may be unable to finance health care, care for dependent children, or provide for family needs. An adult patient's motivation to overcome or compensate for limitations resulting from injury or disability may be greatly influenced by family and work responsibilities or conditions of living.

Health State as a Factor in Nursing

Well-being, general health state, injury, and physical or psychic illness are critical factors in nursing situations, for they are the determinants of the appropriate health care focus and the types of health results sought. Nurses must have information about the general health states of patients as well as information about conditions and events associated with the specific health disorders from which patients suffer.

Information about the patient's health state is obtained from a number of sources: the patient, persons who live with the patient, the patient's physician, the medical history, and the recorded results of physical and other examinations and laboratory tests. Understanding the meaning of such information requires that nurses have knowledge of normal integrated human functioning, pathologic conditions, basic procedures of health evaluation, and the purposes of medical diagnoses and therapy in relation to health and disease. Nurses, in making observations of patients or of records and reports on patients, initially and continuously determine evidence that will enable them to understand patients' health states.

Specifically, the information the nurse seeks will include descriptions of (1) the degree of illness, its causes, and whether it is acute or chronic; (2) obvious injuries or defects; (3) the patient's present behavior patterns (what he or she does or does not do); (4) the effects of disease or disordered function experienced by the patient (including pain, alterations of body temperature, alterations of respiratory and circulatory functioning, gastrointestinal functioning, genitourinary functioning, nervous and musculoskeletal functioning, alterations of the skin and its appendages, and bleeding and anemia); and (5) possible or known effects of the patient's present health state on integrated functioning and effective living.

Nurses must know if the disease or disorder the patient has is one of the common causes of death. Vascular diseases of the central nervous system, acute coronary disease, other heart diseases, and malignancy are leading causes of death. The effect a disease may have on the life of a patient is a factor that affects the outlook and behavior of the patient and family as well as that of the nurse. The effects of a patient's illness on the family are very important in all nursing situations.

The physician's view of the patient's health situation is reflected in the medical diagnosis and prognosis, the recorded medical history, and the results of the physical examinations and laboratory tests. The kind of therapy the physician prescribes and the diagnostic and other measures the physician uses are also significant for nursing.

In nursing situations in which patients are under active medical care, there is need for discussion between the patient's nurse(s) and the physician so that the nurse can determine (1) how the physician views the patient's health situation; (2) the aspects of the patient's medical care regimen that should become parts of the patient's self-care system on a long-term or short-term basis, including monitoring of selected aspects of human functioning; (3) which physician, if there is more than one, has the position of responsibility for integrating and coordinating the patient's medical care; and (4) the projected duration of active medical care for the patient. Only through the conscious and deliberate efforts of physicians and nurses to communicate with each other about the daily care of the patient can nursing care and medical care be coordinated to produce an effective health care system for the patient.

During the initial period of nursing, a patient may be relatively healthy; slightly, moderately, or seriously ill; injured; or suffering from defect or disability. Life experiences, present environmental situation, and interests and concerns influence the patient's view of the health state and the need for health care as well as the patient's readiness or ability to cooperate with health care workers (pp. 180-193).[9] A patient's view of his or her health situation may be related to the characteristics of the disease process itself. There is a process of becoming ill. There are also modes of adaptation to illness and to the recovery process. The disease, the kinds of symptoms, and the rapidity with which they develop help to describe the process of becoming ill.

One physician who studied patients who had cerebral vascular accidents or strokes described the patients as having been plunged within a relatively short time into "a rather unfamiliar and complicated life situation" that "is rapidly changing," a situation in which the "full import and meaning cannot be readily grasped in the initial states." In describing their experiences and reactions in the initial phases of the disease process, the patients' responses demonstrated (1) personality resources, for example, "courage, self-control, patience, and acceptance"; (2) minimization and rationalization of initial symptoms; (3) resignation to the outcome of the illness; and (4) "mounting apprehensiveness and heightened dependency." With strokes, as with other illnesses that can lead to extensive brain damage, there may be unawareness of illness or of deficits such as that resulting from a paralysis. The stroke patient's view of his or her illness during its early phases and the tendency to maximize or minimize difficulties rather than see them realistically were indicators of reactions in later phases of the illness and in the recovery process (pp. 74-76).[10]

In studying diseases and patterns of illness, it is important for nurses and nursing students to learn what has been presently identified about patterns of adaptation. In studies of two types of disabling illness, the following patterns were noted: (1) insightful acceptance, (2) a struggle with conflicts brought on by disability through projection and other psychologic mechanisms, (3) exaggeration of dependency and demands for more help than might actually be required, and (4) a slowly developing depression with loss of motor ability, a sense of failure in coping with events with resultant sadness, and feelings of helplessness that the patient may not recognize initially. Once they are recognized, however, they are not denied (pp. 78-80).[10]

Patients' views of their health situation influence their own roles and nurses' roles in the nursing situation. What responsibility can the patient bear now and fulfill effectively in the future? In light of the patients' perception of and responses to their health situation, what kind of assistance is required to identify the patient role? How can patients be helped to face and accept the demands that illness or injury place on them? Nurses, especially those who have not experienced personal or family problems of a serious nature or who have not been victims of a natural disaster, may not be perceptive about the impact of personal loss or of excessive physical and emotional demands on the individual.

Illness and injury generally impose hardships on people. The outcome of illness and injury may be uncertain; a person is faced with the unknown and may experience anxiety, fear of permanent disability, life-long suffering, or even death. In some instances, patients must make decisions about the kinds of measures they will permit the physician to take. Nurses should be able to envision the meaning that illness or disability and being a patient have for individuals.

If a nurse sees only movements toward health—toward more effective living—without seeing the demands and burdens that injury, illness, and health care place on a patient, the basis for nursing diagnosis and prescription is incomplete. The nursing perspective will be inaccurate, and the nurse will not have a sound basis for proceeding toward the nursing goal of assisting the patient in responsible action in matters of self-care. The patient may be willing to accept care given by the nurse, may demand care from the nurse, or may be uninterested in or even refuse care. Patients may need help in understanding not only their self-care demands but also the rationale for particular self-care requisites or for sets of requisites. A nurse's investigations may reveal that a first task is to help the individual learn how to cooperate in the determination of needs that can be met through nursing.

Health Results

Nurses' investigations of and judgments about the self-care requisites of patients take into consideration the reasons why patients are under health care and the health results to be achieved. The types of health results mentioned previously include the maintenance and promotion of health, including the prevention of disease, defect, and disability; the cure or regulation of disease processes; the preservation or restoration of vital processes; rehabilitation toward effective living in the event of chronic illness or disability; and being able to live and function with some degree of ease and personal satisfaction during a terminal illness.

When patients with health disorders are under nursing care, nurses must have or seek authoritative information about the natural history of specific diseases. The medical literature or physician and nurse specialists with extensive experience in caring for patients with particular diseases are sources. Such knowledge enables nurses to envision the kinds of health results associated with the disease. For example, through fact-gathering activities, the nurse finds that a patient has been diagnosed as having a stone in the right ureter. From observations of the patient and from the physician's notes, the nurse is aware that the pain is severe and the patient is in great distress. The nurse draws on knowledge from anatomy, physiology, and pathology in forming a mental picture of what is presently in process in the patient. The nurse understands the physiologic problem resulting from the presence of the stone and the mechanics related to the possible passage of the stone, considering the size and shape of the stone in relation to the diameter of the ureter and to its tissue structure and physiology. Causes of stone formation and preventive measures come to mind. The nurse draws on his or her knowledge of pain and physiology, psychology, and pathology in making observations and judgments.

From reading the physician's medical orders for the patient and from talking with the physician, the nurse also becomes aware that the physician does not plan at this time to use surgical techniques but will first see if the patient can pass the stone, using drug therapy as indicated. The nurse becomes aware that the patient will be enduring the painful process of passing the stone, with all its distressing effects, and concludes that the desired, immediate health-related results needed by the patient are four in number: (1) elimination of the stone, (2) prevention or control of complications, (3) relief from pain, and (4) reduction of physical and psychologic stress. The nurse knows the distressing effects produced by the passing of stones and is aware of the results to be sought and the kinds of care measures that will be effective while the patient lives through the process of passing the stone. Nurses' knowledge of health, disease, and medical diagnostic and therapeutic modalities should include their points of articulation with nursing. The patient variables, therapeutic self-care demand and self-care agency, provide appropriate linkages.

Patients' Points of View

Patients see their health care situations from their own unique perspectives. Their education, experience, feelings and attitudes about life and people, and knowledge of health care and attitudes toward it color their views. Patients' insights about their own health care needs, the meaning they attach to presenting signs and symptoms, and their awareness of their ability or inability to engage in effective required self-care and to work cooperatively with nurses and physicians is essential information for nurses to have and use in helping patients. Individual nurses should develop approaches that are helpful to them in grasping quickly the views of individual patients about their health care situations and in identifying the interests and concerns of patients.

A woman being interviewed by a nurse-midwife about her obstetric experiences expressed the following views of herself in relation to her first pregnancy: (1) not having knowledge of what to do because of the pregnancy; (2) requiring time to formulate and express questions to ask the nurse and the obstetrician; (3) being able to cope with some but not all of the demands for self-care and self-management during the pregnancy; (4) being in need of learning to live as a woman who is pregnant and who is in labor, to relate to health care professionals, and to provide infant care; (5) being ready or not ready to learn at specific times.* The woman noted that she was well educated, intelligent, and occupationally effective. She was aware of her own limitations for effective action within the health care situations associated with her first pregnancy. She viewed time as a relevant factor.

PERSONAL MATURITY OF INDIVIDUALS, CRITERION MEASURES OF POSITIVE MENTAL HEALTH

Nurses provide nursing to individuals of all ages, demanding that nurses be aware of and understand the meaning of each individual's state of growth and development as well as various aspects of development in nursing practice situations. One aspect of human development not formalized in the nursing literature is individuals' development of their uniquely human qualities and powers in their movement to **personal maturity** and **positive mental health.** "All things being equal, [personal maturity] positive mental health of individuals affects what persons seek to know, what they will question, the roles they are willing or unwilling to take, and what they seek to learn and do for themselves and others" (p. 166).[11] Achievement of positive mental (psychic) health is a life-long endeavor of individuals as each proceeds on his or her path to maturity as a person.

Mental or psychic illness in its various modalities has been described, named, and classified by the American Psychiatric Association. Mental illness and psychic disorders are recognized not only by professionals in the broad field of psychiatric mental health but also by laypeople in communities throughout the world. Health professionals and people in general have less clarity about the behavioral evidence of positive mental health in themselves and in others.

---

*From the record of an interview conducted by Mary E. Fitzpatrick.

A Search for Criterion Measures

My work and that of my colleague Evelyn Mawacke Vardiman (a psychiatric mental health nurse specialist) to isolate criterion measures of positive mental health was brought about by a request to present a paper on "Self-Care and Mental Health, a Nursing Perspective," at the Nursing Mental Health Congress in Palencia, Spain. At this time, data Vardiman collected about the expressed interests and concerns and the problems of daily living of persons with chronic mental illness were being studied. These persons were participant members of a day care center associated with a hospital in an eastern metropolitan area, and these data were collected during Vardiman's tenure as nurse specialist for the center.

Two other factors, factors specific to the behavior of nurses, emphasized the importance of the identification of criterion measures of positive mental health. There was evidence that some nurses failed to recognize or accept the personal maturity of adults under their care, disregarding mentally healthy behaviors such as their statements of fact, their reasoned questions and opinions, or their wanting to know the details of ongoing or proposed care regimens and outcomes sought. There also was evidence of some nurses' lack of attention to, interest in, or inability to differentiate the behavior of persons with mental or psychic illness that were expressions of the affective, cognitive, or personal aspects of the disorder from these persons' mentally healthy behavior. These behaviors included expressions of knowledge that their symptoms were worsening, concern about the untoward effects of their medication, and concern about the probable effects of their behaviors on themselves or others.

In nursing practice situations, the personal maturity of both nurse and patient affect the interpersonal and technologic (clinical) elements of practice. Nurses who are maturing professionally, moving to higher levels of scientific practice, may also be moving themselves to a higher level of personal maturity. Both movements are essential, and each nurse moves at his or her own pace. There is need for nurses to have and use measures to identify and judge their own progress as clinicians. There is also need for nurses to judge their own progress in movement toward the personal maturity that is expressed by behaviors that evidence their essential humanness. Nurses must be aware of and accept the personal maturity revealed by their patients. This is an essential aspect of respecting the person who is the patient. Criterion measures of personal maturity were judged to be important for nurses' use in assessing the maturity of their own behavior and of patient behaviors.

For these reasons, efforts were made to identify criterion behaviors of positive mental health that nurses could use in nursing practice situations. During the search process, the judgment was made that "positive mental (psychic) health . . . refers to modes of human functioning of individuals in life situations that express their uniquely human qualities and personal development as they live and work with other persons in their [families and] communities" (p. 165).[11]*

---

*The endeavor to identify criterion measures of positive mental health readily applicable in nursing practice situations is described in the article from Orem DE and Vardiman EM: Orem's nursing theory and positive mental health: practical considerations, *Nurs Sci Q,* 8:4, 1995.

Taking a Position

In the initial search for criterion measures of positive mental health, the following positions were expressed and accepted.

1. Health can be conceptualized as a state of being, a manifestation of an individual to self and others of features of his or her existence, including circumstances under which he or she exists.
2. Mental health states of individuals affect what they can or will attend to, their powers of appraisal and choice, and their powers to perform and order their actions to goal achievement.
3. "Positive mental health is the operation and expression of the essential humanness of persons." It is the unitary functioning of persons in an essentially human mode revealed to others as specific behaviors (p. 166).[11]
4. Positive mental health of an individual is a compound state including (a) a person's state of awareness of self and what the self enables the person to do privately and in association with others, (b) a person's awareness of coexistence with others as well as separateness from them, and (c) what the person attends to and the person's judgments, decisions, and productive actions in concrete situations of daily living regardless of type of situation (p. 166).[11]
5. Achievement and maintenance of positive mental health requires deliberate effort from individuals in their changing life situations.
6. Positive mental health or functioning in an essentially human mode can be interfered with by somatic or psychic disturbances or by life experiences that cause intense emotional states, for example, fear or grief (p. 166).[11]

Identified Criterion Behaviors of Positive Mental Health

A literature search was conducted to "determine what it was that philosophers, psychologists, clinical psychologists, psychiatrists, and scholars in the broad field of human behavior identify as essentially human qualities and forms of behavior" (p. 166).[11] The selection of behavioral items was guided by three views of humankind expressed by a psychologist and two philosophers (p. 167).[11]

Thirty-eight behaviors were identified, extracted, and grouped in five categories. Each category expressed the behavioral focus of the items of conduct extracted from the literature placed within the category (see box). The categories

---

Categories of Criterion Behaviors of Positive Mental Health

1. Functioning within a veridical (coinciding with reality) frame of reference
2. Functioning to bring about and maintain order in daily living
3. Functioning with integrity and self-awareness
4. Functioning as a person in community
5. Functioning with increased understanding of one's humanity

From Orem DE and Vardiman EM: Orem's nursing theory and positive mental health: practical considerations, *Nurs Sci Q*, 8:4, 1995, p 167.

indicate commonalities among the 38 behaviors. The categories and their numbering do not indicate a developmental hierarchy.

The named behaviors within the categories represent the results of one effort to formalize the time-honored idea that individuals reveal their development as human beings through their behaviors in life situations. The 38 behaviors identified as criteria of positive mental health are offered for study by nurses with respect to their own behaviors and those of their patients in nursing practice situations. Some nurses tend to make global judgments about patient behaviors and fail to view behaviors in their situational context. Nurses, too, may tend to view all their own behaviors as professionally appropriate.

The 38 criterion behaviors are presented by categories. The behaviors are stated in terms of *how I conduct myself* without expression of the "I."

Functioning Within a Veridical Frame of Reference

This set includes five behaviors or principles that guide conduct.
1. Investigate new conditions and circumstances and unusual events that occur within myself or my environment.
2. Seek verification of the validity of my perceptions and perspectives of events and conditions internal and external to me.
3. Recognize misconceptions and misrepresentations of aspects of my bodily structures and functioning or mental functioning and manage the effects of such misconceptions and misrepresentations on myself or others.
4. Investigate and reflect upon the information I have about life situations to identify what is and what is not open to change through appropriate practical endeavor by me or by others.
5. Evaluate the adequacy of my knowledge and the validity and reliability of my skills for task accomplishment in situations of personal and family living or work or play situations.

The five behaviors relate to conscious awareness, to the rational consciousness of men, women, and children who "want to understand, to grasp intelligible unities and correlations, to know what's up, and where they stand"[12] (pp. 322-324).

Functioning to Bring About or Maintain Order in Daily Living

The five behaviors in this group relate to persons' engagement in result-seeking and result-achieving actions of daily living, including self-care and care of others, as well as all other endeavors. The good of order, as described by Lonergan, is recognized and sought (pp. 211-212).[12]
1. Order and prioritize recurring and novel activities of daily living toward the fulfillment of my role responsibilities to result in a sense of accomplishment and satisfaction.
2. Exercise creativity or seek assistance in developing and using a plan(s) to order and prioritize actions when taking on new role responsibilities or in unfamiliar situations.

3. Help members of my family to develop and use plans for ordering and prioritizing result-achieving actions whenever their decision-making powers and processes are developing or when such powers and processes are interfered with by internal or external conditions and factors.
4. Seek to develop, maintain, and adjust habits and routines that ensure that tasks of daily living are accomplished in accord with my role responsibilities, with requisite knowledge and skill, and with the effective and economical use of resources.
5. Keep or bring ways of responding and acting in accord with features and demands of situations of daily living and their meaning for my own life, health, and well-being and for others.

These behaviors are concerned with activities of doing and making within "a field of conscious awareness—empiric, intelligent, rational" (p. 324).[12]

Functioning with Integrity and Self-Awareness

Eight behaviors are identified.
1. Maintain awareness of my own history through recall and reflection.
2. Keep the historical past separate from the existential present.
3. Maintain separateness from and appropriate relationships with other persons, objects, and external events. Do not involve myself with events and things beyond their objective purposes or the reality of these events and things.
4. Develop and maintain myself as one who is not immersed in or dependent on the identities of others.
5. Maintain periods of silence for purposes of reflection on myself to promote self-awareness and self-knowledge.
6. Attend to and make inferences about my own mental processes.
7. Maintain observation of my own behaviors and the behaviors of the persons with whom I interact in situations of daily living and attach meaning to these behaviors.
8. Use humor and laughter to open the way to attaining insights about the realities of myself and others.

The focus here is on the individual as a person who has a self and a mind that he or she uses (pp. 226-227).[13]

Functioning as a Person in the Community

The 10 behaviors in this group are concerned with personal integrity in social relationships.
1. Know my position(s) in the community(ies) of which I am a member and the responsibilities attendant upon the position(s).
2. Maintain myself as a person with sets of roles and responsibilities in the community(ies) of which I am a member.
3. Use my position(s) in the community in a way that contributes to the life of the community and as a means to meet needs of self and others.

4. Bring about and maintain ongoing and mutually satisfying relationships in recurring contacts with others in situations of daily living, including situations in the home, at work, and at play.
5. Sustain attention to persons and matters of interest in the development of concentration toward becoming able to love.
6. Enter into and accept the role responsibilities of being in loving relationships with others in childhood and adulthood.
7. Avoid the use of others as pure instruments toward accomplishment of personal goals.
8. Avoid the purely instrumental use of myself by others toward their goal attainments.
9. Acknowledge and express my recognition of the contribution of others to my life, health, and well-being.
10. Communicate with others through expressive interpersonal actions, including the recounting of needs, feelings, and feeling states.

The 10 behaviors emphasize relationships of friendship and relationships of a contractual character and negate coercive relationships (pp. 445-452).[14] Intersubjectivity and intelligence are implicit in the relationships (pp. 211-216).[12]

Functioning with Increasing Understanding of One's Humanity

The 10 behaviors in this set focus on various aspects of the human condition.

1. Enjoy successes.
2. Seek understanding of my experiences of happiness as fulfillments expressive of my love, as my reaching out to people and things, and as gifts that can help me hold a steady course in life with hope and faith.
3. Endure suffering in those life situations that are inescapable, unavoidable, or cannot be changed but always in congruity with the reality features of these situations and their meaning as related to my life, health, and well-being or their meaning for others.
4. Seek understanding of my experiences of suffering (or those of others) as challenges and tests of my fortitude, affording opportunities for me to come to terms with my life, death, and ultimate end.
5. Seek understanding of illness and other losses within the context of my humanity.
6. Reflect upon my life and the values and meanings that emerge.
7. Recognize situations in which there is need for development of emotional control or other behavioral changes toward task accomplishment, as well as for the well-being of myself and others.
8. Investigate and reflect upon the values that I attach to specific actions, events, conditions, and circumstances.
9. Identify and attach meaning to situations of daily living that I take action to participate in or avoid.
10. Review and appraise the human appropriateness of my priority system or hierarchy of values (spiritual, moral, economic, aesthetic, material, social)

that color my judgments and constitute motivating forces in decision making and action.

The 10 behaviors reflect a progressively higher integration of a person's differentiating human development in his or her life situation. Implicit in the behaviors is movement in character formation and movement toward a developing self-ideal.

The foregoing criterion behaviors of positive mental health specify objects of behavior but not the life situations in which they occur. Nurses' recognition of the behaviors or their absence in nursing practice situations provides one basis for their own judgments and decisions about what to do.

COOPERATION AND COORDINATION IN NURSING AND HEALTH CARE SYSTEMS

The achievement of health results for individuals is based in large part on the capabilities and motivation of health service personnel and their willingness and ability to cooperate and to coordinate their efforts. To *cooperate* is to act jointly in achieving some common goal. A situation that requires cooperation or a joint action of a number of persons sets up a demand that the persons acting together to reach a common goal regulate and combine their efforts so that action will be harmonious and contribute to the achievement of the goal. This regulation and combination of effort is *coordination.*

If several people attempt to work toward a common goal but do so without coordination, duplication of effort, inefficiency, and even failure to achieve the goal may occur. Effective coordination of effort requires that persons involved reach a common understanding of their goal, know their respective roles in its achievement, perform in an agreed manner so that the activities will be properly related to the goal, and communicate developments and changes resulting from their actions whenever such information is necessary for the performance of other roles.

Learning to nurse includes learning to work in cooperation with patients and their families, other nurses, physicians, and other health care specialists. Nursing students and young nurses should have planned experiences designed to aid them in initiating and responding to contacts with other health workers, as well as patients and their families. The language of the health and medical sciences facilitates communication between nurses and other health workers. Terms that are specific to a particular health service may need definition and explanation in interdisciplinary communication. The language of nursing develops as nursing science is developed.

Beliefs of nurses and other health workers about their roles and the roles of others affect their interests and their willingness to function in cooperative relationships in health care situations. Some health workers have little insight about the specific characteristics of nursing and its significance in achieving health results. On the other hand, because of their continuous relationship with a patient, nurses often have considerable knowledge of the roles and contributions of other health workers. Nurses should have skill in representing to physicians, social workers, and others the characteristics of nursing and the nature of the health care contribution it makes in various types of health care situations.

Members of different health services who give help to the same person are sometimes collectively referred to as a health team. A health team is an organized group of health workers who have roles related to meeting the health care needs of a patient or a group of patients. A team does not exist unless there are common goals, cooperative relationships, and coordinated activities. In many health care situations there are no health teams in the usual sense. Frequently, patients are cared for by a number of health workers who cooperate on a one-to-one basis with the patient and with other health workers. An organized health team enables its individual members to see their respective roles in relation to achievement of health results for a patient, to establish a group identity, and to afford authority to and to respect group members in relation to their roles and capabilities.

The formal establishment of a health team may be the only way or the preferred way for giving care or designing and managing care. Team functioning requires time and specialized effort on the part of each person involved. When health teams are not formally organized, cooperation and coordination of effort must be initiated by individual health workers.

Health teams are essential to performing some complex diagnostic and treatment measures. Often some members of these teams work with extremely complex machines or equipment that must be brought into a functional relationship with a patient (e.g., the heart-lung machine during open-heart surgery). Whenever team members work in face-to-face relationships or are linked by highly effective communication devices, coordination of effort is facilitated. Analysis of the roles, relationships, and specific activities of members of a health team (e.g., a surgical team preparing for and performing a surgical procedure for a patient in an operating room) is a helpful exercise toward understanding health team functioning.

Health Care Systems

Variations in nursing situations that are parts of larger health situations arise from the number and kinds of health workers contributing care or service to patients. In some situations there are only nurses and physicians, but in others there are many types of health workers. For example, when persons suffer from an illness of undetermined origin or when medical treatment is complex, a large number and a variety of health workers may be involved. Forms of health care vary from one part of the world to another and, in some instances, within the same country. In the United States, the predominant form of health care is derived from scientific medicine as it has developed in the Western world.

This form of health care has traditionally had as its focus *disease,* which is defined as an abnormal biologic process with characteristic symptoms. The modern concept of disease describes it as a process involving alterations in human structure or functioning including integrated human functioning. The modern concept of disease also includes the concept that a specific disease has more than a single cause (concept of multiple causation). Medical scientists identify, describe, and name unique diseases, that is, distinct pathologic processes. Descriptions include the sequential series of changes that have been observed in individuals suffering from particular diseases.

The increasing knowledge about disease has been complemented by substantial increases of physiologic and psychologic knowledge of value to physicians and other health workers in the diagnosis, treatment, and prevention of disease and in the maintenance and promotion of normal development and functioning. Information about the prevention of disease and the maintenance and promotion of good health has become a part of the general culture. Thus health has come into focus in scientific medicine not just as something to be restored but as a desirable state to be maintained. As a result, the social and economic dimensions of health and health care have been given increased prominence.

At the present stage of its development, scientific medicine includes what has become known as *preventive medicine,* which is defined as "the science and art of preventing disease, prolonging life and promoting physical and mental health and efficiency . . . through intercepting disease processes by community and individual action" (p. 11).[15] Preventive medicine recognizes (1) disease as a process of multiple causation; (2) the relationship of the process to disease agents, living or nonliving; (3) human characteristics; and (4) human responses to internal and external disease-producing stimuli.

The physician is recognized as the practitioner of scientific medicine, whose functions in society include the diagnosis and treatment of disease and its effects. Medical diagnosis, the identification of natural causes and natural effects of disease, precedes treatment. Medical treatment is extended not only to the cure and control of disease processes and the restoration of health and alleviation of symptoms but also to the prevention of disease and to overcoming defects and disability. Physicians in private or group practice of medicine perform these measures for individuals and families. Other physicians may be associated with various organizations, such as hospitals or business and industrial organizations, to supply care to the clients or the members of these organizations and sometimes to their families.

Medical care refers to the care given to individuals by physicians. The term is sometimes used in a broader sense for services to individuals by agencies and members of the various health professions and occupations—hospitals, physicians, dentists, nurses, and pharmacists. Nursing as a health care service is properly referred to as a part of medical care when the term *medical care* is used with this broader meaning. Nonmedical systems of health care exist in addition to the scientific medical care commonly practiced in the United States.

The practice of scientific medicine requires a number of paramedic and technical services. Paramedic services contribute to some one aspect of medical practice. The major paramedic services are physical therapy, occupational therapy, speech therapy, and some of the services of medical social workers. The various paramedic services use specialized diagnostic and treatment techniques requiring skilled personnel.

Nutritionists and dietitians may have important roles in care directed toward the prevention, cure, or control of disease, working with both the physician and the patient whenever dietary treatment is involved. Clinical psychologists also perform functions that contribute to the diagnosis and treatment of mental and emotional disorders through psychologic testing, counseling, and other therapeutic techniques.

In addition to the preceding services, other highly specialized technical services are essential in the physician's use of diagnostic and therapeutic measures. Physicians diagnosing and determining the course of a disease or a disorder and the effects of therapy require not only the efforts of physicians who are specialists in pathology but also the services of chemists, physicists, and clinical laboratory technicians. The physician in his or her medical practice may also require the services of other physicians who specialize in roentgenology (radiologists) and technicians skilled in the use of x-rays and other types of radiation.

"Alternative" (to Western medicine) forms of medical and health care are increasing in use in the United States. Some care measures have their origins in systems of herbal medical care and other forms of care in Eastern medicine, and some have their origin in the folk medicine of our own country.

SUMMARY

The incorporation of the patient variables therapeutic self-care demand and self-care agency into the broad dimensions of nursing practice for individuals is continued. There is a continued development of the substantive structure of the nurse variable, nursing agency in terms of capabilities for understanding and guiding practice in relation to stages of nursing, rules of nursing practice, patients' needs for use of specific helping methods and for types of nursing systems, the organization of nursing design units, and patients' ages, health states, and health care system features.

The content presented is a continued development of stages II, III, and IV in the model (see Figure 13-3) for understanding nursing and developing the practical science of nursing. Linkages of the *element nursing agency* (stage II) with nursing cases (stage III) are identified as well as linkages with models and rules for nursing practice for individuals (stage IV). Models of three types of nursing systems, six nursing design units, and three stages of nursing practice are presented. Rules of nursing practice are presented in relation to the three stages of nursing practice.

The chapter presents a foundation for understanding factors affecting nursing practice.

References

1. Black M: *Models and metaphors,* Ithaca, NY, 1962, Cornell University Press, pp 93-136.
2. Black M: *Problems of analysis: philosophical essays,* Ithaca, NY, 1954, Cornell University Press, p 29.
3. Meyer, RMS, Morris DT: Alcoholic cardiomyopathy: a nursing approach, *Nurs Res* 26:422-427, 1977.
4. Meyer M: Application of the Orem self-care deficit theory to nursing practice. Paper given at a conference on nursing theories: adaptation and self-care, St Louis University Medical Center, October 25, 1978.
5. Taylor SG, Robinson-Purdy AU: Assessing self-management and dependent care capabilities of hospitalized adults and care givers in preparation for discharge, clinical and cultural dimensions around the world, pp. 4-16. Papers and abstracts presented at the first international self-care deficit nursing theory conference, School of Nursing, University of Missouri, Columbia, October 15-18, 1989, Kansas City, Curators of the University of Missouri.
6. *Webster's dictionary of synonyms,* ed 1, Springfield, Mass, 1951, GB Merriman Publishers, p 622.
7. Simon HA: *Sciences of the artificial,* Cambridge, 1969, MIT Press.
8. Weiss P: *You, I, and the others,* Carbondale and Edwardsville, IL, 1980, Southern Illinois University Press, p 50.
9. Knutson AL: *The individual, society, and health behavior,* New York, 1969, Russell Sage Foundation, pp 180-193.
10. Ullman M: Health deviations and behavior. In Orem DE, Parker KS, editors: *Nursing content in preservice nursing curriculums,* Washington, DC, 1964, Catholic University of America Press, pp 74-76, 78-80.
11. Orem DE, Vardiman EM: Orem's nursing theory and positive mental health: practical considerations, *Nurs Sci Q* 8:4, 1995.
12. Lonergan BJF: *Insight,* London, 1958, Longman's Green, pp 211-216, 322-324.
13. Weiss, P: *You, I, and the others,* London and Amsterdam, 1980, Feffer & Simons, pp 226-227.
14. Sorokin P: Social and cultural dynamics, Boston, 1957, Porter Sargent, pp 445-452.
15. Leavell HR et al: *Preventive medicine for the doctor in his community,* New York, 1965, McGraw-Hill, p 11.

CHAPTER 14

The Practice of Nursing in Multiperson Situations, Family and Community

Susan G. Taylor and Kathie McLaughlin Renpenning

394

This chapter identifies the features of nursing practice that must be understood when nurses work in nursing practice situations involving several individuals as the unit of service. Nursing systems in **multiperson situations** are of two basic types: (1) those in which the nursing system is designed for a number of persons who make up a collective or aggregate by virtue of something in common, such as a shared space, situation, or relationship, as well as a common concern that is within the domain of nursing, and (2) **multiperson units,** such as **families** and **communities,** where the unit itself is the object of nursing (often referred to in nursing literature as family-as-client or community-as-client). These variations are illustrated in Figure 14-1.

In this chapter, attention is given to conditions under which existent or developing multiperson collectives or units in society become the object of concern for nursing, classifications of multiperson groups that are meaningful for nursing, and the needed adjustment of nursing practice operations to features of multiperson nursing practice situations.

UNITS OF SERVICE AND KINDS OF MULTIPERSON SITUATIONS

A **unit of service** is the human entity that is the primary focus or object of nurses' attention. It is a complex entity that can be regarded as a whole. The nature of the "whole" is a critical variable in determining the type of nursing system or the characteristics of nursing systems to be designed. *Unit of service* is a term used to designate whether nurses provide nursing to persons as individuals, persons as dependent-care units, or persons in collectives or multiperson units. In the first instance, the individual is the focus or object of nurses' attention; in the last instance, the multiperson unit with its members is the primary focus or object of nurses' attention (see Figure 14-1).

In nursing for individuals or in dependent-care situations, there is one identified person whose therapeutic self-care demand, powers of self-care agency, and existent or projected self-care deficit are the focus of the nurse. When the dependent-care unit is the unit of service, the final objectives of the nursing system are to achieve nursing results for the dependent, not the dependent-care agent. However, these objectives may include helping the dependent-care agent acquire new knowledge and skills. Nursing systems in dependent-care situations—that is, when social dependency is an element of the situation—have some of the attributes of nursing systems for which the individual is the unit of service. However, in addition, the design of the nursing system includes at least one other person and the following additional variables:

- Those associated with the dependent-care system: dependent-care, dependent-care agency, dependent-care demand, and dependent-care deficit
- Select components of the self-care system of the dependent-care agent.

In multiperson nursing situations, the named variables (self-care, therapeutic self-care demand or components thereof, self-care agency, and self-care deficit) of all the members are of concern (see Table 14-1).

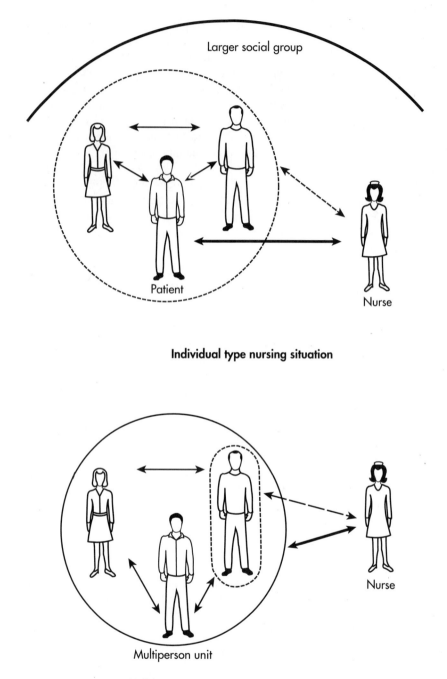

Individual type nursing situation

Multiperson unit type nursing situation

Figure 14-1 The object of the nurse in individual and multiperson nursing situations.

CRITICAL DIFFERENCE BETWEEN NURSING OF INDIVIDUALS, IN MULTIPERSON SITUATIONS, AND FOR MULTIPERSON UNITS

Although humans are described as individuals, separate and unique, they live and survive by a series of interdependent relationships within the primary units of family and community. Because of the nature of human action and relationships, nurses frequently find themselves interacting with several people at one time and in one location, or needing to take into consideration the *other* or *others* of importance to the patient. The consideration of multiperson situations as a different form of nursing than nursing for individuals is legitimated by experiences of nurses and by examination of the way people live and interact.

Nursing system design has its foundation in the contract or agreement between parties to provide and receive nursing (design units A and B, Chapter 13). Design unit A establishes for nurses who is to be nursed, why nursing is needed, and its jurisdiction; design unit B identifies the operational participants in the nursing situation and areas of independence and interdependence. When the nurse establishes that the nursing system to be produced has as its object a multiperson unit of service, nursing operations take on characteristics that reflect that multiplicity of persons and interactions among and between them. When the multiperson unit is the object of nursing, the nursing operations not only reflect that multiplicity of persons and interactions among and between them but also are directed toward the good of the unit as a unit.

When the unit of nursing is an individual, the nurse sees the individual as the one in need of care; the nurse also sees the individual as a member of a family and other groups. Nurses working in hospitals are well aware of the involvement of family in the illness experience of the patient. This involvement may be as intensive as providing much of the care for the patient or as minimal as social visits and phone calls. The attention of family members, friends, or acquaintances may enhance the patient's condition, or it may be a hindrance to the well-being of the individual. If the family members are placing demands on the patient that divert the patient's energy, there may be a negative effect on recovery. In a home care situation, family and friends may be the essential element in maintaining a balance between solitude and social interaction for the patient.

The nurse who cares for patients in the home environment experiences more directly the importance of the context of the family or social unit and the impact of that environment on the patient. These experiences of nurses lead to the consideration of groups not only as a setting within which care of the individual occurs or as basic conditioning factors but also as units of service.

A multiperson unit is made up of more than a single person and regarded as a whole, as "we." The size of a multiperson unit may range from two to some undetermined upper limit. In a multiperson unit, noting that each individual has his or her own set of operations and requisites is important; the identification of these is important to understanding the functioning of the whole, the unit. Nevertheless, understanding the operations and requisites of each individual does not provide understanding of the functioning of the whole. Relationships must be identified and understood, including relationships of unit members to one another and to relevant persons outside the unit. The action systems generated by persons in the unit (self-care, dependent-care, and other systems of daily living) must be identified and relationships specified.

Each person in the unit of service has a therapeutic self-care demand and developing, developed, or declining powers of self-care agency. The health and well-being of each are subject to the effects of the interactions between and among the persons in the situation and the system of living within the unit, with the good operation and welfare of the unit as nursing considerations. There exists within the family and other interactive multiperson units a care system with many subsystems. This care system has developed over time to meet the therapeutic self-care demands of the individual members through role allocation and interaction and some combination of independent and interdependent actions.

RATIONALE FOR NURSING FOR MULTIPERSON UNITS, FAMILIES, AND COMMUNITIES

As previously stated, the acceptance of families and other groups as units of service of nurses can be legitimated by nursing experiences and knowledge of the way people live and interact. There is a philosophic basis as well. Human beings grow and develop in relation to other persons. "The Self exists only in dynamic relation to the Other . . . the Self is constituted by its relation to the Other; that it has its being in its relationship; and that this relationship is necessarily personal" (p. 17).[1] The interdependence of human beings leads us to understand that the well-being or functionality of the unit can be an end in itself. Not only are we concerned with the health and well-being of the individuals who function within social units but also we recognize that there is a level of well-being that goes beyond that of the separate individuals to include the quality of interaction and the outcomes of those interactions on the unit as a whole. When the unit of service is a multiperson unit, the nurse's objective focus is the unit and the individuals comprising it. There is interaction between the self-care systems of the various members of the multiperson situation, and the concern of nursing includes the therapeutic self-care demand of those persons. The nurse may work with individuals within the unit, knowing that the health and well-being of individuals will contribute to the welfare of the unit. Likewise, the nurse may work with the collective group, knowing that the welfare of the unit may contribute to the health and well-being of the individuals who make up the unit. Nurses may serve persons both as individual units of service and as parts of a multiperson unit when certain conditions prevail. For example, the nurse may be serving the chronically ill older family member as an individual and as a part of the multiperson unit of the family.

There is much in the literature of other disciplines, such as sociology and psychology, on multiperson units. Family systems theory has categories of family types. A variety of groups form, and people come together for a variety of purposes. People who are not related as family may reside together for extended periods, such as in group homes. Multiperson situations may include the simple to complex affiliative "we," with relationships between individuals,[2] and the unrelated aggregation of individuals with no personal relationship, such as the "we" in an airport terminal or patients on a nursing unit in a hospital.

In developing theory about nursing systems for multiperson units and in projecting models for practice and designs for nursing systems, the nature and meaning of the relationships (or lack thereof) must be understood. An important aspect of this concerns whether there are "direct or impersonal relations." Direct relations are those in which individuals have a personal knowledge of one another. Impersonal relations exclude this condition; they are relations between persons who are not personally known to one another.

CRITERIA FOR IDENTIFICATION OF MULTIPERSON NURSING SITUATIONS

Although nurses interact with patients, families, and other groups in many different multiperson situations, there are two basic types of situations: those with a direct personal relationship among the members of the unit and those with an impersonal relationship. The characteristics of the multiperson situation (Table 14-1) condition the nursing system that can be established. The relationships between and among members of the group set the limits for the system (design units A and B), the interpersonal aspects of the nursing situation, and the technologic aspects of the care system.

Factors that have a major influence on the development of relationships and consequently on the development of nursing systems form the basis for the classification system. The type of structured unit affects the type of relationship the nurse can anticipate. It makes a difference if the structured unit is a family with direct personal relationships or a group that came together for a shared purpose who do not personally know one another. The enduring factor conditions the commitment of the members of the unit to interdependence and shared problem resolution, and those units that endure are likely to have a higher level of interdependence. Those persons who live together develop care systems that reflect the residential closeness and the increased time spent in proximity. Criteria for identification of multiperson situations as a unit of service are described in the box on p. 402.

Very often in family and community nursing practice situations, the nurse begins working with an individual but in so doing collects data about family and community variables. In analyzing this data it may become evident that the self-care system of the individual is heavily influenced by family and community conditioning factors that need to be addressed. At this point, two nursing systems may be required, one in which the individual is the unit of service and one in which the multiperson unit of family or community becomes the unit of service.

There are multiperson situations with impersonal relations, as in unstructured groups, in which case the nurse may interact with more than one person at a time

Table 14-1 Characteristics of Individual and Multiperson Nursing Situations

Type of Nursing Situation	Therapeutic Self-Care Demand and Self-Care Requisite	Characteristics		Purpose of Nursing
		Action Limitation and Action Requirement		
Individual	The therapeutic self-care demand is constituted from some mix of universal, developmental, and health deviation requisites.	There are all types of health-derived or health-related limitations for engagement in care.		To develop or regulate the exercise of self-care or dependent-care capabilities. To compensate for action limitations so that the therapeutic self-care demand will be met effectively and continuously.
Multiperson unit Community groups, including work group situations	Some self-care requisites are common to all persons who constitute the group. Methods for meeting these self-care requisites are developed and have a known degree of effectiveness. The environment in which group members work or live affects the nature of the common self-care requisites as well as the methods for meeting them.	Action limitations are limitations of interest, motivation, knowledge, or skill on the part of group members. There is a requirement for organized, cooperative effort to bring about the conditions and acquire resources to meet self-care requisites common to group members.		To promote the development or exercise of essential self-care or dependent-care capabilities. To promote habitual performance of essential measures of self-care or dependent-care under known prevailing conditions. To bring about the development and maintenance of cooperative efforts essential for group welfare.

| Family or residence group situations | The interrelatedness of members and their living environment affects the values of the self-care requisites of individual family or group members. Meeting the therapeutic self-care demand of one or more individuals affects if and how the therapeutic self-care demands of other members can be met. | Action limitations are limitations of interest, motivation, knowledge, and skill on the part of group members. There is a requirement for organized, cooperative effort to meet the therapeutic self-care demands of individuals within the group and to promote the well-being of the group as a unit. | To promote development by family or group members of the capability to view the family or group as a unit of structure and operation. To promote the development or exercise of essential self-care or dependent-care capabilities. To promote the development of the capability on the part of some or all group members to (1) plot out the interrelatedness of the therapeutic self-care demands of members, (2) design a plan for meeting individual and group needs, and (3) secure and maintain the required human effort and material resources. |

Criteria for Identification of Multiperson Situation as Unit of Service

1. There are two or more persons in direct relationship with a personal interaction (intersubjectivity) existent or possible between members of the unit with the potential for intersubjectivity between the nurse and one or more or all members of the unit.
2. The existence of a multiperson care system. **Multiperson-care systems** are those courses and sequences of action performed by the persons in multiperson units for the purpose of meeting the self-care requisites and the development and exercise of self-care agency of all members of the group and to maintain or establish the welfare of the unit. The existent care systems for individuals are interactive. The subsystems of the multiperson system are the self-care systems of the individuals. The units of operations within multiperson units are the existent, emerging, developing self-care operations and dependent-care operations, operations relative to development and exercise of self-care agency with the end being the health and well-being of members of the unit, providing a developmental environment for all and the effective and economic functioning of the whole.
3. There must be some internal (within the unit) condition that affects knowing and meeting the therapeutic self-care demands of one or more of the members of the unit, affecting the health and well-being of one or more or all members of the unit. A part of the internal condition could be the degrees of interaction described in terms of extent and intensity, role allocation or role assumption.

---

but which would not be considered a multiperson unit. The use of television to present information to large numbers of people, while an effective use of media, does not qualify those persons influenced as a multiperson unit. The larger society within which we live and work does not necessarily qualify as a multiperson unit. This is not to diminish the importance of nurses' concerns about health-related issues as affected by the larger society. It should help to clarify the roles and functions of the nurse in different situations. Nurses have responsibilities, legitimate roles in multiperson situations that are not multiperson units of service per se. The nurse who is providing nursing to a multiperson unit of service uses interpersonal and group processes to affect the self-care systems of one or more of the individuals in the unit so that the welfare of the unit is enhanced. This is done within an personal-interpersonal nursing care system. The nurse who is concerned with the health of the public, those persons who constitute the large society, will use public health nursing theory and interventions, including monitoring, surveillance, mass education, immunization, quarantine, and community development. These differences are clarified in the section on communities.

CATEGORIES OF MULTIPERSON-CARE SYSTEMS OR NURSING SYSTEMS

Type One Multiperson-Care Systems

Care systems in multiperson units of service for classification type one are structured unities formed from individualized self-care and dependent-care systems. Given two or more existent care systems with care agents or designs for new or adjusted systems that place new demands on care systems, it is possible for nurses or members of the unit to (1) examine individual systems, (2) identify real or potentially desirable or undesirable points of articulation among the systems and between the systems and other operations of daily living, and (3) identify the needs for resources, availability of resources, and time and place frames of reference. The individual care systems with their articulations are the parts, the subsystems from which a multiperson-care system is constituted. Care systems as here described contribute to the health, human development, and well-being of members of the unit. They are enabling for fulfillment of responsibility for the units as a whole, including community responsibilities.

Type Two Multiperson-Care Systems

When persons in the unit do not live in daily continuous intersubjectivity with one another but come together in a developmental environment on a periodic basis to achieve goals related to their own self-care or dependent-care for others, another kind of care system exists. Care systems in type two multiperson units are (1) nurses' general designs for self-care or dependent-care and for the exercise or development of self-care agency or dependent-care agency to meet care requisites or developmental needs common to members of the unit and (2) nurses' and members' actions to generate learning systems to individualize and adjust elements of the general design to each member's situation.

When the patient is an individual who is a member of a structured, enduring social group, the nurse has the responsibility for ascertaining which persons form a functional unity and need to be a part of the design of the nursing system, as described by Orem's design unit B (see Chapter 13). Unless the nurse identifies the group as a multiperson unit of service, the nurse does not have direct obligations to the members other than those incurred as a part of the design of the nursing system for the individual.

When the members of the unit of service do not live together continuously, their coming together will affect the self-care requisites of the members for some limited time. The interrelatedness is a function of coming together, sharing some common requisites and mutually agreeing to work on shared tasks or goals. There is a requirement for organized, cooperative effort to bring about the conditions and acquire the resources to meet self-care requisites common to group members. Because the unit is less enduring, the nurse, while capitalizing on the cooperative efforts to meet the common requisites must also attend to the development of the self-care, self-management system of each individual as they will be moving away from the structured group.

Type Three Multiperson-Care Systems

Care systems for persons who meet as a group at specific times (type three) are composed of persons who have similar types of self-care requisites, with a need to acquire knowledge and skills that will enable them to meet particular composed of their therapeutic self-care demands. The interrelatedness of the individuals in the unit initially may be impersonal; the members become acquainted as the nurse uses functional group processes and knowledge about group dynamics in working with the group. Nurses must develop skill in being able to see persons in groups both as individuals and as group members. The focus is on the development of a learning system. In most instances, the primary type of nursing system would be supportive-educative.

Other Categories of Multiperson-Care Systems

In addition to these categories, a number of other descriptors can be applied, based on the nature of the care systems in place within the unit and the kind of nursing system required. The care system in place within the group might be partly or wholly compensatory care for one member, with the care being provided by other members. There are primary and secondary caregivers. The care system may be collaborative, complementary, compensatory, or custodial. There are many systems that are mixed, with a partly to wholly compensatory nursing system in place for one member of the group and a supportive-educative nursing system in place for the rest of the members of the unit. These systems, however configured, are action systems, and as such they need to be created by the persons involved.

Collaborative Care Systems

The collaborative care system has been described by Geden and Taylor. This system is made up of the interaction of the individuals' self-care systems, as shown in Figure 14-2.

The collaborative care system is thought to be a unique whole, with each member having demands and making contributions to the system. "Inherent in the collaborative care system is the concept of shared work, resulting in negotiated roles for integrating and performing actions to meet the requirements for care. The negotiation includes identification of the therapeutic self-care demands (individual and interactive) and the selection of actions based on individuals' capabilities for taking such action,"[3] as shown in Figure 14-3.

"While the pattern or distribution of actions may vary, the collaborative care system requires both members to make a contribution to the system of care. For instance, a couple may choose one member to be a primary decision-maker about self-care and another may provide the material resources. This is unlike a dependent-care system wherein one person acts on behalf of another and there is no requirement that the dependent person actively negotiate his/her own care" (p. 330).[3] In a collaborative care system, when "one person becomes ill and is no longer able to collaborate in the production of care, the other is confronted with

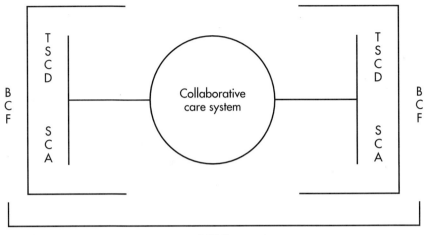

Figure 14-2 The collaborative care system. *BCF,* Basic conditioning factors; *BCF-C,* Couples basic conditioning factors; *SCA,* Self-care agency; *TSCD,* Therapeutic self-care demand. From Geden E, Taylor SG: Theoretical and empirical description of adult collaborative self-care system, *Nurs Sci Q* 12:329-334, 1999.

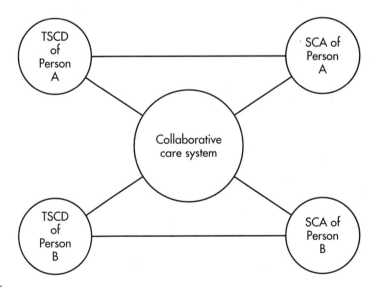

Figure 14-3 Shared working of the collaborative care system. *SCA,* Self-care agency; *TSCD,* Therapeutic self-care demand. From Geden E, Taylor SG: Theoretical and empirical description of adult collaborative self-care system, *Nurs Sci Q* 12:329-334, 1999.

the need to take on those self-care actions to meet the demands no longer met through the collaborative care system" (p. 333).[3]

SOME COMMON FEATURES OF NURSING PRACTICE IN MULTIPERSON NURSING PRACTICE SITUATIONS

Despite the many kinds of multiperson nursing practice situations, there are some common features of nursing practice within those situations. These commonalities are presented as they relate to the dimensions of nursing systems: social contract, interpersonal features, and technologic features.

Social Contract Features

The common characteristic of the social contract between nurse and members of the multiperson unit is a function of the multiplicity of persons with whom the nurse must establish objectives. The multiperson unit exists or comes together for some shared purpose. The nurse works with the various members of the group, together or separately, to determine the scope and limitations of the nursing responsibilities (design unit A). The nurse often uses processes of negotiation, collaboration, and group interaction to clarify the objectives, roles, and responsibilities of the persons involved. The nature or characteristics of the unit are a major factor in determining the extent of the social contract, the strategies the nurse uses in determining jurisdiction and limits, and other social contract features. When there are direct, personal relationships among the members of the unit, such as in a family, the nurse must have an understanding of and sensitivity to the personal interactions and functioning of the family or personal systems, the meaning of relationships, and the interactive dimensions of the care systems of members of the unit.

Within these various situations, there may be instances when the nursing focus shifts from the unit to the individual. The first consideration in designing a nursing system is the clarifying the functional relationships of persons involved and establishing the contractual responsibility of the nurses. The nurse must determine if the obligation for care, or the object of care, is the individual—an identified patient—or the multiperson unit. If the former, the family members and other individuals in the situation are incorporated into the nursing system in ways that meet the objectives of care for the individual.

Another commonality in determining the role and scope of responsibilities in a nursing situation is the awareness of the function of culture. Cultural variations in family and community structure and function affect the allocation of roles and responsibilities associated with self-care, dependent-care, and nursing. The particular cultural value and behavior regarding the family and community and the essential roles within the family and community may determine whether the nurse interacts with the patient as an individual or interacts with the family or community as a multiperson unit of service. For example, if the cultural norm is such that the wife-mother has the responsibility for decision making about the care systems for all family members and the husband-father is a passive recipient of care, it is likely the nurse will use a multiperson unit approach. In other cultures where the autonomy of the individual is paramount and there is a high degree of self-responsibility, the individual is more likely to be the unit of service. Antecedent knowledge about culture in general and certain cultural group norms and mores is necessary for designing nursing systems.

Interactional Features

In multiperson units of service, a common feature of the interpersonal dimension of the nursing system is the simultaneous interaction by the nurse with two or more persons. There is a personal interaction (intersubjectivity) existent or possible between members of the unit, with potential for intersubjectivity between the nurse and one or more or all members of the unit. This requires that the nurse use group process methods as well as individual communication strategies in establishing the group, in identifying the nursing focus, and in designing and implementing nursing systems.

Technologic Features

Technologic features of nursing systems in multiperson units extend beyond those used to regulate the therapeutic self-care demand and self-care system of the individual members of the group. In the framework of the theory of nursing systems in multiperson situations of practice, group processes and interactions and community development processes may replace or be added to the interpersonal system that is created and develops between nurse and patient when the individual is the unit of service.

The focus is on the interrelationships of self-care systems and other conditions of living, one to another. The nurse who is providing nursing to a multiperson unit of service uses interpersonal and group processes and community development processes to affect the self-care systems of one or more of the individuals in the unit so that the therapeutic self-care demands of the individuals are met and the welfare of the unit is maintained or enhanced. The methods of helping used by the nurse for multiperson units of service are generally the provision of a developmental environment, support, guidance, and teaching. The nurse may act for or do with an individual member or members of the unit.

As noted earlier, multiperson-care systems are those courses and sequences of action that are performed by the persons in multiperson units for the purpose of meeting the self-care requisites and the development and exercise of self-care agency of the members of the group. The subsystems of the multiperson-care system are the self-care and dependent-care systems. The units of operations within multiperson units are the existent, emerging, developing self-care operations and dependent-care operations, operations relative to development and exercise of self-care agency, with the end being the health and well-being of members of the unit, providing a developmental environment for all and the effective and economic functioning of the whole.

For the unit to be the object of the nurse's attention, there must be some internal (within the unit) condition that affects knowing and meeting the therapeutic self-care demands of one or more of the members of the unit affecting the health and well-being of one or more or all members of the unit. A part of the internal condition could be the functionality or dysfunctionality of the basic family system, the distribution of power in the community, the communication patterns in use within the unit, the stability of the unit, the existence of self-care limitations on the part of members of the unit, limited resources to meet the self-care demands of the members, and so forth. The nursing system for the unit will consist of the actions taken in cooperation with the members of the unit to meet the self-care requisites of one or more or all of the members of the unit or to regulate the development or exercise of their self-care agency or dependent-care agency, at the same time maintaining the functional integrity of the unit.

Nurses may serve persons both as individual units of service and as parts of a multiperson unit when certain conditions prevail. For example, the nurse may be serving the chronically ill older family member as individual and also as a part of the multiperson unit of the family. Inherent in this is that there is within the unit some identified (identifiable) action system inadequacy based in the self-care demands and self-care agency of one or more of the members of the unit or in the interaction of systems.

NURSING PRACTICE IN FAMILIAL TYPE NURSING SITUATIONS

Descriptions of Familial Type Situations and Types of Nursing Cases in Familial Type Nursing Practice

The definitions and perceptions of family vary by culture and social group. Family may be defined as a system or unit of interacting persons related by marriage, birth, or other strong social bonds, with commitment and attachment among unit members that include future obligations and whose central purpose is to create, maintain, and promote the social, mental, physical, and emotional development of each of its members. For some, the label *family* is limited to those related by blood or marriage; others take a more extensive view and include other strong social bonds as an adequate basis for the title *family*. In this chapter, all those social units that meet the definition as given will be considered familial type situations. Relationships within a family are direct and personal, close and intimate, to almost solitary living on the part of some members of family. The interactions are characterized as interdependent, with aspects of dependence and independence as related to developmental stages and health states of the members. The degrees of interdependence, dependence, and independence may also vary by culture.

There are three basic types of familial situations of interest to nurses: family (1) as a basic conditioning factor conditioning an individual's requirements for care and ability to provide care for self; (2) as structure (setting) for dependent-care unit(s); and (3) as a unit of service. When the nurse anticipates developing a nursing system that includes the family, the first step is to determine the unit of service. The question to be answered is: Will the nurse be responsible for providing nursing to an individual who is a member of a family, to a dependent person who has a caregiver within a family, or to the family as a unit?

Family as Basic Conditioning Factor

When an individual is the unit of service for the nurse, the family has meaning to the nurse as a factor that conditions the self-care system, the therapeutic self-care demand, and the self-care agency of the patient. The family system within which the individual is functioning is a major factor in setting the parameters of the requirements for care and the development of effective systems of care for the individual who is the patient. Self-care is learned within the family. The specific values of self-care requisites are conditioned by the family. For example, the size of the family, family expectations of the individual members, and the resources available for individual family members all have a conditioning effect on the self-care requirements and the means of meeting them for an individual. The person raised in a large family may have very different requisites for solitude and social interaction than does the person raised in a small family and may need to develop different action strategies to meet demands for solitude. The family may be a resource available to be used for and by the patient in managing his or her care requirements. Conversely, in some situations the family may be seen as having a negative effect on the health and self-management of the patient. Patients, members of their families, or others who are acting for patients may or may not be interested in the need or psychologically able to accept the need for collaboration with nurses or the need for being active participants in their own self-care or the care of their dependents (p. 230).[4]

Family as Setting for Infant and Child Care, Dependent-Care Systems Associated with Health Deviation Type Care

Dependent-care can be considered a specialized family operation that requires management. The family is seen as the setting that conditions the dependent-care system and within which dependent-care systems are produced. The kind of care needed varies according to the nature of the dependent-care unit and the reasons for the dependency, which may be related to age, developmental state, or health state. Dependent-care associated with health deviations may range from providing custodial care to actively participating in a complex care system. When a dependent-care system is needed because of health deviations, specific factors that condition dependent-care agency include the severity of illness, the complexity of the technology in use or to be used, the intensity of the dependent's suffering, the meaning of the dependent-care relationship, and the care agent's tolerance for involvement in personal care measures for others. The quantity and quality of dependent-care assistance required by an individual is a function of the complexity of the individual's self-care demand and the nature of the self-care limitations. Types of dependent-care systems include parent and minor child,

---

Family Functions of Primary Concern to Nursing

1. The socialization of family members as self-care and dependent-care agents.
2. The recognition of therapeutic self-care demand of individual family members and the development of strategies to meet these demands including:
   (a) awareness of changes occurring in persons and environment.
   (b) knowledge of conditioning effects of these changes on the health state of family members.
   (c) knowledge of ways of meeting therapeutic self-care demands of family members and skills and motivation to meet these.
   (d) awareness of the conditioning effect of the roles and interrelationship of family members on the therapeutic self-care demands and self-care abilities of each individual family member.
3. Access to, control, and management of resources needed to meet therapeutic self-care demands and health care needs of family members.
4. The integration of the aspects of self-care and dependent-care into an overall satisfactory plan of living and development for the family.

adult-adult, and the adult child and elderly parent. The nature of the relationship that exists between the dependent person and the caregiver is a major conditioning factor in the establishment of the dependent-care system.

Family as Unit of Service

From a nursing perspective, the family as the unit of service is based on the premise that the **family has certain functions related to self-care** and dependent-care of all its members that exceed or are different from meeting each individual's self-care requirements. The basis for this is the recognition that a family has a unity constituted from its members that leads to structure and functions that are substantially different from those of the individual member. Within the framework of self-care deficit nursing theory, there are certain family functions that are of primary concern to nursing.[5] These functions are outlined in the preceding box.

Examples of Familial Type Units of Service

A number of familial type units have meaning for nursing (see box on p. 411). The meaning for nursing is derived from the fact that the structure of the unit or the stage of development of the unit in some way affects meeting the therapeutic self-care demands of the individuals or carrying out other functions of the family.

Familial-Type Units of Service

Families with different structures
  Nuclear families
  Extended families
  Multigenerational families
  Split families (some members reside together)
  Blended families
  Adult-only families
  Single-parent families
Families by developmental stage
  Child-bearing families
  Child-rearing families
Families with altered health states
  Families with sick children
  Families with sick adults
  Adult or adolescent child caring for adult parent
Familial-type situations
  Transitional living groups

NURSING PRACTICE OPERATIONS IN FAMILIAL TYPE NURSING PRACTICE SITUATIONS

Nurses who work effectively in **familial type situations** must be able to take and maintain a *nursing* focus as distinguished from the focus of social worker or family therapist. In designing nursing systems, the nurse must have a clear idea of the object of the action system to be produced. When the object of the system is a multiperson unit, the self-care systems of the individuals become the subsystems. The more clearly the nurse understands the dynamics of the interrelatedness (or lack thereof) of the individuals and the effect of living conditions on the person(s) involved, the more appropriate will be the design of the nursing system. The relations may be direct or indirect, personal or impersonal, and of varying intensity and extent. All of these condition the design and production of the nursing system. An essential first step in the design of nursing systems for multiperson units of service must be the determination of what is: the roles of members, their existent and changing relations, the elements and adequacy of self-care systems and articulations between the individual systems and other aspects of daily living, and the structural and functional integration within the unit, the intent of action being the well-being of the unit as well as that of its members.

Diagnostic Operations

Individual as Unit of Service

When the individual is the unit of service, the primary assessment question related to family system elements is: Do and how do family system factors condition the patient's self-care requisites, methods of meeting self-care requisites, and self-care agency? A second question is: To what extent can, will, or should the family members be involved in the care of the patient? The nursing diagnosis, when the individual is the unit of service, is related to the nature of the self-care deficit of the patient. Prescriptions may include actions to be taken by family members to accomplish the goals of meeting components of the therapeutic self-care demand of the patient and the regulation of self-care agency.

Dependent-Care Unit as Unit of Service

When the unit of service is the dependent-care unit, whether that unit is composed of the whole family or a part of the family, the assessment includes the family as the source of the basic conditioning factors affecting both the dependent and the responsible person or caregiver. It is necessary to distinguish the family as a factor that conditions the dependent-care system from the family as unit of service because the primary objective of care in dependent-care systems is the therapeutic self-care demand of the dependent one, not that of all family members.

Assessment and diagnosis include the determination of the therapeutic self-care demand of the dependent, determination of the nature of the self-care agency of the dependent, and the determination of the care capabilities or dependent-care agency of the caregiver(s). The nursing diagnosis is the statement of the dependent-care deficit expressed in terms of the caregivers' limitations for action as they relate to helping the dependent. Included in this diagnosis is the statement of the nature of the self-care deficit of the dependent. For example, the dependent patient may be limited in ability to perform the complex actions required to care for a tracheotomy. The spouse, as caregiver, might be diagnosed as limited in ability to assist the dependent in caring for the tracheotomy because of fear of injuring a loved one and lack of experience with providing personal care to another person or to a particular person.

In most instances, meeting the caregiver's therapeutic self-care demand is not an objective of the nursing system; however, the care system that is prescribed must take into account the caregiver's need to care for self at the same time he or she is providing dependent-care. The nurse would assess the caregiver's therapeutic self-care demand and self-care agency as factors that condition the caregiver's ability to provide the care as well as conditioning the meeting of a dependent's requirements for care. From the perspective of the nurse, the stability of the dependent-care unit is a major factor in prescribing the care system for the dependent. If there is a different caregiver each time the nurse interacts with the patient, as in a home visit, the dependent-care system needs to be reevaluated; adjustments must be made to account for the variations of ability of dependent-care agents and the impact of the varying caregiver's abilities on the dependent person.

Family as Unit of Service

The condition that establishes the basis for nursing the family as a unit would arise when the functioning of the family unit is being affected by actions taken or not taken to carry out functions related to self-care or dependent-care of family members (internal condition criterion). As noted earlier, the nurses' decision about conditions that justify identifying the multiperson unit include "a need for protection and prevention, regulation of a hazard; need for environmental regulation; need for resources" (p. 296-299).[4]

The nursing database would include the calculated therapeutic self-care demand for each individual family member, the quality and nature of the self-care agency and dependent-care agency of each family member, and the current system (and its adequacy) for meeting the therapeutic self-care demands of the family members, within the context of the family system. Of special concern is the interrelationship between the self-care requisites and self-care abilities of the individual family members and the resulting interdependence in providing for the care of each other. The assessment questions of primary interest when the family is the unit of service are: Is the family system functioning in a manner such that the four functions related to self-care are being adequately met or does family functioning interfere with meeting the health-related therapeutic self-care demands of some or all of the family members? What are the interrelationships of the self-care and dependent-care systems within the family?

Knowledge about family systems is essential antecedent knowledge for nursing. There are four dimensions to be assessed:

1. Individual subsystems
2. Family interaction patterns
3. Unique characteristics of the whole
4. Environmental field considerations

The individual subsystems to be assessed are the self-care systems of each of the individual family members. The interaction patterns include the dependent-care systems that have been established to meet the therapeutic self-care demands of the dependent family members. In addition to the dependent-care systems, there may also be other collaborative or compensatory arrangements between family members that have been established or have evolved to ensure that the therapeutic self-care demands of each other are met. These interaction patterns, along with the way the family is carrying out the functions related to self-care of members, constitute the unique characteristics of the whole. Environmental field considerations are analogous to assessment of the basic factors that condition both the requirements for self-care and self-care agency and include such factors as sociocultural orientation, health state, health care system elements, and family system elements.

Nursing diagnostic conclusions are related to the family focus on the four identified functions and the effects of meeting the therapeutic self-care demands of individual family members on other members and on family structure and function. Nursing for families is a function of the current or projected therapeutic self-care demands of individual family members, their self-care agency and dependent-care agency, and the effects of meeting the therapeutic self-care demands of individual family members on other members and on family structure and function. When the family is the unit of service, nursing diagnostic statements include reference to the individuals' self-care deficits and dependent relationships, as well as reference to the functions of the family. In the design of the nursing system, concern shifts from the self-care requisites and abilities of each individual member to the roles and interrelationships within the family and the impact of these interrelationships on the self-care demands and self-care agency of each of the family members. Examples include the articulation of self-care systems of husbands and wives, the articulation of care systems for children, and the interpersonal behaviors of family members.

Prescription and Regulatory Operations

Identifying the family as the unit of service suggests that the nurse has specific obligations to each and every member of the unit and that the objective of care—the reason for nursing involvement—is the well-being of the whole unit as manifested in the meeting of therapeutic self-care demand and regulation or development of self-care agency of individuals in interaction. Prescription and regulatory operations are congruent with this obligation. In some instances the best interest of one individual may be subordinated to the interest of the whole family. Although it may be best for the elderly grandmother with a chronic disease to be kept in the family home, the impact of meeting the therapeutic self-care demand of the grandmother may be having a very negative effect on the family's health and well-being. If the elderly grandmother is the nurse's patient, the nurse's obligation to family members might be limited to communication of types of self-care limitations occurring and projected; if the environment in which the care is being provided (e.g., the home) begins to be inadequate for the care of the patient (grandmother), the nurse's obligation is to the grandmother. This would require the nurse to evaluate the environment and make adjustments to see that the patient is well cared for. It is quite possible that the actions taken in this situation would be similar to those in the first, but it is also possible that they would be quite different. In both examples, the nurse might recommend that the grandmother be moved to a nursing home. In the second example, the nurse might recommend a different pattern of personal care that would require family members to alter their schedules so they would be able to meet the grandmother's needs. The family might acquiesce and continue to subordinate their needs and wants, either willingly or unwillingly. The care system established for a family composed of adults living together is significantly different from the system established for adults who do not live together. For example, the adult daughter may have care responsibility for her mother. Because they do not live together, the daughter cannot be directly involved in the productive operations of self-care by the mother. If there is a need for compensatory care, it will require the assistance of a third person.

The following situation is presented as an example. The Burke family is composed of a mother, father, and two siblings, one of whom is chronically ill. During a home visit, the nurse assessed the individual members and the family system elements and noted that the mother was spending all her energy meeting the therapeutic self-care demand of the ill child and the well sibling and not attending to her own care. The father was meeting his own demands but was not able to assist in care of other family members. Mrs. Burke was experiencing deficits in maintaining an adequate intake of food, a balance between rest and activity, and a balance between solitude and social interaction. As a result, she was not meeting affectional needs with her husband. He was not participating in meeting the dependent-care needs of the children or in assisting his wife to meet her self-care and other personal needs. Affectional functions of the family have been disrupted because of the dependent-care and self-care situations.

This family situation, then, constitutes a legitimate nursing situation in which interventions are directed toward the mother's self-care deficits and the ill child's self-care demands. Appropriate interventions might range from helping to increase or enhance the father's dependent-care abilities directed toward the wife and children, arranging for home health care help for the mother, or even removing the ill child from the home setting to decrease demands on the family. If, after these self- and dependent-care demands are met, the affectional functions of the family remain disrupted, the situation would likely require the assistance of a family counselor rather than nursing.

NURSING PRACTICE IN COMMUNITY TYPE SITUATIONS

Expanding understanding of the determinants of health, changing health care delivery systems, the interdisciplinary nature of those systems, and efforts to deliver quality health services for all while containing costs lead to the requirement for new models descriptive of nursing within the community health system. Community nursing practice has expanded over the years to include home care as well as traditional public health nursing. The increase in number and kind of community health care services, shortened hospital stays, and the emphasis on home care require us to expand our conceptualization of community nursing.

The perceived decline in infectious disease and the rise in the relative importance of other illnesses and chronic diseases have led to the development of a new paradigm, which accepts that the occurrence of disease within a population can be studied at multiple levels, including populations, individuals, organs, tissue, cells, and molecules. Within this perspective there is a holistic view of disease and recognition of the need for a multidisciplinary approach to health-related matters. In addition, the emergence of **community participation** in multilevel studies implies working across disciplines and with the community itself in defining variables, designing instruments, and collecting data that reflect the ecologic reality of life in the community as people experience it.

Nurses in the community have a distinct and important service to offer. The contribution of nursing to promoting and maintaining the health and welfare of the populations being served is enhanced when nurses in **community type situations** are able to take and maintain a nursing focus, as distinguished from the focus of other community health workers.

In community type nursing situations, nurses are continuously concerned with the relationship between and among community variables and the health and well-being of persons for whom they are providing service. Nurses work with:

1. Individuals within the context of family and community and within a particular environment
2. Individuals and their caregivers in a dependent-care system, which is also within the context of family and community within a particular environment
3. Groups in the context of the community within a particular environment
4. Community of persons in relation within a particular environment

All nursing occurs within an interdisciplinary context. As professionals with a particular knowledge base and set of skills, nurses are in a position to establish the scope and boundaries of the domain of nursing and to contribute a nursing perspective to each situation. Development of such a perspective requires that nurses have a clear conceptualization of the characteristics of the health profession, nursing. This perspective, when added to that of other health professionals within the interdisciplinary environment, enriches the understanding of health-related matters and of the dimensions of health care and service.

The goals of community nursing include health promotion, protection, prevention, and access. Prevention includes primary, secondary, and tertiary prevention. Primary prevention focuses on the root cause of the problem and targets the population in the stage of susceptibility before the onset of a health problem. Primary prevention includes monitoring and management of environmental factors that are hazardous to health and conducting early intervention, such as immunizations and provision of reproductive health services with the goal of reducing morbidity. Secondary prevention seeks to identify risk behaviors and reduce negative health outcomes through early detection, including screening programs, and through behavior modification such as behavior change counseling and education. Tertiary prevention focuses on the medical and nursing treatment of disease to ameliorate symptoms. Although this type of prevention from a community perspective is not always considered "prevention," it includes the treatment of communicable disease to prevent spread of the disease and management of chronic disease to limit morbidity.

Labonte[6] describes the "new" health practices reflected in policies following development by the World Health Organization of the Ottawa Charter,[7] in which health is defined as a resource for living and health promotion conceptualized as concern about the creation of living conditions in which a person's experience of health is increased.[8] The focus of health promotion moved from "strictly medical and behavioral health determinants, to health determinants defined in psycho-logic, social, environmental, and political terms. Empowerment, or the capacity to define, analyze and act upon problems in one's life and living conditions, joins treatment and prevention as important health care professional and health agency goals."[6]

COMMUNITY AS A MULTIPERSON UNIT OF SERVICE

Within the perspective of community as a multiperson unit of service, there are various ways to conceptualize community. Community may be conceptualized as a conditioning factor. In addition, Kirkpatrick[9] suggests that community can be represented by any one of three metaphors. These include an atomistic-contractarian model, an organic-functional model, and a mutual-personal model. Regardless of which conceptualization or metaphor represents one's view of community, from the perspective of self-care deficit nursing theory, community nursing is concerned with self-care systems, self-care practices and the relation-ship of community to those variables. Taylor and McLaughlin[10] have suggested the **functions of community in relation to self-care** (see following box).

Community as Conditioning Factor

When the goal of nursing is to alter the conditioning effect of community variables on the person variables of self-care agency and therapeutic self-care demand, the community becomes a multiperson unit of service. The self-care systems of single persons and of individuals as members of the multiperson units making up the community and the community variables become interacting components. The nurse in such situations must be able to think about populations, conceptualizing the components of therapeutic self-care demand pertinent to members of the population, evaluating the development and effectiveness of self-care agency of community members, and relating the conditioning effects of community variables to the significant components of the therapeutic self-care demand and to the production of self-care.

The health service system that is constructed is an interdisciplinary one in which the actions of nursing are directed at community elements with the goal of

---

Functions of Community in Relation to Self-Care

1. Facilitating meeting the therapeutic self-care demand and dependent-care demand of community members
2. Facilitating development and/or protection, and exercise of self-care agency
3. Controlling environmental hazards and/or assisting community members to over-come the effects of such hazards
4. Monitoring the health of members and preventing the spread of infectious diseases

altering the conditioning effect of community systems and variables on health and the person variables, facilitating action to meet the therapeutic self-care demands of community members, or facilitating the development and exercise of self-care agency of community members (see box on p. 417). The strategies used include community development, group processes, political processes, and communication. The processes for data gathering and the methods of analysis are derived from nursing, epidemiology, public health, sociology, psychology, political science, community development, communication, anthropology, and others, as well as medical science. Providers of health care services use various processes to identify and categorize populations and subpopulations for the purpose of meeting the health requirements of a community. These processes include:

1. Applying epidemiologic techniques for identifying populations at risk
2. Employing public health expertise to identify needed community programs
3. Utilizing community development strategies for identifying the community perspective on health-related priorities and needs

When the subpopulation in need of health-related services has been identified, use of self-care deficit nursing theory provides a structure for examining the relationship of community systems and structures to self-care systems and self-care practices and identifying the role nursing can play in design and delivery of such services. Analysis of this sort is useful for clarifying the parties to the contract. The parties may include one or all of the following: individual persons, groups, or the community at large. Nursing does not act alone but in concert with other disciplines. However, the contribution or particular view of nursing within the interdisciplinary environment is in relation to the proper object of nursing. The community nursing practice model (Figure 14-4) illustrates the variables of concern to nursing and their relationships and provides direction for structuring the nursing component of the interdisciplinary care system.

The Atomistic-Contractarian Model: Community as Aggregate

In this model, community is conceptualized as an "aggregation, a collection of atoms, each driven by self-interest" (p. 30).[9] From the perspective of this model I would require that both you and I are immunized to protect me from any communicable diseases you might have and vice versa. Within this conceptualization, data may be collected at the individual level and/or at the community level, and analysis and intervention may take place at either or both levels.

For example, data may be collected about the number of individuals who know about the relationship between safe sexual practices and AIDS but who do not practice safe sex. Analysis may involve looking at the relationship between individual and group variables, such as exploring the peer values related to safe sex. Prescription may be at the individual level, through design of education programs to help persons know how to practice safe sex, and at the community level, with the provision of ready access to condoms.

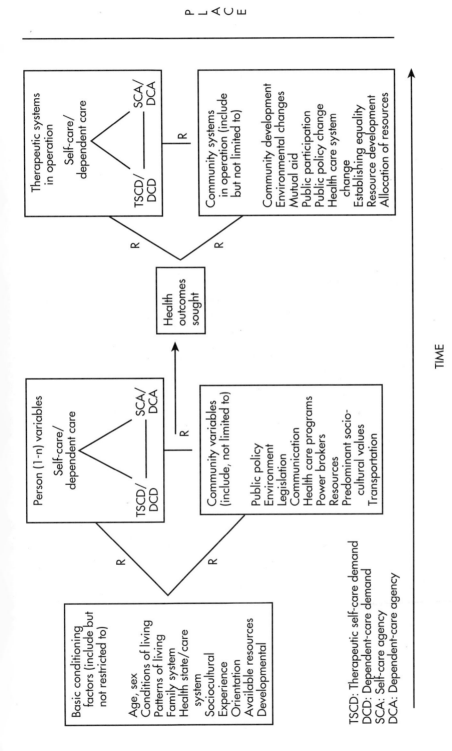

Figure 14-4 A structural community nursing practice model derived from self-care. (Adapted from Taylor SG, McLaughlin K: Orem's general theory of nursing and community nursing, Nursing Science Quarterly 4:153-160, 1991.)

The Organic-Functional Model: Community as a Functional Entity or System

From this perspective the whole is the primary focus, and community is viewed as an entity. Within this perspective, the community is an organism. "Organisms display a kind of structure in which higher levels subsume and control lower levels while remaining dependent upon and in constant interaction with them" (p. 65).[9] This model is reflected in the use of general systems theory to understand the concepts and interrelationships of group and community.

Viewing community from this perspective, nurses are concerned with the question: Are community systems functioning in a manner such that the functions of community in relation to self-care are being achieved? (See box on p. 413.) To answer this question, they would review data relating to self-care systems and community systems in operation. For example, self-care systems in operation for persons of limited income often include community soup kitchens or food lines. These contribute to meeting several components of therapeutic self-care demand: maintaining a sufficient intake of food and maintenance of a balance between solitude and social interaction. The focus of nursing would be on the actions required and the abilities of the person(s) to meet components of the therapeutic self-care demand (in particular, to maintain a sufficient intake of food, to provide care regarding elimination, to maintain a balance between solitude and social interaction, to promote normalcy, and to overcome factors that interfere with development). Included in this would be concern of the knowledge about availability of the service, capability and motivation to access the service, and quality of the food provided. If the limitations for acting were related to community elements or quality of food, or environment were not adequate in relation to the components of the therapeutic self-care demand, the nurse prescription may include using community development strategies or political processes to accomplish needed changes.

Mutual-Personal Model: Community as Persons in Relationship

From the perspective of the mutual-personal model, relationships are central. Treatment of other persons does not come from self-love but out of the realization that I cannot be what I am without another person. The self is fulfilled only in I-thou relations. The idea of community within this perspective is not limited to persons who can be in direct contact with one another but to persons who "have mutual access to one another and are ready for one another" (p. 143).[9] This representation of community is reflected in the literature in discussion of healthy cities and health promotion in which changes in health are brought about through public policy and legislation and other strategies to facilitate healthier life-styles as well as education.[7]

After the individuals making up the community have been identified, nursing should focus on their goals and values about health-related self-care, the relationship of interactions within the community to self-care, factors limiting persons' ability to meet their health-related self-care goals, interactions and relationships that would facilitate development and exercise of self-care abilities, and resources required. Within this view the nurse integrates in the prescription community development strategies that focus on building *community* and empowering community members to act on their own behalf.

STRUCTURING THE NURSING COMPONENT OF HEALTH CARE SYSTEMS IN THE COMMUNITY

Health care systems as action systems do not exist until they are created, and they are created for a specific purpose: the management of health-related concerns. The nature of the system varies with the persons making up the system, the outcomes to be achieved, and the value system of the community, including its willingness to allocate resources. A nursing system is a component of the health care system. Recognizing the interdisciplinary nature of the health care system and community nursing, the nursing system should be designed using a nursing model that is articulated with those of other health care professionals and incorporates public health models. Such a model is presented in this chapter. Structuring the nursing component includes determining what services are required and what resources are available so that these can be brought together in such a manner as to achieve the desired goals. The process begins with identifying the variables of concern to nursing and their relationship, describing the population from the perspective of nursing, defining the nursing practice operations, identifying and describing the articulation of the nursing system with other components of the health care system, and determining and allocating the roles of persons involved in the overall health care system.

A COMMUNITY NURSING PRACTICE MODEL

Community nursing practice from the perspective of self-care deficit nursing theory embodies this thinking about health care systems and the desired outcomes of health promotion and disease prevention. Although the nursing focus is derived from the proper object of nursing, the inability of persons to maintain the quantity and quality of required self-care, the nurse in the community is required to think beyond the values of the specific variables of therapeutic self-care demand and self-care agency of individuals. The nurse must be able to think of those variables in relation to populations, community, and community systems in operation, and the relation of these to the person variables.

In the community, health care professionals work in terms of trying to understand relationships. Nursing is particularly concerned with the relationships among the person variables descriptive of self-care and community variables that have an impact on those person variables.[10]

Figure 14-4 is helpful in depicting the scope of concern of nursing and in diagrammatically representing the relationship of the person and community variables of concern to nursing. This figure forms the basis for discussion of structuring the nursing component of health care systems in the community.

Describing the Population for Nursing Purposes

The variables of concern to nursing are identified in Figure 14-4. The population description is developed from data related to these variables. In describing a population for nursing purposes, the administrator or planner must determine what data are available in the system and what data are needed. In addition to the epidemiologic and medical data to evaluate health risks that are present, information about self-care limitations is also required. Allison and McLaughlin-Renpenning[11] developed the structure derived from self-care deficit theory and reproduced in the following box on p. 422 describing a nursing population.

Nursing Practice Operations

Nursing practice in community involves the nurse constantly collecting and analyzing data about individuals, families, groups, and communities. Nursing practice operations include identifying the unit of service, being aware when data are being collected to design a nursing system for a particular unit of service and when the data are for the purpose of identifying the conditioning effect on health and self-care or other variables. This is particularly complicated when multiperson units are involved. The classification of multiperson units and description of categories of care systems previously described are useful to help clarify this thinking. This step is important to understanding the role of nursing, the boundaries of the nursing service, and the relationship of nursing to other disciplines.

Diagnosis and Prescription

Questions of Concern

In community nursing practice, two related questions guide the diagnostic and prescriptive phase for the nurse. The first is: What are the health outcomes or changes sought? As previously mentioned, prevention of disease, injury, disability, and premature death are major desired outcomes, along with promoting quality of life and well-being. Underlying these desired outcomes is the control of health services costs while ensuring universal access to these services. The second question is: What category (or categories) of health care system(s) is (are) appropriate in this situation to achieve the health outcomes or changes sought? Data about the person variables and the community variables are collected. Data sources may be persons, studies, statistical information, and so on. These data are examined to estimate the relationship among the community variables and self-care system(s). Based on this estimation, a decision can be made that the health care system(s) appropriate in the situation should address individuals, families, groups, a subpopulation, and/or the community at large. In deciding what data to collect, what meaning to attach to that data, and the appropriate interventions, community nursing brings together nursing theory and related theories and sciences such as epidemiology, public health theory, community development, sociology, economics, health administration, law, politics, management, and environmental sciences. The nursing system may be for the specific

A Structure for Categorizing Data in Describing a Population for Nursing Purposes

1. Basic Conditioning Factors
   1.1 Personal
       1.1.1 Age
       1.1.2 Sex
       1.1.3 Residence and environmental factors
       1.1.4 Family system factors
       1.1.5 Sociocultural factors including education, occupation
       1.1.6 Socioeconomic factors
   1.2 Patterns of living
   1.3 Health state and health care system factors
       1.3.1 Medical diagnosis
       1.3.2 Nurse-determined conditions
       1.3.3 Patient's description of health state
       1.3.4 Family member's description of health state
       1.3.5 Health care system features: disciplines, services, and care
   1.4 Developmental state in relation to meeting developmental self-care requisites
       1.4.1 Patient's goals and view of future
       1.4.2 Objective appraisals regarding developmental potential
       1.4.3 Self-management capabilities considering health state, conditions of living
       1.4.4 Factors necessary for or adversely affecting self-management
2. Therapeutic Self-Care Demand
   2.1 Actions associated with universal self-care requisites
       2.1.1 Maintenance of a sufficient intake of air
       2.1.2 Maintenance of a sufficient intake of water
       2.1.3 Maintenance of a sufficient intake of food
       2.1.4 The provision of care associated with elimination processes and excrements
       2.1.5 The maintenance of a balance between activity and rest
       2.1.6 The maintenance of a balance between solitude and social interaction
       2.1.7 The prevention of hazards to human life, human functioning, and human well-being
       2.1.8 The promotion of human functioning and development within social groups in accord with human potential, known human limitations, and the human desire to be normal
   2.2 Developmental self-care requisites
       2.2.1 Provide and maintain an adequacy of materials, such as water and food, and conditions essential for development of the human body at stages when foundations for bodily features are laid down and dynamic developments occur

Adapted from Allison SE, McLaughlin K: *Nursing administration in the 21st century: a self-care theory approach,* 1998, Sage Publications, pp 73-78. Reprinted by permission of Sage Publications. Categories of data 1 to 5 and data items express conceptual and reality elements of self-care deficit nursing theory described and explained in this and earlier editions of *Nursing: Concepts of Practice.*   *Continued*

2.2.2 Provide and maintain physical, environmental, and social conditions that ensure feelings of comfort and safety, the sense of being close to another, and the sense of being cared for

2.2.3 Provide and maintain conditions that prevent both sensory deprivation and sensory overload

2.2.4 Provide and maintain conditions that promote and sustain affective and cognitional development

2.2.5 Provide conditions and experiences to facilitate beginning and advanced skill development essential for life in society including intellectual, practical, interactional, and social skills

2.2.6 Provide conditions and experiences to foster awareness that one possesses a self and of being a person within the world of the family and community

2.2.7 Regulate the physical, biologic, and social environment to prevent development of a state of fear, anger, or anxiety

2.3 Health deviation self-care requisites

2.3.1 Seeking and securing appropriate medical assistance

2.3.2 Being aware of and attending to the effects and results of pathologic conditions and states, including effects on development

2.3.3 Effectively carrying out medically prescribed diagnostic, therapeutic, and rehabilitative measures

2.3.4 Being aware of and attending to or regulating the discomforting or deleterious effects of medical care measures performed or prescribed by the physician, including effects on development

2.3.5 Modifying the self-concept (and self-image) in accepting oneself as being in a particular state of health and in need of specific forms of health care

2.3.6 Learning to live with the effects of pathologic conditions and states and the effects of medical diagnostic and treatment measures in a life-style that promotes continued personal development

3. Self-Care Agency

3.1 Self-care limitations, capabilities

3.1.1 Knowing

3.1.2 Decision making

3.1.3 Performing self-care

3.2 Power components of self-care agency

3.2.1 Ability to maintain attention and requisite vigilance with respect to self as to conditions significant for self-care

3.2.2 Controlled use of physical energy for self-care

3.2.3 Ability to control the position of the body and body parts for self-care

3.2.4 Ability to reason within self-care frame of reference

3.2.5 Motivation for self-care

Adapted from Allison SE, McLaughlin K: *Nursing administration in the 21st century: a self-care theory approach,* 1998, Sage Publications, pp 73-78. Reprinted by permission of Sage Publications. Categories of data 1 to 5 and data items express conceptual and reality elements of self-care deficit nursing theory described and explained in this and earlier editions of *Nursing: Concepts of Practice.*

A Structure for Categorizing Data in Describing a Population for Nursing Purposes—cont'd

3.2.6 Ability to make decisions about care of self and to operationalize these decisions

3.2.7 Ability to acquire technical knowledge about self-care from authoritative sources, to retain it, and to operationalize it

3.2.8 A repertoire of cognitive, perceptual, manipulative, communication, and interpersonal skills adapted to the performance of self-care operations

3.2.9 Ability to order discrete self-care actions or action systems into relationships with prior and subsequent actions toward the final achievement of regulatory goals of self-care

3.2.10 Ability to consistently perform self-care operations, integrating them with relevant aspects of personal, family and community living

4. Dependent Care Agency
   4.1 Dependent care capabilities and limitations
       4.1.1 Knowing
       4.1.2 Decision making
       4.1.3 Producing dependent-care
   4.2 Power components of dependent care agency
5. Foundational capabilities and dispositions
   5.1 Conditioning factors and states affecting capabilities and dispositions
       5.1.1 Genetic and constitutional factors
       5.1.2 Arousal state
       5.1.3 Social organization
       5.1.4 Culture
       5.1.5 Experience
   5.2 Selected basic capabilities
       5.2.1 Sensation: proprioception and exteroception
       5.2.2 Learning
       5.2.3 Exercise or work
       5.2.4 Regulation of the position and movement of the body and its parts
       5.2.5 Attention
       5.2.6 Perception
       5.2.7 Memory
       5.2.8 Central regulation of motivational, emotional processes
   5.3 Knowing and doing capabilities
       5.3.1 Rational agency
       5.3.2 Operational knowing
       5.3.3 Learned skills: reading, counting, writing, manual, reasoning, verbal, perceptual
       5.3.4 Self-consistency in knowing and doing

Continued

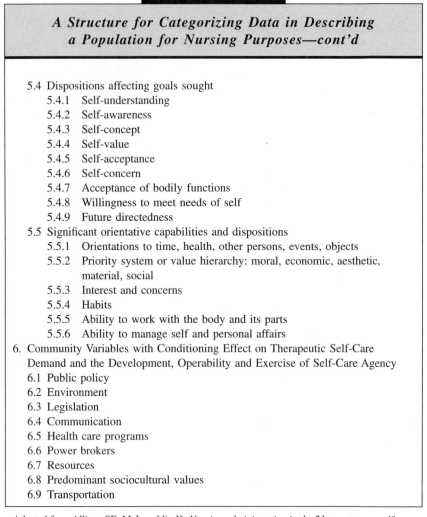

**A Structure for Categorizing Data in Describing
a Population for Nursing Purposes—cont'd**

5.4 Dispositions affecting goals sought
    5.4.1   Self-understanding
    5.4.2   Self-awareness
    5.4.3   Self-concept
    5.4.4   Self-value
    5.4.5   Self-acceptance
    5.4.6   Self-concern
    5.4.7   Acceptance of bodily functions
    5.4.8   Willingness to meet needs of self
    5.4.9   Future directedness
5.5 Significant orientative capabilities and dispositions
    5.5.1   Orientations to time, health, other persons, events, objects
    5.5.2   Priority system or value hierarchy: moral, economic, aesthetic, material, social
    5.5.3   Interest and concerns
    5.5.4   Habits
    5.5.5   Ability to work with the body and its parts
    5.5.6   Ability to manage self and personal affairs
6. Community Variables with Conditioning Effect on Therapeutic Self-Care Demand and the Development, Operability and Exercise of Self-Care Agency
    6.1 Public policy
    6.2 Environment
    6.3 Legislation
    6.4 Communication
    6.5 Health care programs
    6.6 Power brokers
    6.7 Resources
    6.8 Predominant sociocultural values
    6.9 Transportation

Adapted from Allison SE, McLaughlin K: *Nursing administration in the 21st century: a self-care theory approach,* 1998, Sage Publications, pp 73-78. Reprinted by permission of Sage Publications. Categories of data 1 to 5 and data items express conceptual and reality elements of self-care deficit nursing theory described and explained in this and earlier editions of *Nursing: Concepts of Practice.*

purpose of providing nursing or may be a part of a larger interdisciplinary system concerned with the overall health and welfare of the community. Both types of systems may be operational at the same time.

Estimation of the Values of the Person Variables

The person variables that are of interest to the nurse are:
1. The characteristics of the self-care or dependent-care systems
2. The nature of the therapeutic self-care demand or dependent-care demand

3. The state of development of self-care agency or dependent-care agency and the extent to which it is being exercised or can be exercised

These variables are all influenced by basic conditioning factors: age, sex, developmental state, conditions of living, patterns of living, family system factors, health state, health care system factors, sociocultural organization, available resources, and experience. Each of these conditioning factors singly and in combination affects the value of the variable, making its expression particular to the individual at a specific point in time. When individuals become part of multiperson units, expression of each variable is influenced by the interaction and interpersonal relationships of persons making up the unit. Such expression is also influenced by the interrelationship of the therapeutic self-care demand and the self-care agency of each person making up the unit (Taylor, 1989).[10]

Hemstrom[12] illustrates this process in a description of the development of a community health nursing experience with a complex aggregate client for BSN completion students at a private university. Working in collaboration with the neighborhood group, a representative sample of the population was selected and interviewed to assess their concerns. Data were summarized, inferences drawn, and problems amenable to nursing intervention were identified and prioritized.

Estimation of Values and Meaning of Community Variables

Community variables including resources available, environment, public policies, legislation, communication networks, health services, and power brokers have been identified as conditioning self-care practices and the exercise and development of self-care agency. Nurses collect data about the identified variables, explore relationships, and use nursing and related theory to help attach meaning to that data in reference to the proper object of nursing. This step may be exclusively a nursing activity, or it may be interdisciplinary. The outcome of this process is coming to some conclusion about "what is," with nursing contributing information in relation to the proper object of nursing and the integration of this nursing-specific meaning into the broader interpretation of the situation.

Identification of Health Outcomes or Changes Sought

In structuring a nursing system, it is necessary to identify the health outcomes sought or changes required. These reflect the perspective of members of the community and their valuing of health promotion; primary, secondary, and tertiary prevention; control of costs of health services; and universal access. The design of any intervention system requires understanding the end toward which the process is directed. The selection of strategies, control, and evaluation is dependent on health outcomes or changes sought or required. The identified outcomes and selected strategies may be at the level of the individual or at the community level.

Design and Planning

The processes of design and planning for community nursing require that nurses be able to think from a population perspective, as well as able to relate the conditioning effects of community on the individual self-care system(s). The design and the associated plan for accomplishing the goals to be achieved are a function of the interrelationships among the health outcomes sought, community systems in operation, and therapeutic systems in operation. When the community is the unit of service, the therapeutic systems in operation are the dependent variable, as well as the source of data to determine the extent to which the goal of health for all is being achieved. The community systems in operation are the variables to be manipulated to achieve the desired goals.

Therapeutic Systems in Operation

The therapeutic systems in operation are the collective self-care systems of the persons making up the population of concern. These include the composite of the therapeutic self-care demand of all of the persons and the composite knowledge, capabilities, and motivation to perform self-care. They are conditioned by the community systems in operation.

Community Systems in Operation

Community systems are necessary for the maintenance and functioning of a community. Some of the community systems in operation that are interrelated with the therapeutic systems in operation and on the health outcomes sought or changes required include management of the environment, public participation, mutual aid, public policy and government, health services, resource management, and education.

Regulatory and Therapeutic Operations

Results Sought

As in all nursing practice, the results sought through the regulatory operations of nursing practice in community situations include:
1. Continuously meeting the therapeutic self-care demand or some components of the same of all members of the community
2. Regulation or development of the powers of self-care agency
3. Protection of self-care abilities or protection for future development

The Variables of Concern

The strategies to achieve the results very often focus on community variables and community systems in operation. When these are the focus of concern, the care system may be interdisciplinary, with nursing contributing a nursing perspective and other disciplines contributing their unique perspective.

In the practice situation, the diagnostic and prescriptive operations and the regulatory operations often have a circular pattern, with the extent and intensity of nurse-patient interaction varying over time. As well, the unit of service that is of interest may change from an individual one to a multiperson one, and the care system may change from a nursing system to an interdisciplinary system as more information becomes available.

Evaluation of Health Outcomes: A Control Operation

Evaluation of health outcomes—the health of all persons and the functioning of the community—is an important regulatory operation. The evaluation may be formative and/or summative. It is focused on the desired outcomes, the data gathered, the accuracy of the analysis, the regulatory and therapeutic operations used, and the extent to which the goal of health for all is achieved.

A CASE STUDY

The following example is an illustration of community nursing that is consistent with the view presented in this chapter. Survey data are used to determine "what is" and to provide direction for changes required. The focus and contribution of nursing within the interdisciplinary team in the community are outlined. Strategies for change are directed at the individual and at the community at large.

In 1987 the Ottawa-Carleton health region launched a community-based primary prevention called "Heart Beat" that targeted the whole population.[13] The data from two community surveys indicated that heart disease was a leading cause of death and disability in the region and that 80 percent of residents in the area had at least one modifiable risk factor for heart disease. Within the interdisciplinary team designing and delivering the program, the role of nurses was twofold:

1. To raise awareness of the relationship between life-style and the health of individuals and families (relationship of conditioning factors, therapeutic self-care demand, and self-care practices)
2. To strengthen motivation, skills, and confidence of people in relationship to life-style choices (development and exercise of self-care agency)

A number of strategies were used to bring about awareness of the need for change and support to change. These included contests to motivate teenagers to quit smoking; portable stations set up in the workplace, malls, and community centers to measure cholesterol, blood pressure, and body mass index and to assess life-style; health fairs and community presentations on related topics; bilingual self-help kits to help individual identify barriers to behavior change and to develop strategies to overcome these barriers; and information about community resources. In addition to these strategies related to individual behavior, self-help groups were developed. Attention was directed at the physical and social milieu of the community, as the nutrition division worked with local restaurants to provide "heart smart" food, point-of-purchase messages were provided in grocery stores, and workplaces were encouraged to provide fitness facilities and no-smoking environments. Volunteer groups were mobilized to assist in delivery of these programs, and development of support and self-help groups provided a means for involvement of community members and input from them. When the article was written, the follow-up community survey was planned but still to be done. However, as an initial follow-up, a telephone survey of 1000 adults indicated the number of people over age 18 who smoked dropped from 32% in 1984 to 20% in 1989.

A COMMUNITY PARTICIPATION MODEL

Understanding factors that facilitate and interfere with community participation becomes important to nursing when the community is the unit of service. Sawyer[14] noted that nursing has a commitment to social justice and equity. Many authors of nursing articles have asserted that nurses are ideally suited to social action, and this commitment is evident in the concept of community participation.

Several articles support that the way a community participates depends on environmental factors: demographic, economic, political, and sociocultural factors. Sawyer[14] asserted that programs using community participation that have been touted as successful internationally have common elements. These successful programs have supportive environments in terms of demographic, economic, political, and sociocultural elements. In addition, Courtney and colleagues[15] confirmed that respecting and considering these contextual factors as integral to community participation are essential to creating and sustaining participation.

In many articles, however, various terms were used interchangeably to express the concept of community participation, such as community involvement, community empowerment, and community partnership.[14,16-18] Gamm[19] proposed three types of partnerships in advancing community health:
1. Community action partnerships, in which the partnership forms to address a specific problem or pursue a specific opportunity
2. Community organization partnerships, in which a set of organizations in a similar service sector agree to collaborate for mutually agreed-upon goals
3. Community development partnerships, in which a partnership attempts to increase participation by people and organizations in collaborative activities that advance the community on multiple fronts or that contribute to community assets and services in multiple areas

In addition, Gamm[19] suggested that when creating partnerships for community health and carrying out health-improvement activities, leaders should be aware of and respond to four key dimensions of accountability: political accountability, commercial accountability, clinical and patient accountability, and community accountability.

Furthermore, Courtney and associates[15] proposed steps and strategies in the partnership process as follows:
1. Exploring potential partners
   a. Familiarizing yourself with individual, family, or community
   b. Facilitating dialogue
2. Inviting to partner
   a. Risk taking
3. Commitment to role change
4. Partnership action
   a. Initiating partnership action
   b. Working phase of partnership action
   c. Evaluating accomplishments and renegotiating roles and goals

Factors influencing community participation are summarized in the community participation model presented in Figure 14-5.

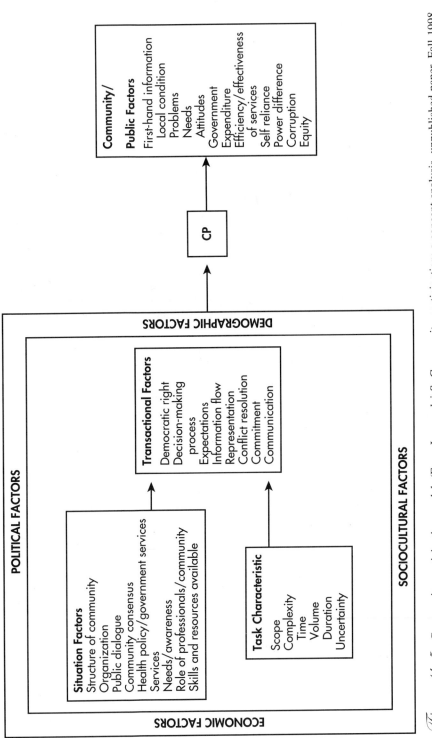

Figure 14-5 Community participation model. (From Isaramalai S: Community participation: a concept analysis, unpublished paper, Fall 1998, University of Missouri, Columbia.) *CP,* Community Participation.

SUMMARY

A nursing system does not exist until it is deliberately constructed. The construction of a nursing system within the greater health care system in multiperson situations requires that nurses be able to think about nursing in relation to groups, the community, and populations, as well as individuals. A requirement of the practice of nursing in multiperson situations is identification of the unit of service and an understanding of the service called nursing, including the proper object of nursing, the domain, and boundaries of the service. In addition, nurses must develop an understanding of the interdependence of the person variables of self-care, therapeutic self-care demand, and self-care agency, with family and community variables and systems in operation.

Nursing practice in family and community type situations may involve individuals as single persons or individuals as members of a group for which the object of nursing is the individual. It may also involve a multiperson group as a unit of service. A significant feature of the design of nursing in multiperson situations is identification of the unit of service. This identification is essential to development of the contract to provide and receive nursing. There are variations in nursing operations that are a function of the unit of service, as group processes and interactions are added to the interpersonal interactions and processes.

In family and community type situations, data may be gathered at the level of the individual, the family, or the community, with the object of nursing being the individual or the multiperson unit. In some instances, there may be separate but related nursing systems in operation at the same time, with the individual as unit of service for one nursing system and the multiperson unit as unit of service for another.

When the community is the unit of service, the care system is generally a multidisciplinary system. Self-care deficit nursing theory provides direction for explicating the relationship between community variables and systems in operation and person variables and therapeutic systems in operation in relation to self-care. The theory also provides direction for defining and describing the roles and responsibilities of nursing within the interdisciplinary care system.

References

1. Macmurray J: *Persons in relation,* New York, 1961, Harper and Brothers, p 17.
2. Weiss P: *You, I, and the others,* Carbondale, 1980, Southern Illinois University Press, pp 270-287.
3. Geden E, Taylor SG: Theoretical and empirical description of adult couples collaborative self-care systems, *Nurs Sci Q* 12:329-334, 1999.
4. Orem D: Nursing: concepts of practice, ed 5, St Louis, 1995, Mosby, pp 230, 296-299.
5. Taylor S: An interpretation of family within Orem's general theory of nursing, *Nurs Sci Q* 2:131-137, 1989.
6. Labonte B: *Health promotion and empowerment practice frameworks,* Toronto, 1993, Centre for Health Promotion.
7. World Health Organization: *Health promotion: development of discussion frameworks in the WHO Regional Office for Europe,* Geneva, 1988, World Health Organization.
8. Hartwick G: Developing health promoting practices: a transformative process, *Nurs Sci Q* 46:219-225, 1998.

9. Kirkpatrick FG: Community: *A trinity of models,* Washington, DC, 1986, Georgetown University Press, pp 30, 65, 143.

10. Taylor S, McLaughlin K: Orem's general theory of nursing and community nursing, *Nurs Sci Q* 4:153-160, 1991.

11. Allison SE, McLaughlin Renpenning K: *Nursing administration in the 21st century: a self-care theory approach,* Thousand Oaks, Calif, 1998, Sage, pp 73-78.

12. Hemstrom M: Application as scholarship: a community client experience, *Public Health Nurs* 12:279-283, 1995.

13. Sullivan LC, Carr J: Promoting healthy hearts, *Can Nurse* 86:28-30, 1990.

14. Sawyer L: Community participation: lip service? *Nurs Outlook* 43:17-22, 1995.

15. Courtney R et al: The partnership model: working with individuals, families, and communities toward a new vision of health, *Public Health Nurs* 13:177-186, 1996.

16. Brownlea A: Participation: myths, realities and prognosis, *Soc Sci Med* 25:605-614, 1987.

17. Hildebrandt E: Building community participation in health care: a model and example from South Africa, *Image: Nurs Scholarship* 28:155-159, 1996.

18. Sekgobela M: Community participation: the heart of community health, *Nurs RSA Verpleging* 1:30-31, 1986.

19. Gamm L: Advancing community health through community health partnerships, *Health Care Manage* 43:51-67, 1998.

CHAPTER 15

Nurses

This is the final chapter in a work developed around the needs of people for nursing and nurses' production of nursing to meet such needs. Emphasis has been placed on nurses' knowing nursing as a field of knowledge and a field of practice and on nurses' ability to think nursing and to produce nursing for individuals and groups.

The self-care deficit theory of nursing with its constituent theories of self-care, self-care deficit, and nursing systems and their conceptual constructs have been presented in terms of their usefulness in nursing practice and nursing science endeavors. They have been represented as frames of reference for understanding nursing, as pointing to the concrete realities of nursing practice situations and to the kinds of data required for making nursing judgments and decisions, and as providing constructs for subsuming and organizing patient, nurse, and other situational data and attaching nursing meaning to it.

434

More specifically, the conceptual constructs of the theories and the relations among them have been presented in terms of their use in the development of the practical science of nursing and in the identification and development of applied nursing sciences. This is in accord with the premise that nursing as science would have the form of a practical science and a set of applied sciences.

Persons educated in nursing and qualified to practice nursing may or may not be engaged in the production of nursing or in its design for individuals and multiperson units. Nurses engage themselves in a mix of occupations within nursing but think of themselves as members of the profession of nursing.

This chapter presents a descriptive summary of the preparatory education of nurses. It considers the education of nursing practitioners, the preparation for movement into nursing research and other fields, and the mix of roles of professionally qualified nurses. Prior to this, the work of providing nursing for populations in need is addressed, with attention to the essential work of nursing practitioners and nursing administrators. There is an initial and brief consideration of the occupational and professional interests of nurses.

OCCUPATIONAL AND PROFESSIONAL CONSIDERATIONS

The term *occupation* is used to refer to the work, the kind of activity, that persons who trained for it seriously engage. These persons habitually engage in the activity but not always as a means of earning a livelihood.

The term **profession,** like the term *occupation,* is used to refer to work pursuits. In this sense, it signifies fields in which individuals pursue years of study and training, achieve qualifying professional degrees from institutions of higher education, are tested to determine fitness to practice, and in some fields are licensed to practice. In nursing, the term *profession* in this sense is the basis for distinguishing nurses prepared for entry to the beginning professional level of nursing practice who move themselves to become advanced professional practitioners from nurses prepared in technical programs preparatory for nursing. *Profession* is also used in the sense of all the persons engaged in a field of practice that requires the named qualifying characteristics.

Nurses must face and accept the matter of differences in their interests, differences in education preparatory for nursing, and differences in their work or career orientations to nursing and begin to be concerned about their contributions to the survival and advancement of nursing as a human service in communities. What each nurse does and does effectively within one or some combination of occupational fields makes a contribution to the continued existence and acceptance of nursing in human society.

The professions exist in societies so that members can identify, resolve, and solve or mitigate specific types of human problems of members of the society. In nursing the problems are ones that arise from the subjectivity of men, women, and children to health-derived or health-associated deficits for self-care or dependent-care of persons who must care for themselves or be taken care of by others. This is the domain about which professionally qualified and professionally advanced nurses must continue to acquire knowledge through nursing practice, scholarly endeavors, and nursing theory formulation and development; validate knowledge through reserach; and develop and validate technologies of practice. The areas of theoretically and practically practical nursing knowledge are distinguished; and nursing knowledge, as it develops, is structured around the identified areas in Figure 8-3. The forms of the applied nursing sciences emerge.

Because a profession perpetuates itself and seeks to advance itself toward helping societies in resolving and solving existent as well as emerging human problems within its domain, each profession has members engaged in (1) providing professional services that are in accord with existent and emerging needs of populations; (2) the education of new members with qualifications, in the numbers required to provide services, and in advanced education for present members; and (3) the development of the practical and applied sciences specific to the domain of the profession (see Figure 4-1). Thus, it can be seen that all of nursing's occupational fields are essential for the survival and advancement of nursing in societies throughout the world. The international and intercontinental associations and collaborations among nurses continue to increase.

Professions ideally are characterized by movement to fulfill their reasons for existence in societies. The health service professions are confronted with both demands for continuing development of their sciences and technologies and with demands for change associated with varying conditions in the populations to be served. The demands for development and change in nursing are great and continue to increase.

Nurses over the years have exhibited reluctance to take and maintain control over essential qualification of persons for the practice of nursing, to identify and represent to others the domain and boundaries of nursing, to establish what nurses with a range of qualifications should do in health care situations, and to maintain the domain and boundaries of nursing. Failure of nurses to attend to the features of nursing as a profession will continue to be reflected in inadequacies of education and training for nursing practice and in the absence of nursing science in nursing courses. Interpersonal content such as content on caring and communication are important in preparatory educational programs for nurses, but such content does not express why people need and can be helped through nursing. That some people require nursing is assumed by nurses in many educational programs. But why specific individuals in some life situations require nursing and can be helped through nursing is unexpressed.

Nurses in the United States and in other countries of the world are confronted with change. What nurses do today to fulfill the reasons for the existence of nursing and to maintain nursing's domain and boundaries will determine the movement required from future generations of nurses. It should be a developmental movement and not a movement of continuing repair.

It is important that nurses have the freedom to bear the responsibilities of nursing practice. Nurses should understand the depths and breadth of their capabilities for nursing practice and their own legitimacy as nurses in concrete situations of practice. Nursing students and nurses should critically examine where they fit within the occupation and profession of nursing. Distinguishing roles and role responsibilities of persons prepared through different forms of work preparatory education should be understood by nursing students. How one moves in occupational-professional fields for the most part is determined by where one begins.

THE EDUCATION OF NURSES, AN OVERVIEW

Schools of nursing have proliferated in the United States since the first schools were opened in 1873. Nursing education during the early period of its development was promoted by interested lay or professional people, often associated with hospitals. Pioneer schools of nursing were modeled at least in part after the Nightingale School associated with Saint Thomas's Hospital in London (pp. 7-9),[1] which was opened in 1860 under the sponsorship of Florence Nightingale and financed through the Nightingale Fund (pp. 225-238).[2] Since World War II, nursing has entered the so-called scientific age. Education for nursing has expanded to include a broader base in general studies, in the humanities and behavioral and social sciences, and in leadership and management. Traditional biologic and medical science content remains in nursing programs, sometimes with considerable expansion and restructuring of emphasis.

With the ever-increasing knowledge of humanity and the complexity of health care and medical technology, there has been a concomitant demand for nurses prepared at the university level. In addition, the enactment of social legislation (Medicare and Medicaid) has greatly increased the need for nurses and for personnel who assist them in providing and managing nursing. The number and types of workers who serve by providing self-care assistance has increased rapidly since 1940. Not all workers are prepared or licensed as nurses. Nurses are limited by external and internal factors in what they can do to meet nursing requirements in a community. Limiting factors include time, prevailing conditions, interests, values, and abilities of the nurses of a community. Effective organization of nursing services is essential both in the provision of nursing and the maintenance of satisfaction among nurses. Modern nurses are no less capable than nursing leaders of the past. Finding ways to meet and keep up with changing requirements for nursing is the task of and a challenge to each nurse. Nurses have a substantial part in the process of moving communities toward standards of nursing practice that ensure safe and effective nursing. No other group can perform this task for nurses. Nurses, collectively, have a responsibility for the quality of the services they provide in a community.

Members of younger generations of nurses have an education that has been enriched with modern science and technology and general studies. The young nurse may be in the formative stage of the art of nursing, but his or her foundation for its development may exceed that of nurses with years of nursing experience. Techniques and practices in current use are evaluated and sometimes questioned by younger nurses and nursing students. This is the role of each new generation, for in this way nursing practice is refined and enriched. Because practices tend to become fixed or institutionalized, they are not easily changed, but without developmental change stagnation and deterioration of nursing effectiveness occur. Young nurses and nursing students should seek knowledge of valid but unrecorded nursing techniques from more experienced nurses who have attained nursing widsom from thoughtful and effective nursing practice. Nurses who have developed techniques and have evidence of their effectiveness should contribute this information to the developing body of nursing knowledge. Developing, validating, and recording techniques of nursing practice are important tasks in the continued development of a body of nursing knowledge.

Nurses have been educated for limited roles in nursing in the United States. This is done in other fields and is a mark that a service is being extended to more and more persons. The content and length of programs of nursing education should vary according to the roles for which different types of nurses are being prepared. In the delivery of nursing in communities and in institutions, the contribution that each type of nurse is to make to nursing should be defined, and provision should be made for coordinating efforts in the interests of both patients and nurses. Division of the work of nursing among several types of nurses without providing for the coordination of effort and results leads to chaos. The demand for nurses who are effective in appraising the needs of individual patients for nursing and in designing systems of nursing assistance is increasing, along with the demand for nurses who can effectively supervise nurses who are prepared for limited roles. Changes in nursing education and changes in nursing practice are interrelated.

Nurses must be able to fill their positions in a spectrum of health care services developed around technologies of health care and health care problems. The nurse is not a solitary worker. The days when only physicians and nurses made up health teams is over. Expansion of the spectrum of health services places demands on nurses for coordinating actions with persons from an increasing number and variety of health services. The specific character of nursing activities is closely related to the kinds of health problems that prevail in the community. For example, communicable disease, serious injuries from industrial accidents, and chronic illness result in needs for different types of nursing actions and care systems. Communities vary in the combinations of health problems that prevail, although certain health problems are common to all communities. The character of nursing activities is also affected by the way in which patients can be helped. The requirements of persons who are ill and are patients in hospitals or nursing homes sometimes result in heavy demands for continuing care by nurses and other types of personnel. Community health centers and health maintenance organizations bring an increased demand for nursing that emphasizes guidance and instruction in therapeutic self-care and help to patients so that they can identify and manage internal conditions that interfere with their self-care actions. Some industrial and business firms employ nurses full-time to serve their employees' health needs. These nurses may give direct assistance to employees as the need arises, but they are primarily concerned with preventive measures related to the health and well-being of the firm's employees and their families. Many governmental, health, and welfare agencies also employ nurses in a variety of health-related activities. Regardless of the kinds of health and other problems that determine the specific work of the nurse, he or she is always recognized as a specialized worker with a distinctive social position and pattern of behavior. It has been indicated that the nurse's role in society focuses on (1) the maintenance of those self-care activities that individuals continuously need to sustain life and health, recover from disease and injury, and cope with the effects of disease and injury and (2) self-regulation of the individual's self-care capabilities.

Nursing students and nurses entering practice want to learn to nurse with effectiveness and in a way that is satisfying to persons nursed and to themselves. Because nursing is offered within social groups as an available human service, nurses must develop and advance in their knowledge of nursing and become skilled performers of the operations of nursing practice. These achievements are not possible without sound preparatory education for entry into nursing practice.

The membership and status or position of individual nurses in the occupation and profession of nursing depends on their educational preparation, type of license or certification to practice, and experience and recognition of practice capabilities by colleagues and peers. Education for nursing is work preparatory.

FORMS OF EDUCATION FOR NURSING

The form(s) in which nursing education should be offered continues to be questioned and is at times a public issue. The terms **professional, technical,** and **vocational** are emotion-arousing terms for some nurses. Past and present self-appointed experts on nursing practice and nursing education often did not and do not know or seek knowledge about the proper role functions of persons with different forms of work-preparatory education, or they disregard them as too difficult to implement. Persons tend to ignore or oversimplify the social, scientific, and economic rationales that legitimate the use of various types of workers in nursing.

Three forms or types of work-preparatory education are accepted in the United States. These usually are named as follows:
1. Vocational and vocational-technical
2. Technical
   a. Low-level technical
   b. High-level technical or technologic
3. Professional

Sometimes, and to confuse the matter, all forms of work-preparatory education are referred to collectively as vocational education. The forms of work-preparatory education serve different purposes and traditionally have been justified on the basis of economic considerations for the society and for individuals who pursue the specific forms of work-preparatory education.

Persons enrolled in work-preparatory programs ideally view themselves and are viewed by others as engaged in a form of personal development that is enabling for skilled performance within a selected occupational field. The time designation for achievement of skilled performance may be set as *upon program completion* or *after a stipulated period of apprenticeship under experienced individuals in the field.* In nursing, it is usually necessary for individual nurses to design and work out plans for their own apprenticeships. Career pathways in nursing are not well developed.

Centers of Organization of Work Preparatory Programs

Types of work-preparatory education have different centers of organization and use different principles in the selection and organization of knowledge and learning experiences. The centers of organization of educational programs and rationales for program development are shown in Table 15-1.

Professional nursing programs preparatory for *entrance* to practice and for *movement* toward the professional (scientific) form of practice have as their organizing center human beings and the range of types of conditions and problems of persons who can benefit from nursing (form A in Table 15-1). Programs preparatory for entrance to practice subsume under form A the essential sets of process operations of nursing practice, the recurring types of problem situations for which there are developed valid and reliable technologies for

Table 15-1 Forms of Work Preparatory Education by Organizing Centers and Rationales

Form	Center	Rationale
A	Conditions and problems of human beings that constitute the special domain of nursing	The proper object of nursing is identified, and nursing is established in a society. The practical science of nursing is being developed. Individuals elect to prepare themselves to practice nursing, obtaining and maintaining a scientific base for practice in the nursing sciences and in nursing-related disciplines. Individuals elect to advance nursing as both a field of practice and a field of knowledge.
B	Recurring types of problem situations in the field of nursing practice and developed, validated technologies for identification, resolution, and solution of specific questions within the problem situation	Recurring types of problem situations in nursing are identified, described, and explained. Technologies of high validity and reliability are formalized. Individuals elect to do detailed technical work as outlined in standard operating procedures or as detailed by an expert practitioner. Individuals elect to perfect and to advance techniques of practice.
C	Work operations that can be safely selected out from a larger set(s) or series	Work operations can be isolated without adversely affecting the whole set or series of actions considered as a dynamic, coordinated system. Individuals elect to do repetitive, circumscribed work.

achieving nursing results (form B in Table 15-1), and the related work operations necessary for result achievement. These programs also provide the science foundation for movement to a professional (scientific) level of practice with advanced science requirements.

True technical programs have as their centers recurring types of problem situations of persons who are seeking or are receiving nursing and the developed, validated, and reliable technologies for the identification, resolution, and solution of nursing practice problems (form B in Table 15-1).

Programs true to the vocational mode are organized around specific tasks or work operations that can be separated out from larger sets of series of operations without loss of effectiveness or production of adverse results within the whole system of action (form C in Table 15-1).

The variations in the work focuses of persons prepared in the three types of work preparatory programs are shown in Figure 15-1. The illustration shows the interrelations of the three focuses within a single schematic situation of practice. It is easy to imagine the kinds of problems, errors, omissions, and outright harm to persons under care that arise in complex nursing situations when either a vocationally or technically prepared person is placed in a position of responsibility for the whole nursing situation without specific guidance and direction from a nurse who is functioning at the professional level of practice.

Nursing education in the United States from the period of its inception and initial growth has been beset with problems related to (1) the form in which it is

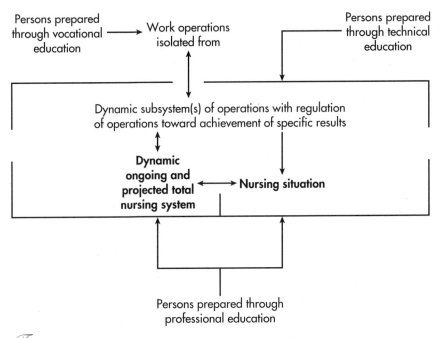

Figure 15-1   Focuses of persons prepared in types of work-preparatory programs.

offered and (2) its control by service agencies such as hospitals or by educational institutions. Nurses as well as the whole occupation and profession of nursing have been and continue to be adversely affected by issues of reform and control of nursing education.

The question of how individuals with different forms of work-preparatory education fit into the occupation and profession of nursing remains to be answered in some educational and service settings. Clear answers to the question should be sought and used to ensure the welfare of individuals who enroll in the programs and individuals who seek nursing or related services. Table 15-2 may be of some help in sorting out role differences. In the table, general roles associated with types of work-preparatory programs are developed as roles and role responsibilities in nursing and in the personal care of individuals. Students in various types of work-preparatory programs have a right to precise information about the social, economic, and occupational features of the programs in which they are enrolled. Sometimes these features are glossed over or misrepresented, or enrolled students are unable or unwilling to deal with information about them. It is reasonable to expect that students will be helped to understand how specific types of work-preparatory programs will enable them to fill specific roles in the occupation and profession of nursing.

Skilled Performance

Skilled performance by persons in nursing and other fields requires development and perfection of *perceptual skills* in receiving and processing sense information, the maintenance of alertness, and action to control factors that adversely affect attentiveness and vigilance. Skilled performance also demands *requisite knowledge for signal recognition,* that is, recognizing events that call for action, attaching meaning to signals singly or in combination, or making judgments that vagueness prohibits positive identification and that more information is needed.

For skilled performance in practical endeavors, individuals ideally psychologically structure or organize their knowledge in forms that can be readily drawn on as they (1) identify and observe the reality features of practice situations, (2) make judgments about features that can and should be changed or regulated, (3) make judgments and decisions about availability of appropriate and validated techniques for so doing, (4) make decisions about what kind and degree of change or regulation will be sought in specific features using techniques with high or low or no established validity and reliability, and (5) proceed to do and manage the work of changing or regulating features of the situation. How nursing students and nurses psychologically structure knowledge about nursing and nursing-related fields is affected by the forms of their work-preparatory education and by the organization of nursing content and nursing-related content within their educational programs.

Skilled performance by a person in an occupational or professional field demands *motivation* to act for quality in performance, sustained endeavor, and management of self and work operations to achieve results within an effective

Table 15-2 Roles and Role Responsibilities Associated with Forms of Work-Preparatory Education

Form of Education	General Role	Role Responsibility	Occupational-Professional Role
Vocational	Aide	*Nursing:* Performs assigned tasks selected out from the work operations of an ongoing nursing system *Self-care or dependent-care:* Performs tasks that are parts of systems	Aide to a nursing practitioner or a technically prepared nurse Aide to persons who are responsible for and are managing: 1. Their own self-care systems 2. Dependent-care systems for dependent adults or children
Vocational-technical or technical	Technician	*Nursing:* Operationalizes, maintains, and manages dependent-care systems of therapeutic quality for helpless or near-helpless persons under stable conditions and circumstances Conducts and manages subsystems of operations within a dynamic nursing system under control of a nursing practitioner	Practical or vocational nurse working with guidance and instruction from a nursing practitioner Technically prepared nurse working under standardized procedures or functioning as assistant to a nursing practitioner
High-level technical	Technologist	*Nursing:* Uses validated and reliable techniques in operationalizing and regulating dynamic subsystems of operations toward achievement of specified results in nursing systems, self-care systems, and dependent-care systems	Technologically prepared nurse with following functions: 1. Provides nursing, working within established protocols 2. Performs as associate of a nursing practitioner 3. Contributes a nursing component to ongoing self-care or dependent-care systems

Continued

Table 15-2   Roles and Role Responsibilities Associated with Forms of Work–Preparatory Education–cont'd

Form of Education	General Role	Role Responsibility	Occupational-Professional Role
Professional:			
1. Qualifying for entry to practice	Professional entry level of practice to experienced level of practice	Uses validated and reliable techniques in designing, operationalizing, and regulating dynamic nursing systems, including regulation of all subsystems	Nursing practitioner working within established protocols
		Operationalizes and regulates subsystems of operations within dynamic nursing systems, using validated and reliable techniques	Associate or assistant to a professional nursing practitioner
2. Advanced	Professional-scientific level of practice	Provides nursing diagnosis, including collecting data to the point needed for considered professional judgments	Professional nursing practitioner
		Provides creative design of nursing systems and subsystems of work operations	
		Provides design of techniques for attaining nursing results, in the absence of validated techniques	
		Operationalizes and manages nursing operations in complex nursing situations	
		Provides nursing consultation	

time frame without harm to self and others and without waste of time or materials or human energy. Because all fields of endeavor demand performance of some *range of types of work operations,* skilled performance requires the mix of skills necessary to perform specific work operations. Skills include perceptual motor skills, manipulative skills, verbal skills, and reasoning skills. Work operations can be typed according to the predominant skill or mix of skills required in their performance. Result and purpose achievement demand unification of actions to constitute a coordinated dynamic system. Skilled performance, therefore, demands knowledge of the fit of one work operation, one set of actions, within the larger framework of actions.

Knowing Nursing's Domain

As previously represented, adequate preparatory education and training for nursing practice includes nursing courses that are organized around why people require nursing and how they can be helped through nursing in certain life situations. The self-care deficit theory of nursing, its constituent theories, and their conceptual constructs have been used effectively in the organization and development of nursing content in preparatory programs for nursing practice. Valid, reliable, and conceptually developed nursing theory provides nurses with a mode of thinking about nursing, with an orientation to practice, with knowledge of the powers of nursing agency that they must develop and exercise, and with a language for communication about nursing.

Nurses who are effective practitioners of nursing recognize when persons are in need of nursing, but they may not be able to express with clarity the bases for their recognition of need. Inability to express what nurses do when they nurse and why they do what they do characterized many graduates of nursing programs in the United States into the last quarter of the twentieth century.

Nursing developed and continued to manifest the characteristics of a task-oriented occupation rather than a profession with a focus on human beings with discernible requirements for nursing.

As the need to make nursing available to more and more people was recognized in the beginning period of modern nursing, attention became focused on the *action domain of nursing practice.* Components of the action domain of the nurse often were expressed (1) as *recurring tasks* that were performed by nurses according to standardized procedures, that is, routine courses of action and specifications for task performance and (2) as rules to which nurses should adhere. Nursing as *taught* in nursing schools and programs became task-oriented rather than person-oriented. It was up to the individual nursing student and nurse to seek understanding of the personal and interpersonal aspects of nursing and incorporate these into practice.

Knowing nursing is a personal achievement of women and men who develop themselves to become and be able to practice nursing. Antecedently (before practice) acquired theoretical nursing knowledge enables the search for the answers to previously posed questions that nurses ask when they enter into the life situations of others. Knowledge of the human sciences is essential for nursing practice when properly articulated with nursing facts and points of theory. It is the descriptive and explanatory knowledge of the elements and relationships of nursing practice situations that identifies points of articulation with facts and points of theory from the human sciences as well as from the practical science and the applied sciences of medicine.

Theoretical nursing knowledge from authoritative sources is not to be memorized, but rather understood, conceptualized, and made dynamic in practice situations. Knowledge that gives guidance and direction to action is dynamic in the knower, the nurse. Development of understanding of the features that nursing has in common with other human services, including other health services, is conducive to developing insights about and forming images of the general features of nursing practice situations. Inquiry into nursing as a helping service and inquiry into nursing situations in which persons are taken care of should contribute to nursing students' and nurses' understanding of the most general personal and interpersonal features of nursing situations.

The historical emphasis on *tasks and procedures* within the *action domain of nursing practice* seems to have stilled or overruled nurses' interest in the questions: What gives rise to human requirements for nursing? Why can people benefit from nursing? Nurses' failure to attend to these questions resulted in an absence of agreement among nurses about what nursing is and is not. As a result, the question of *what tasks nurses should perform* continues to arise whenever boundary questions between nursing and medicine or nursing and some other field of practice arise. For example, the lack of clarity about the practice domain of nurse practitioners is essentially a boundary problem, the solving of which requires insights about how human requirements for nursing differ from human requirements for medical care. As long as a majority of nurses are willing to define boundary problems in terms of tasks and procedures, nursing cannot be properly moved to fulfill its human and social mission. Tasks separated from the human and environmental factors, conditions, and circumstances that specify why and when and by whom they should be performed *provide no basis for understanding nursing as care or art or as knowledge that grounds the nurse's art.*

As a new century begins, social conditions in the United States should cause nurses to recall the social conditions in Europe and America during the nineteenth century. The physically and mentally sick and the poor and destitute are still with us in hospitals and other care facilities, in their homes, and on the streets. The chronically ill as well as the acutely ill, the aged and the aging, and the young with impaired structural or functional integrity can benefit from many forms of care, including nursing. The "trained nurse" of the nineteenth and early twentieth centuries made a difference in society. Perhaps more interest on the part of nurses in why people need and can benefit from nursing would help nurses to better focus their attention and orient their actions so that they can produce more enduring effects and results for persons under their care. Some nurses have thrown off the tasks showered on them from other practice fields and are in a position to advance nursing as a practice field. Nurses who do this are addressing the human and social problems that are associated with needs of people for nursing.

Nurses who have mastered and use the self-care deficit theory of nursing and who contribute to its refinement and further development have noted changes in themselves and in other nurses. One experience that nurses express is an increase in their sense of self-value or self-worth as nurses. Other positive changes expressed by nurses over the years since the theory has been in use were compiled in 1987.[3] Changes in the listing have not been subjected to validation procedures. They are offered as an indication of what nurses have expressed in relation to their own or other nurses' use of the self-care deficit theory of nursing.

- Nurses develop their personal styles of practice within the domain and boundaries of nursing set by the theory.
- Nurses focus on providing nursing to persons whose legitimate need for nursing is established through the criterion of the existence of health-derived or health-related self-care deficits. Stereotyping is eventually eliminated.
- Nursing diagnoses become more valid and are expressed within a nursing frame of reference.
- Therapeutic self-care demands and ways to protect and to regulate the exercise or development of self-care agency are determined and prescribed. Nursing care systems are designed.
- Nursing documentation increases and improves.
- There is an increase in and upgrading of the kinds of referrals made by nurses, including referrals to nursing specialists.
- Nurses (and physicians more slowly) recognize the need for nursing discharge of patients separate from medical discharge.
- There is movement toward nurse-managed clinics.
- Nurses recognize that they have a theoretical base that serves them in performing the professional function of design of systems of nursing care. The design function is retained by and specific to the professional person.
- Nurses through their design of systems of nursing bring into focus their own role responsibilities and role functions, as well as those of other nurses, their patients, and members of patients' families who are dependent-care agents.

Such practice changes are most likely to occur in health service enterprises in which nursing administration views the self-care deficit theory of nursing as one means to aid in efforts to ensure the continuing provision of effective nursing to populations served by the health care enterprise.

NURSING CASES

Nursing cases are concrete instances of persons requiring and receiving nursing because of health-derived or health-related self-care deficits. Each nursing case has a history of events that precipitate requirements for nursing, events that occur during the period of being nursed, events that precipitate change from one system of providing nursing to another, and events that terminate the provision of nursing.

Nursing practice features of nursing cases fall roughly into two groups. Operational features are broadly grouped as societal, interpersonal, and technologic features. These features identify, in analogous terms, the players in the drama of nursing and their places in families and the larger society, what the play is about, the roles of each player, relation of players to one another, the time-place localization of players, the playing out of roles by each player. Second are characterizing features of the players themselves and their environments. In the real world of nurses, nurses' patients, and nursing operations, distinguishing features of individuals and their environments are associated with a number of factors named *basic conditioning factors*. In the case example of Mrs. Doe (Chapter 12), health state and the imposed pattern of living were major conditioning factors. Basic conditioning factors also affect nurses and their power of nursing agency.

Practicing nurses must have the capabilities to identify and organize information about patients in each nursing case in terms of its societal, interpersonal, and technologic meanings for nursing. They must have detailed, authoritative, antecedent knowledge about *basic conditioning factors* and their relevance to individuals and their properties and powers and to the behavior of individuals singly or in groups. Nurses' knowledge of basic conditioning factors ideally is both theoretical and experiential. For example, nurses know from the fields of human development and human behavior specific developments that are associated with different periods of the human life cycle. They know from the fields of sociology, cultural anthropology, and economics that there are life-style differences and differences in the availability of resources in social groups within societies. But nurses also know from their practice of nursing the features that some patients probably would have in common with other patients, for example, the well-developed manipulative skills of male veterans of a particular war who live in rural areas and are farmers and mechanics. Nurses, for example, also know from experience the effects of high-stress, high-demand households on patients, and what is and is not possible for nurses to do to help them maintain an adequate system of self-care. Nurses learn and document what nursing adjustments help educationally deprived persons with arrested cognitive development before such adjustments and technologies can be validated and become a part of practically practical nursing science.

Nurses who enter into the life situations of others who are in need of nursing are professionally obligated to accept these persons and become informed about them and their conditions and circumstances of living. Empirical knowledge is sought not only from the views of "taking care of" and "helping" but from the view of nursing science, theoretically and practically practical nursing sciences, including views provided by the articulating life sciences.

What nurses seek to know about persons under their care is limited to information relevant to their nursing. Observations of nurses are guided in each instance of nursing by their antecedent theoretic and empiric knowledge of nursing as it is generally or specifically relevant to the patient. There is a nursing basis for nurses obtaining particular kinds of information and not other kinds of information in each instance of nursing practice.

Nurses must be able to attribute nursing meaning to information obtained and to use it as the basis for making nursing judgments and decisions. All information, both relevant and irrelevant, about patients is held in confidence. According to its nature, information may be referred back to the patient, the patient's significant others, or to the physician or other health worker whenever the information is specific to their domains. In the latter situations nurses may help patients convey the information, record it in the official patient record, or communicate it verbally in emergency situations.

Information About Nursing Situations

Nurses, if they are to produce nursing beneficial to their patients, must have knowledge of the broad parameters of patient's health states and their health care situations. This holds for even those situations in which nursing has a very restricted area of jurisdiction. To aid nursing students in acquiring knowledge of the broad dimensions of individuals' health care situations, the following organization of information is suggested.

Area one—Age and gender of person

Area two—Health care focus (groups 1 to 7); general health state, related requirements for preventive health care and health promotion care

Area three—Persons' complaints and evidence of physical or psychic suffering

Area four—Medically diagnosed pathology of organic or psychic functioning; associated symptomatology; and effects on the person's behavior and management of self and personal affairs

Area five—Medical diagnostic and treatment modalities and protocols for use

Area six—Disfigurement; transitory, permanent; subjectivity to structural or cosmetic correction

Area seven—Disability: physical, psychologic including emotional control and cognitional functioning; technologies for overcoming the associated action limitations

Area eight—Paramedic protocols for care

Area nine—self-management capabilities and limitations

Information that would be subsumed under the nine areas is relevant to nurses' prediagnostic investigations of the presence or absence of a deficit relationship between powers of self-care agency and their being able to know and meet the component parts of their therapeutic self-care demands. All areas, for example, may provide information necessary for nurses to make judgments about the values of the universal and developmental self-care requisites, obstacles to meeting them, and valid methods for meeting them. Areas three through eight provide information about existent or emerging health-deviation self-care requisites. Area nine provides information about how persons can manage themselves in a stable environment or in a changing one.

Nursing Cases and Nursing Science

Three general categories of nursing cases are recognized: **wholly compensatory, partly compensatory,** and **supportive-educative.** The general categories of nursing cases are in accord with the three modalities of nursing practice described in Chapter 8. The three broad categories of nursing cases are analogous to the identification of medical cases as *medical* or *surgical,* based on the broad modalities of medical practice. Within these general categories both in nursing and in medicine, subsidiary types of cases are identified, for example, by health state or health disorders or by age and developmental state.

Medical classifications of medical cases should be understood by nurses, but medical classification cannot be substituted for nursing classification because of the differences in the proper objects of the two professions.

In specific situations where persons require and receive nursing, the features selected to identify types of nursing cases do not exhaust the kinds of information (as previously indicated) that nursing should seek and use as nurses design and produce nursing for individuals. The selected features that describe types of nursing cases are aids to nurses in their development of nursing science (1) in identifying the enduring and characterizing features of nursing cases and the natural history of their development and progress (stage III; see Figure 8-3) and (2) in the area of develoment of nursing diagnostic, prescriptive, and production models for identified types of cases (stage IV; see Figure 8-3). The following is a suggested identification of critical features of each of the three general categories of nursing cases. The features are specifics about patient variables or identify basic conditioning factors. The features singly or in combinations could be used to identify subcategories of the three general types of cases.

CRITICAL FEATURES OF THREE GENERAL CATEGORIES OF NURSING CASES

A. Wholly compensatory nursing cases are characterized by
    1. Absence of or extremely limited self-awareness and self-management capabilities
    2. a. Complete deficit for performing self-care measures because of undeveloped or nonfunctional self-care agency
       b. Deficit for performing all self-care measures that require manipulative movement because of imposed medical restrictions on activity
       c. Not attending to self or engaging in self-care without continuous direction and supervision
    3. Composition, complexity, and stability of the therapeutic self-care demand and its essential and critical components as related to the health care focus
    4. General health state and health care focus
    5. Age and gender
B. Partly compensatory nursing cases are characterized by
    1. Degree of operability of self-management capabilities
    2. Composition, complexity, and stability of the therapeutic self-care demand in relation to developed and operational power of self-care agency
    3. Age and gender
    4. General health state and health care focus
C. Supportive-educative nursing cases are characterized by
    1. Developed and operational powers for self-management within stable or changing environments

2. Limitations of knowledge and skill with respect to meeting a specific self-care requisite(s) (a self-care regimen) within an environmental context

3. Seeking increasing competency to know and meet his or her therapeutic self-care demand in time and over time or to direct another and cooperate with another in meeting elements of the therapeutic self-care demand

Nurses' ability to observe and their development of insight about nursing cases within the larger configuration of person's health care situations is a first step toward developing bodies of knowledge about nursing cases. The next step is nurses' noting similarities and differences in nursing cases and their development of classification of cases. Identification of the features of a number of clear-cut or typical cases of a particular type and the range over which these features may vary in concrete instances is movement toward the development of an empirical area of nursing science, namely, nursing cases and their natural history, stage III (see Figure 8-3).

Specialization of Nurses' Practice

All nursing practitioners specialize their practice in some way and to some degree. Common ways for specializing work in any field is by place of practice, time of day, and nature of the work done. Nurses use these ways, of course, but it is by type of nursing case that nursing practitioners tend to specialize their work of nursing. There is no one way of classifying nursing cases or specializing nursing practice. Nurses use and have used the areas or combinations of areas suggested for analysis of broad health groups. The trends of specialization in nursing are toward cases with distinct types of requirements for nursing associated with some combinations of self-care requisites and related self-care limitations.

THE PROVISION OF NURSING TO POPULATIONS

The term *population* is used here in the sense of the number or body of individuals belonging to the class of individuals who require nursing and who should be helped through its provision. Both nursing practitioners and nurses who function in nursing administration are essential in ensuring the provision of nursing to populations in need of this health service. Nursing practitioners function hour-to-hour or day-to-day or less frequently in the design and production of nursing for a case load of patients. Practitioners bear nursing responsibility for all persons constituting their case loads, however the case load is defined.

Nursing administration is defined as the body of persons who function in situational contexts to collectively manage courses of affairs enabling the provision of nursing to the population currently served by an organized health service institution or agency and to populations to be served at future times. To achieve this goal, administrators exercise powers given them by the governing bodies of institutions or agencies, the purpose of which are accomplished in whole or in part through nursing. Nursing administration in its various situational contexts within a health service agency or institution is an executive or a managerial organ within the formal structuring of positions and role responsibilities.

The situational contexts in which persons who constitute nursing administration hold positions and function are identified in terms of distance from governing boards and chief executive officers or institutional administrators measured against distance from nurses engaged in the production of nursing for individuals or groups. Nursing administrators located in positions directly concerned with ensuring the day-to-day, minute-by-minute production of nursing for a subpopulation of a larger population (as on a hospital unit) often combine in one position the functions of nursing practitioner and operational unit administration. This holds not only for residence care institutions but also for home health care agencies, where nurse agency administrators function to provide nursing consultation within their areas of nursing specialization.

When nursing practitioners in private practice serve patients in their own offices or in patients' homes, there is a coming together of the case load of patients and the nursing population being served. Nurses in private practice must fulfill practitioner responsibilities as well as administrative responsibilities.

Provision of nursing to populations demands both nursing practice models and nursing population descriptions and models. Both have as their foundation valid descriptions of nursing cases and classifications of nursing cases that are useful to nurses in making inferences about nursing requirements (see Figure 8-3).

Nursing Practice Models, Population Descriptions and Models

Development of practical science includes the stages of synthesis of nursing practice models (stage IV) and the stage of description of nursing populations and synthesis of models for providing nursing to populations (stage V) (see Figure 8-3).

A practice model is a carefully worked out design for the structure and formation of a nursing system or a segment of a nursing system for a type or subtype of nursing case when one or both patient variables (therapeutic self-care demand and self-care agency) have (or can be predicted to take on) certain qualitative or quantitative characteristics. A well-known example of nursing practice model is the design for nursing during the preoperative, intraoperative, and postoperative stages of nursing for persons undergoing major surgical treatments. Practice models are also illustrated through Joan E. Backscheider's work with educationally deprived adult clinic patients with *limitations of operative knowing* (one of the foundational capabilities and dispositions of self-care agency) (pp. 219-229).[4] Persons who think concretely and cannot deal with abstractions can be helped through nursing to master a regimen of self-care when this specific self-care limitation and its meaning for develoment of instructional systems for them is recognized by nurses, and appropriate instruction and other forms of help are instituted. The basis for use of a valid regulatory model is accurate diagnosis of limitations of operative knowing in persons under nursing care. Backscheider developed the foundations for a diagnostic model and an instructional model about what, when, and how to do care measures every day for oneself. The essential component of the instructional model is a communication element. Instructional models include content about self-care measures to meet components of therapeutic self-care demands and the courses of action to be performed. In nursing situations of this type, the self-care systems of patients often are articulated with partly compensatory periodic nursing systems. Backscheider's models are examples of (1) diagnostic and (2) instructional-developmental models addressed to the patient property of self-care agency.

Although practice models can be found in the nursing literature, many nurses use their own known only to themselves. Formalization and validation of practice models is work that can and should be done in nursing practice settings.

Population descriptions developed by nursing administration differ from the detailed nursing cases developed in stage III of practical science development (see Chapter 8). The description of populations to be provided with the health service nursing must be adequate for answering questions about the quality and amount of nursing required by time periods to serve the population of the agency. Nursing administrators should consider various approaches to description to find one that yields only essential information for judgment and decision making about kinds and numbers of nurses essential for the provision of nursing. The description also should yield information about both the physical and psychologic demands on nurses who nurse members of described subpopulations.

Nursing administrators can review the kinds of data about patients currently and consistently available in the health care enterprises they serve. Nursing implications of available data can and should be identified. Moving from what is available to what is essential may save time, effort, and resources. One goal of nursing administration should be the immediate availability of descriptive nursing information about the types of nursing cases in the population being served and projected populations. Nursing administration requires knowledge of developments in preventive health care and in medical diagnosis and treatment, the prevalence of types of diseases and injuries in the community and the major causes of death in the community, and changes in features of the community's health care system. The implications of this knowledge for nursing should be worked out in detail. Maintaining knowledge of what a community needs and what a health care enterprise can do in meeting a community's requirements for nursing is an essential task of every nursing administrator.

Models for the provision of nursing for populations are production design models that relate nurses by qualification and nurse teams and case loads to subpopulations served by health care enterprises. The design of systems of nursing for individual patients has been represented as a responsibility of nursing practitioners. Designs for ensuring the effective production of nursing for a nursing population being served by a health care enterprise is a function of nursing administration.

Nursing Services in Communities

Many communities in the United States and elsewhere expect nursing to be available on a community-wide basis. The pattern for nursing as a community service to individuals and families was set in the United States during the latter part of the 19th century. That pattern has changed since the developmental years, but modern nursing practice can be traced back to the three types of nursing service identified as hospital nursing, private-duty nursing, and district nursing.

What quality and quantity of nursing service are available to a modern community? What are the costs involved in providing this service to the community? What must patients pay for nursing, and how and where can they obtain this assistance when it is required? These important questions must be answered, partly by the citizens of the community and partly by nurses. Nursing, like the other services established in a community for the health, welfare, and safety of its citizens, must be planned for, maintained, and developed in keeping with community needs. If a community is to have nursing available, it must have nurses. Each community, therefore, must answer the question: How can this community fulfill its needs for nurses?

The strength and effectiveness of nursing as a health service in the community depends on the values of the community. The provision of nursing makes heavy demands on community resources. Many persons in a community need nursing at the same time—in their homes, in hospitals and clinics, in nursing homes and homes for the aged, in child-care institutions and clinics, and in a variety of other facilities providing health service. A community may require large numbers of nurses to supply the demands for nursing that exist at the same time, and often in the same place, throughout 24 hours of each day and each day throughout the year. From both the community's and patients' point of view, nursing is a costly service and frequently may be in short supply. A community that is convinced that nursing is an essential health service will be more likely to engage in activities and programs necessary for providing nursing than will the community that holds no such conviction. In addition, many communities face the problem of finding candidates for nursing careers and preparing them for nursing practice.

The types of nurses needed and the educational facilities available for preparation for nursing practice also must be considered in providing adequate nursing in the community. Before World War II, nurses were educated almost exclusively in schools maintained and controlled by local hospitals. The level of preparation for all nursing personnel was essentially the same. Since that time, the increasing demand for nurses, periodic shortages of nurses, and the increasing complexity of health care have resulted in the preparation of persons for work in nursing in all the existing forms of occupational education and training. The number and qualifications of persons employed to provide nursing often differ from the required number of nurses qualified to give nursing.

Nurses' failure to develop or implement standards of nursing practice at the local community level has resulted at times in ineffective nursing and undesirable conditions of practice. Licensed nurses may not be prepared, able, or willing to design, provide, and manage systems of nursing assistance for patients and to supervise other nurses and auxiliary workers who contribute to the daily provision of nursing for individuals. Nursing practitioners often are not present or are so infrequently or remotely available that patients have little or no contact with them. As a result, technically prepared nurses, practical nurses, and nursing aides are placed in positions they are unprepared to fill.

The growing interest of American nurses in the development and implementation of standards of nursing practice to enhance the quality of nursing provided in community health agencies and hospitals should bring about improved conditions for both the consumers and practitioners of nursing.

The development of criterion measures of nursing care, along with instruments and procedures for use in measuring the quality of nursing provided in a health care facility, is making an important contribution to nursing. The previously mentioned work of Horn and Swain and their associates is an example of such work. Continued effort to ensure that the nursing provided in particular settings is in accord with patients' self-care deficits is needed. This effort, however, should be accompanied by efforts to ensure that qualified nurses have time to engage in nursing diagnosis and prescription and in the design, production, and management of effective nursing systems for individuals and groups.

The settings in which nursing is provided vary by types of health care agency. The setting affects both nursing administration and nurses' practice of nursing. The place where a patient is nursed is a variable that requires consideration. Place is of importance for several reasons. Some of the reasons can be best expressed as questions. Is the patient away from his or her usual place of residence and from an accustomed environmental setting? If so, what is the patient's outlook? Is the experience producing stress, accepted, or even conforting to the patient? A patient's response to being a patient in a hospital, an extended care facility, a nursing home, a community health center, a clinic, or an outpatient department of a hospital is influenced by his or her knowledge and attitudes regarding health care and to what is being experienced.

Although they provide modern diagnostic, treatment, and rehabilitation facilities, hospitals may become so routine-oriented that individual patients and their need for nursing are submerged by routine practices. The task of each nurse in a hospital nursing situation is to make certain that each patient is provided with nursing care that conforms to the nature of and reasons for the patient's self-care deficit and that the hospital system is adaptable to the nursing system for the individual patient. Routines are necessary, but they are not necessarily valid or justifiable if they interfere with the accomplishment of health goals and nursing goals for patients.

Other resident care facilities, such as extended care facilities and nursing homes, present some of the same advantages and disadvantages to nursing that the hospital presents. Routine service, large numbers of persons to be given care during the same time period, inadequate numbers of nurses, nurses with inadequate preparation, or the absence of nurses often militates against effective nursing in extended care facilities and nursing homes. Courtesy, kindness, and help from nurses and others in assuring patients that health care facilities and services are for their benefit are important in securing effective use of community facilities.

Other community facilities, such as clinics or day or night care health centers, serve patients who are at home for some part of the day. Nursing care of patients who come to these centers must take into consideration the possible need to adjust factors in the home environment to the patient's system of self-care or the need for the patient to make adjustments to the home situation. Hazards of travel, the time required for travel, available modes of travel, and costs require consideration.

Patients who are given nursing care in their own homes are in their accustomed environments. The environment is new for the nurse, however. A nurse who nurses patients in their homes may be a staff member of an agency that provides home care services. The agency may be a community health agency or a hospital that provides home care services. Such nurses have available to them equipment provided by the agency and may call on the agency for other types of health care services needed by persons receiving nursing.

Persons who are in permanent or temporary residence in health care institutions such as hospitals, who may require nursing as well as other forms of health care, will require a range of services due purely to their status as residents. Figure 15-2 identifies services that health care institutions, such as hospitals and nursing homes, should provide for persons under health care, health care providers and other workers, and visitors. Whenever and wherever numbers of persons come or are brought together in common facilities (e.g., clinics), preventive public health services are essential for their protection. Ideally, an institution will maintain a supportive and developmental environment for all who come within its walls. The responsibility for the continued provision and maintenance of preventive public health services rests primarily with health care institution executives and administrators. All residence care and health care workers and other personnel, however, as well as patients and visitors, should participate in the fulfillment of this responsibility. Public health services are concerned with the protection of populations.

ORGANIZATION FOR NURSING—NURSING ADMINISTRATION AND NURSING PRACTICE

No population or subpopulation of persons in need of nursing can be provided with nursing in the absence of cooperation between a competent nursing administration and competent nursing practitioners. Persons who fill these roles have distinct but related responsibilities. Both groups generate or should generate

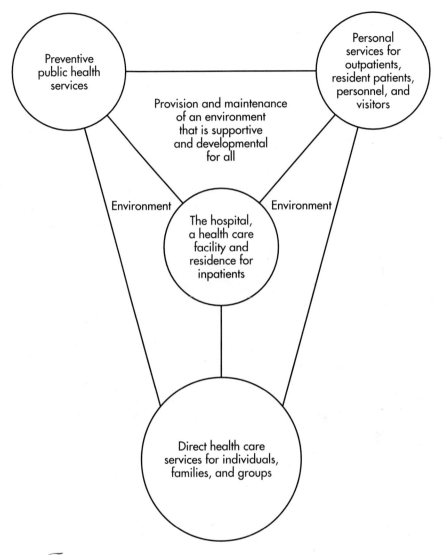

Figure 15-2   Service operations of hospitals and health care facilities.

"systems of consciously coordinated personal activities or forces" (pp. 72-75).[5] The activities of nursing practitioners are for the nursing of individuals or groups and for coordination of their actions with those of other nurses and other health care providers. The activities of nurses in nursing administration are for gathering and analyzing data descriptive of a nursing population or subpopulation and for ensuring that nursing practitioners and assistants with the nursing willingness and qualifications are brought into cooperative interrelationship and into nursing relationships with members of the population served through the provision of nursing. Administrators and practitioners coordinate their activities to fulfill their respective functions. They come together as working groups in the formulation of standards of care and rules of practice for providing nursing to the population served and in developing criterion measures for measuring the quality of nursing provided.

Nursing one individual over time is quite different from the day-to-day provision of nursing to two or more persons during the same time period. The practitioner of nursing focuses on the patients within his or her case load as individuals to be nursed. The complement of individuals to be nursed by a single nurse with or without assistance during the same time period is determined according to some governing principle or plan used by health service institutions or agencies that have provisions for offering nursing as one of their health services. The complement of persons for whom a health service agency has contracted to or is in the process of contracting to provide nursing or agrees to admit on an ad hoc basis for purposes of receiving nursing (and other health services) is the focus of nursing administration.

The nursing administrator focuses on populations or subpopulations that have requirements for nursing and can benefit from nursing. Whereas the nursing practitioner focuses on individuals with diagnosed health-derived or health-associated self-care deficits in their time-place localizations, nursing administrators must ensure that existent and future populations are provided with nursing. The nursing practitioner provides nursing. Nursing administration knows members of populations real or projected in terms of types and configurations of requirements for nursing, not as individuals, except when questions of adequacy of nursing arise. Nursing practitioners know the members of health agency populations they are to nurse as individuals whose nursing requirements are specific to them and must be diagnosed. **Population** is used as a class word—a word used to refer to all the people served or to be served by a health care institution or agency.

The Functions of Nursing Administration

Persons in nursing administration have nursing-oriented functions concerned with achievement of the broad health care–providing purpose of the health service institution or agency. They also have executive and managerial functions specific to their location in the health care institution of which they are a part.

Nursing-Oriented Functions

To function effectively, nurses who fill positions in nursing administration must have antecedent and continuously developing knowledge about nursing and about the organized enterprise that offers nursing as a community service. Knowledge requirements for nursing administrators include at a minimum the following:

- Organized knowledge of the practical science of nursing, theoretically and practically practical nursing science
- Knowledge of practice models for nursing persons with types and configurations of requirements for nursing, validated and emerging models
- Knowledge of forms of education preparatory for nursing practice, including preparation of nursing specialists and legal qualification for practice
- The purpose of the institution or agency of which they are an organic part
- The extent to which and the manner in which nursing contributes to the continuing attainment of the institution's or agency's purpose
- The nature and extent of their received powers to manage courses of affairs that ensure the continuing provision of nursing to a population or a subpopulation served by the agency or institution
- Knowledge of the domain and boundaries of nursing in concrete practice situations, as well as the domain and boundaries of health professionals whose work articulates with nursing

In their positional locations within organized health service enterprises, nursing administrators use their knowledge of nursing and nurses (as well as other kinds of knowledge) to do the following:

- Produce nursing descriptions of populations or subpopulations served by identifying and classifying combinations of factors associated with self-care deficits and factors relevant to contractual and interpersonal features of nursing practice
- Analyze the nursing descriptions to make judgments about the types of nursing practice models that would have to be juxtaposed or interlaced in the production of nursing for members of populations with the described types of self-care deficits
- Estimate the time requirements for nursing and the periodic or continuous nature of required nursing systems and the amount and quality of nursing effort required
- Consider desirable and undesirable locations for members of populations with types and configurations of requirements for nursing
- Consider (1) the capabilities that nurses must have to practice nursing for members of populations with types and configurations of requirements for nursing and (2) desirable and undesirable mixes of nurses and assistants to nurses in the provision of nursing
- Consider and work with nursing practitioners in developing and testing desirable case loads for nurses or combinations of nurses and assistants, considering both number of patients constituting a case load and the mix of patients by the types and configurations of their nursing requirements

Executive and Managerial Orientations and Operations*

The foregoing nursing-oriented executive functions of nursing administration as well as associated managerial operations are understood within the larger framework of the functional systems of service enterprises developed in Chapter 4 in the section titled Service Enterprises and in Figure 4-2.

Nurses through their production of nursing in the role of nurse perform one of the essential operational functions of a health service agency, but they also contribute to the executive and governing functions through what they do in the effective production of nursing. In the role of employee, nurses direct appropriate contributions to governing and executive functions. These contributions should be elicited and facilitated by nursing administration.

Nursing administration contributes to the operational function of the production of nursing through the suggested nursing-oriented functions. These six functions provide the groundwork of administrators' executive functioning at their various locations in health service enterprises and for making appropriate contributions to the governing functions. Nursing administration is charged with knowing what nursing is required by the subpopulations and populations served and with bringing about and maintaining conditions that will ensure its production. Nursing administration is charged with:

- The creation of functional wholes as organizational members fulfill their role responsibilities; this involves the proper ordering of persons and material resources; a patient unit within a hospital where nurses work together and with nursing administration, collaborating with other health professionals, is an example of a part of a larger functional whole.
- Ensuring that current decisions and actions about ways and means to provide nursing for a population and its subpopulations are in harmony with future requirements for the production of nursing and for the survival or growth of the health care enterprise.

In fulfillment of these responsibilities, nursing administration performs the work operations of (1) objective setting in relation to the population to be served through nursing and to the health care enterprise; (2) analysis and organization of work to achieve objectives; (3) establishing standards for selection of nurses, assistants to nurses, and other support personnel; (4) motivating and communicating; (5) producing designs for measuring performance and results; and (6) measuring performance and results.

The Functions of Nursing Practitioners

In hospitals or in other resident health care enterprises, nurses function in the same situational contexts as other health professionals who provide direct health services for patients. Also operating in these situations are persons filling positions that provide residence services such as housekeeping, food service,

---

*Some ideas presented in this section are further developed in Orem DE: In Henry B et al., editors: Nursing administration, a theoretical approach, Dimensions of Nursing Administration, Cambridge, 1989, Blackwell Scientific Publications.

maintenance service, and temperature and air control services. Nursing administrators and practicing nurses must know and protect the domain and boundaries of nursing as a field of practice and at the same time coordinate nursing activities with other health services and with residence services. Boundary maintenance is required when patients are not in residence in health care settings, but the requirement may be less extensive.

Nurses are in resident health care agencies and in outpatient clinics of hospitals or public health clinics to provide nursing. They are not there to serve as clerks or receptionists or to take patients from one place to another unless nursing is required during the process of moving the patient. To justify their presence in health care enterprises, nurses must be nursing oriented; to be nursing oriented is to be patient oriented. Nurses must be able to practice nursing but also able to represent nursing to patients, families of patients, other health workers, nursing administration, executive officers of the enterprise, and, when necessary, to members of governing boards. The ability to communicate about nursing and what is required to produce it under prevailing and changing conditions and circumstances is an essential quality of nurses functioning within health care enterprises.

Production of Nursing

Nursing may be provided to individuals continuously or periodically over some duration of time. The continuous provision of nursing is envisioned most readliy in settings such as intensive care units or in therapeutic environments for mentally ill individuals. The continuous provision of nursing means that the nurse is with or immediately available to persons under care. The nurse is an essential human element in the environment of the patient. It does not mean that nurses are continuously engaged in doing something for or with persons under continuous nursing care. The periodic provision of nursing is envisioned most readily in terms of patients' visits to nurses in nursing clinics, in nurses' offices, or nurses' home visits to patients. The duration of visits varies.

Time requirements vary when nursing is continuously provided in order to know and meet patients' therapeutic self-care demands, regulate the exercise or development of patients' self-care agency, and maintain or bring about a state of patient well-being. The subtypes of wholly compensatory nursing systems described in Chapter 13 are all time demanding, but in different ways. Patients' lack of stability along dimensions of human functioning and the complexity of and lack of stability in the therapeutic self-care demands of patients makes additional time demands on nurses.

The periodic provision of nursing usually occurs within the design of partly compensatory and supportive-developmental nursing systems. The nature of and reasons for patients' self-care deficits are indicators of time requirements. The age, state of maturation, conditions of living, interests and orientations, and potential for extending and developing their self-care agency are other indicators. Backscheider identified factors or combinations of factors associated with both time requirements for nursing and kinds of nursing results for an adult nursing clinic population (pp. 215-218).[4] The factors were expressed by Backscheider as "deficits for action" and included limitations for participating with nurses, limitations in actual provision of self-care, and limitations for extending and deepening self-care agency. The deficits were expressed as (1) action deficits in "operative knowing," as evidenced by patterns of concrete thinking; (2) motivational emotional action deficits, as evidenced by patients from "high-stress, high-demand households"; (3) action deficits in consistency of performance and self-discipline; and (4) a deficit for action associated with quality of the health orientation, limitations of time, and location of care in the individual's priority schedule or value hierarchy.

In the production of nursing when nursing systems are periodic, nurses in leadership roles for production of nursing care may work alone or with nursing assistants. These nurses may need and seek nursing consultation for both self and the person under nursing care. Nursing consultation should be available. When periodic nursing systems articulate with dependent-care systems, nurses, as well as nursing assistants, work with the dependent-care agents who may be members of the patient's family or friends. Nursing consultation may be needed to facilitate more effective relationships or to help individual dependent-care agents with specific nursing-relevant matters.

In the production of continuous systems of nursing over the 24 hours of each day, more than one nurse is needed. The number of nurses is determined by the hours of nursing of each nurse and the arrangements with respect to the presence and responsibilities of nurses in nursing leadership roles. The role responsibilities of nurses who provide nursing at different time periods to the same patient are sometimes ill defined. Failures of nurses to engage in nursing diagnosis and nursing prescription and to produce nursing that is in accord with known requirements can result in harm to patients and constitute malpractice. Nurses who care for the same patient at different times during the 24 hours of each day should function as a team. Such teams, when composed of nurses working at three different times periods, must overcome the difficulties of not meeting face to face at the same time and must ensure that there is essential agreement about stable elements or about how to handle changing elements in the design for the nursing system they are following and producing. Coordination of effort is not in opposition to the creative practical endeavors of each nurse.

The production of nursing demands the presence of nurses who know patients and their requirements for nursing. Nurses cannot know how patients can be helped through nursing in their time-place localizations if they are not with them. Nurses who do not engage in nursing diagnosis of patients have no basis for designing systems of care that reflect patients' requirements for nursing. In health care enterprises, because of free days for nurses and other reasons, there should be at least two nurses who know each person under nursing care. Although the foregoing statements may be judged as unrealistic, they are conditions to be worked toward by nursing administration. Nurse-nurse relationships in providing nursing for a subpopulation of patients during the same time period is of critical importance to both nurses and nursing administration.

Professionally Realistic Nurse Teams

Team is used here in the sense of two or more nurses with different role responsibilities contributing to the nursing of persons constituting a single case load. Two types of teams are identified.

In the first type, the nurse in the governing and leadership role is an advanced, experienced nursing practitioner. The other nurses are qualified for entry to the professional level of practice of nursing who are gaining nursing experience under the guidance and direction of the advanced nursing practitioner. They are being introduced to increasingly complex nursing practice situations where diagnostic, prescriptive, and regulatory nursing operations are performed in conjunction with or are reviewed by the advanced nursing practitioner.

The role responsibilities of the nurses vary with the complexity of the nursing requirements of patients and the nursing systems to be produced for them. Nursing consultation may be required. The assignment of nursing assistants to the nurse team is based on the number and kinds of care measures that need to be performed regularly for persons constituting the case load that can be safely separated out for performance from the total system of regulatory or treatment nursing being produced by nurses (see Figure 15-1).

This type of nurse team is indicated when patients' requirements for nursing are very complex, with some degree of instability of patients' therapeutic self-care demands and where nurses educated for entry to professional level practice are provided with a way to move toward this level of practice.

In the second type of nurse team, a nurse in the governing or leadership role is highly knowledgeable and experienced in the nursing of patients with particular and well-described types of self-care deficits. Other nurses working with this nurse would be technically prepared nurses, with ranges of experience depending on the types of cases within the case load. Diagnostic and prescriptive operations would be primary role responsibilities of the nurse in the governing and leadership role, with time-specific contributions from technically prepared nurses. These nurses would be involved primarily with the continuing provision of treatment or regulatory nursing for patients constituting the case load. The assignment of nursing assistants would be based on the presence of the conditions identified for the first type of team.

This type of nurse team is indicated when patients' requirements for nursing are predictable within limits over some duration of time and when the technologies used in the production of nursing have a high degree of validity and reliability. This type of nurse team may require nursing consultation when special problems arise.

The suggestions about two types of nurse teams are made in light of the absence of career pathways for nurses prepared for entry to professional-level practice and in light of the failure in some practice settings for nursing administration to differentiate the role responsibilities of professionally from technically prepared nurses and to safely separate out role responsibilities of vocationally prepared nursing assistants from total systems of nursing in production. Refer to role responsibilities of home health aide in the type of nursing case described in Chapter 12.

Time Requirements for Nursing

Nursing practitioners and nursing administrators should continuously acquire information about time requirements for nursing, given particular types of nursing cases. Both must have the empirical knowledge and the nursing science base for using time requirements for nursing as a basis for planning for the production of nursing care.

Time requirements for nursing vary with the nature and causes of patients' self-care deficits associated with their therapeutic self-care demands and their self-care capabilities, their developed self-management capabilities, and their personal maturity and interests. Time requirements may also vary with patients' conditions of living, their family system elements, their potential for extending and deepening self-care agency, methods of helping nurses used, and the arrangement of nurse and patient roles that are generative of particular types of nursing systems.

Attention is directed to variations in therapeutic self-care demands and self-care agency and to variations associated with the continuous and the periodic provision of nursing to individuals under the care of nurses.

Variations in Therapeutic Self-Care Demands

A therapeutic self-care demand has been described as a nursing prescription for the self-care measures to be performed to meet identified sets of self-care requisites—universal, developmental, and health-deviation (see Chapter 10). A person's therapeutic self-care demand is one of the two patient variables of nursing systems, the other being the patient's ability to engage in self-care, that is, self-care agency. A person's therapeutic self-care demand varies with age, developmental state, health state, and other factors.

Variations in therapeutic self-care demands of members of a nursing population and variations in the demands of individuals from time to time may be identified and described in terms of (1) the particular values of each one of the universal self-care requisites, (2) the particular values of the developmental requisites, and (3) the presence of health-deviation self-care requisites and their derivation, for example, from a pathologic process, as medically prescribed and associated with medical diagnoses or treatment measures, or as associated with regulation of the effects of medical diagnostic and treatment measures. Given particular values of specific self-care requisites, variations in therapeutic self-care demands may result from the complexity of processes for meeting requisites, methods and from the measures of care (action systems) necessary for using selected methods.

Two possible variations in the mix of self-care requisites exist: (1) a combination of universal and developmental requisites and (2) a combination of universal, developmental, and health-deviation requisites. The seven types of nursing situations classified by health care focus (see Chapter 9) suggest these two variations. Whenever the life cycle focus prevails, there is a mix of universal and developmental requisites. For example, in the event of mental retardation or other forms of retarded development with the absence of injury or overt disease processes, there would be a need for adjustments in the values of the universal and developmental requisites and for the use of appropriate methods for meeting them, for example, the selection and use of appropriate instructional methods and educational experiences and the appropriate regulation of living conditions to foster the patient's personal development, including involvement in self-care.

In the remaining six types of nursing situations, health-deviation requisites are present in addition to universal and developmental requisites. These six types of nursing situations also vary according to (1) the number and kinds of health-deviation requisites and the relationships among these requisites and (2) the degree to which the normal values and ways of meeting the universal and developmental requisites are changed.

For example, when persons have the condition that has the medical name of *chronic congestive heart failure,* the patient's health care focus, if it is therapeutic, is on self-management and meeting specific self-care requisites directed toward the regulation of the burden on the heart and toward the prevention of complicating conditions. Under the care of physicians and nurses and with assistance from family members, patients:

- Remain on a prescribed amount of bed rest
- Maintain a posture that prevents dyspnea
- Engage in some exercise, avoiding exertion that results in dyspnea
- Take precautions against contracting infections
- Act to regulate stress-producing conditions
- Control sodium intake and use prescribed medications to regulate excretion of body fluids; monitor for effects and results
- Use prescribed medications to regulate cardiac functioning; monitor for effects and results
- Monitor for known complications and general sense of well-being or illness

This set of health-deviation self-care requisites includes ones that are essentially adjustments in the universal self-care requisites. The regulatory contribution to a person's well-being made by meeting each health-deviation self-care requisite and the interrelationships among the requisites must be understood by nurses if they are to help patients in managing themselves and in understanding and meeting their therapeutic self-care demands.

Nurses should have knowledge about recurring disorders of human structure and functioning, including knowledge of their natural history, to understand the associated health-deviation self-care requisites. This knowledge includes how the values of some or all of the universal self-care requisites may be affected. Specific pathologic processes usually affect the values of some but not all of the universals. When a disease becomes generalized (e.g., cancer) or when a person is critically ill, nurses must operate with continuing awareness that all the universal self-care requisites may require continuing adjustment.

Variations in therapeutic self-care demands of individuals also result from the presence of factors that affect the choice of methods for meeting universal self-care requirements (and other requisites). Age, gender, states of development and health, and personal interests and concerns give rise to such factors. Methods selected for meeting each universal self-care requisite must be adjusted to certain conditions; for example, in maintaining a sufficient intake of food, the condition of being an infant or a child requires methods that are effective for feeding infants or young children. A selected method must be able to surmount interfering factors, as in feeding by gavage when a person of any age cannot swallow.

Patients may also suffer conditions that interfere with the natural processes associated with meeting some or all of the universal self-care requisites, especially the requisites for maintenance of sufficient intakes of air, water, and food and for care related to excretory processes (see Apendix C). Interference may be external to the individuals, for example, the quality of the atmosphere as related to air intake. In relation to food intake, interferences may be personal, as with food preferences or avoidance of certain foods on the basis of cultural or religious proscriptions. Interferences with food intake also may be, for example, because of structural anomalies such as cleft palate or disturbances of the neural mechanism of the swallowing reflex. In such situations, methods for meeting universal self-care requisites must be able to surmount interfering factors. Sometimes this requires methods derived from medicine, for example, the use of the *surgical method of introduction of tubes and needles into the body.* Examples include feeding by gavage, feeding intravenously, and emptying the bladder by catheterization.

In summary, time requirements for nursing (or for self-care) vary with the basic composition of persons' therapeutic self-care demands, that is, with (1) composition by types of requisites, universal, developmental, health-deviation types; (2) the number of developmental and health-deviation requisites; for example, persons who suffer from one or two or more diseases or health disorders may have health-deviation self-care requisites associated with the regulation of each disease entity or with regulation of its effects; (3) the complexity of the methods or technologies used to meet the requisites; and (4) the sets of operations or care measures necessary to use the method or technologies in meeting each requisite. Nurses who provide nursing to particular nursing subpopulations can estimate with considerable accuracy the time requirements for production of care.

Variations in Self-Care Agency

In nursing practice, the capability of patients to engage in self-care can be assessed according to three scales: developmental, operational, and adequacy (pp. 203-210).[4] In taking this type of diagnostic approach to making judgments about the self-care agency of patients, nurses seek to determine the following with respect to self-care:

- What individuals have learned to do and do consistently
- What individuals *can* and *cannot do* now or in the future because of existing or predicted conditions and circumstances

- Whether what individuals have *learned to do* and *can now do* is equal to meeting all the current or projected demands on them to engage in self-care, that is, to meeting their therapeutic self-care demands now or at some future time

Because self-care is learned behavior, nurses must take into account the readiness and capabilities of individuals for extending or deepening their abilities to engage in self-care. Variations in the self-care agency of patients, as previously suggested, can be understood and examined in relation to:

- Self-care measures that patients know how to perform and usually do perform (repertoire of self-care practices, usual components of their self-care systems)
- Action limitations that restrict the performance of what patients know how to do with respect to self-care (limitations that interfere with the performance of the operations required for the decision-making and productive phases of self-care)
- Self-care measures to be performed to meet known self-care requisites for which patients have or do not have requisite knowledge, skill, or willingness (adequacy or limitation of knowledge, skills, and techniques, or willingness to meet known self-care requisites using particular care methods)
- Patients' potential for extending or deepening their knowledge of self-care and mastering the techniques necessary to perform required self-care measures that are not within their existing self-care repertoires (potential for further developments to extend or deepen self-care agency)
- Patients' potential for consistent and effective performance of new and essential self-care measures, including the integration of essential self-care measures into the self-care system and daily life

To accumulate and validate knowledge about variations in the self-care agency of nursing populations, it would seem practical to approach the five possible variations separately. In particular nursing situations, nurses should consistently investigate the first three variations. If there is a lack of adequacy (third variation), the fourth and fifth variations, dealing with patient potential, should be investigated.

This section on organization for nursing is a partial basis for understanding what should be attended to in the formation of standards of nursing care and in the development of criterion measures for determining the quality of nursing provided to individuals and groups accepted for care. Efforts toward quality assurance without a base of information about the existent nursing requirements of members of a population or subpopulation are at best questionable.

EDUCATION FOR PROFESSIONAL-LEVEL NURSING PRACTICE AND RELATED ENDEAVORS

The survival and advancement of nursing as a human health service with a formalized and developing science base depend on the presence and functioning of nursing practitioners prepared in accord with standards for professional-level education and practice. Standards for this form of education vary from one professional field to another and sometimes from country to country within the same field. In the United States the establishment and continued presence of established programs of nursing education in the professional form have been opposed and thwarted by forces inside and outside nursing. Such forces continue to operate to the detriment of society and intelligent women and men who want to practice nursing and pursue careers in nursing.

Nurses prepared through the professional form of education should be prepared after experience in nursing practice situations to move themselves to the expert level of clinical nursing practice and to specialization of practice. With adequate graduate-level preparation in universities and experience in nursing practice, they can move to the part-time or full-time practice of nursing science in the form of scholarly endeavors, theory development, nursing research, or technology development and validation.

Professional-Level Education

Authentic programs of education qualifying for entry into professions include three components: a preprofessional component, a professional component, and a continuing education component within the professional field. Professions differ in the composition of the preprofessional component and when and where it is pursued. They also differ in the length and composition of the professional component.

Preprofessional components in the health services professions include:
- Course sequences in the liberal arts and humanities
- Course sequences in the basic sciences or in disciplines of knowledge necessary for pursuing courses in the professional component, for example, general biology is basic to pursuing courses in physiology

The professional components include:
- Courses in the sciences and disciplines of knowledge foundational to and essential for pursuing courses in and understanding the practical and the applied sciences of the professional field; in nursing, for example, courses in human development are necessary for understanding developmental self-care requisites, modes of thinking by developmental stages, and how to operationalize methods of helping by developmental stages
- Course sequences in the professional field including the theoretically and practically practical nursing sciences and the applied sciences, and instructional experiences in clinical practice

The continuing education component of professional education in the health service professions addresses demands on practitioners to keep abreast of scientific developments, technologic developments, and clinical rules of practice to be followed in diagnosis and treatment of types of cases. Developments that should affect the work of practitioners arise from the work of scientists and the work of advanced clinical specialists in the profession. Continuing education is also designed to keep members of the profession abreast of changes in the health service needs of populations served and relevant environmental and social conditions associated with needs for practice changes.

These broadly expressed components of professionally qualifying education are one indication of the complexity of education for the professions. Diversity of disciplines of knowledge and the need for systems of organization of content based on the function the organization of content is designed to serve are primary concerns of program developers.

Mastery of the subject matter areas of a discipline involves a process of knowing that includes not only content but also a style of thinking. Content includes concepts and their relationships. The thinking style of a discipline is established by the modes of inquiry and the level of data leading to (1) the insights expressed by the concepts and to (2) relationships among concepts.

Professional-Level Education for Nurses, Considerations

In development of programs of professional education for nursing practice, understanding the fields and areas of knowledge of the practical science nursing provides rationales for the selection of foundational courses. The points of articulation between subject matter areas of nursing science and foundational courses should be made explicit through teaching. The question of what is an adequate sequence of courses in nursing must be answered before making final decisions about foundational courses.

A major problem in education for entry to nursing practice is the development of courses in the professional field that are constituted from subject matter that is nursing. All too often courses that carry a nursing title are primarily made up of content from the biologic, behavioral, and medical sciences. The offering of an adequate sequence of nursing courses is a major undertaking unless course designers are guided by a general concept of nursing and their understanding of nursing as a practical science linked to applied sciences.

Nurses and nursing students should understand that the nursing sciences are but one of at least seven fields of knowledge that treat of nurses and nursing. The fields as previously identified are:

- Nursing social field—dimensions of nursing as an institutionalized service in social groups under fixed and changing social, cultural, economic, and political conditions
- Nursing, a profession and occupation
- Nursing jurisprudence, or nursing and the law
- Nursing history
- Nursing ethics
- Nursing economics
- Nursing sciences, the practical and applied nursing sciences

Each one of the seven identified fields has its distinct structures and modes of inquiry. Some of them are constituted from a number of areas of knowledge. The modes of inquiry specific to the first six fields are those of the disciplines that are named in titles, for example, law, history, ethics, and economics. The first two—nursing's social field and nursing, a profession and occupation—are associated with a number of social and behavioral sciences.

The nursing sciences, the practical and applied nursing sciences, are the critical components of professional-level education for nursing. The failure of nurses in the United States to understand the nature of nursing science and to accept their professional responsibilities for its development continue to affect the quality of and sometimes the existence of professional-level education for nursing.

Each of the seven fields of knowledge named can be developed as a distinct discipline or as an applied field. How they are introduced in preparatory programs for entry into professional-level nursing practice should be determined by how each field of knowledge affects professional level nursing practice. Nursing science is central to the technologic features of nursing practice and through its conceptual structure points to needs for content from the other fields. The social, including occupational, dimensions of nursing must be considered. The legal, ethical, and economic features of nursing cases and nursing practice situations must be developed.

Schools of nursing in universities have the responsibility for identifying what they can and will contribute to the development of nursing science and to the other named fields of knowledge about nurses and nursing. The development of the practical and applied nursing sciences is hindered by the absence of an explicit consensus and clear-cut positional view in the nursing profession about why nursing exists, what its object is, and what its domain and boundaries are. The reasons why people need nursing must be linked to nursing's interpersonal features.

University faculties of nursing, nurses in nursing administration, nursing practitioners, and individual nurses who teach nursing must have the courage to take a position about why people need nursing and about what nursing can and should be. Dale Walker, in her expression of a nursing administration perspective on use of self-care deficit nursing theory, refers to Vivian Dee's crediting Dorothy Johnson with the statement "To openly use a nursing model is risk taking behavior for the individual nurse; for a nursing department to adopt one of these models . . . is risk taking behavior of an even higher order" (p. 252).[6]

Taking a position about nursing in terms of its proper object and its domain and boundaries is taking a position about the *concrete origins of nursing in persons who require and can be helped through nursing.* Nurses continue to develop, explore, and accept or reject theories of humanity, theories about internal phenomena in the lives of individuals, theories about human reactions and interactions, and theories about health promotion and preventive health care systems. These are not general comprehensive theories of nursing but narrower or sometimes broader conceptualizations that may be integral or adjunctive to nursing, not descriptively explanatory of it. The self-care deficit theory of nursing as developed in this text has been accepted by nursing practitioners, by nursing curriculum designers, by teachers of nursing, and by nursing researchers and scholars as a valid general comprehensive theory of nursing. It also has been denigrated and rejected by some nurses since its inception.

The mastery of a general comprehensive theory of nursing is a first step for nursing students who want to become able to maintain awareness of the relationship between what they know and what they do as nursing practitioners. The conceptual elements of a general theory of nursing constitute one essential aid for nursing students who want to (1) know what to attend to and observe in nursing practice situations; (2) develop appropriate nursing imagery, for example, about what will occur if nursing is not provided when particular combinations of conditions exist; (3) characterize and name what is observed; (4) attach more general as well as nursing meaning to what is observed; and (5) know the limits and the range of possible courses of action that are open to nurses and nurses' patients under types and combinations of prevailing conditions and circumstances.

Thinking nursing and seeing and conceptualizing the whole structure and dynamics of nursing situations to the degree necessary for understanding them is distinct from viewing nursing as skilled performance of standardized sets of operations or skilled performance of tasks separated out from larger dynamic systems of operations. Nursing practice demands that nursing practitioners understand systems of work operations and defined tasks both in terms of the specific results that each one brings about and in terms of their contributions to the attainment of specified nursing goals for persons under nursing care. The product of the *actions* of nurses, their patients, and those who assist in task performance is or should be a unified, dynamic, and continuing system of action (a nursing system) through which patients' demands for self-care of a therapeutic quality are met and their capabilities of engaging in self-care are regulated. Nursing practitioners ideally see their role responsibilities in terms of the wholeness of nursing situations and in terms of the design, production, and management of dynamic, effective nursing systems.

Exercise

Exercise in Recognizing Subject Matter by Disciplines of Knowledge

1. Select one class period within a nursing course in which you are enrolled. During this class period identify the kinds of subject matter focused on by the teacher and students during the class period as:
   a. Nursing content
   b. Content from other fields that is relevant to nursing
2. Distinguish nursing content to the degree that you can according to location in one of seven fields of knowledge about nurses and nursing identified in this chapter. If you identify nursing content as a part of nursing science, locate it in Figure 8-3 within one of the fields of nursing knowledge represented in the figure.
3. Name the sciences or disciplines of knowledge to which non-nursing content belongs.
4. To the degree that you can, identify how content from non-nursing disciplines is linked to nursing content.

Another kind of knowledge must be considered in relation to education qualifying for nursing practice. This is *personal knowledge* arising from direct insights into self and others in personal relations. Phenix (pp. 193-211)[7] considers personal knowledge as a distinct sphere of knowledge.

Nurses in practice situations relate as persons to individuals under their care and to other involved individuals. The intersubjectivity of persons in practice situations may result, within the capabilities of individuals and the limits of time, in some personal knowledge of self and the other on the part of each involved individual. Furthermore, both nurses and patients need to reflect about capabilities for action and about feelings and emotions experienced.

A number of disciplines investigate and contribute to the accumulation of knowledge about personal relations and personal knowledge of self and others. The work of Peplau,[8] Orlando,[9] and Travelbee[10] and other nurses contributes to this sphere of knowing from the perspective of nursing practice. This is a field of knowledge that should be developed as an applied science that would be associated with nursing practice and nursing cases within the practical science nursing (see Chapter 8).

Personal knowledge as described by Phenix[7] is an essential component of the cognitional orientation of nurses. Knowledge of what is being experienced by individuals within nursing practice situations is essential experiential knowing. The intersubjectivity of nurses and persons under their care is a given condition of nursing practice, as is the contractual relationship between nurse and nurse's patient. The maturity and personality organization of each nurse should be enabling for the nurse's relating of self to others on a person-to-person basis and at the same time enabling for working with them within a contractual relationship toward the attainment of nursing results.

Persons who institute, promote, and finance formal preparation for nursing practice should recognize that nursing is a theoretically and empirically grounded practical endeavor. Even in the early 21st century, not all persons recognize or accept that the deliberate actions of nurses in practice situations must be grounded in previously mastered knowledge and technique, based on insights accumulated through experience in practice situations, and immediately guided by acquired current factual information about the reality of each practice situation that rounds out the structured commonsense knowledge that nurses have gained through experience.

Each nursing practitioner must be able to approach, communicate, collaborate, and work with persons under care and with persons who are legally responsible for the individuals under care. But each nurse must be able to make right judgments and decisions about actions to be taken in each situation of practice in the achievement of objectively based and desired nursing results. Persons who enter into situations of nursing practice with knowledge limited to routinely performed tasks or technologic subsystems of care to be operationalized and maintained are not prepared to design and produce or manage comprehensive systems of nursing for individuals and groups in complex practice situations.

Work Combinations of Nurses

Nurses who are educated for entry to professional practice in universities or senior colleges often continue their education in graduate-level nursing programs in universities. Practitioners who continue their education as students of nursing tend to become clinical nursing specialists in some area of nursing practice. This includes primary care and family nursing practices. Or nurses move themselves to become qualified to develop specific areas of nursing science. Technically prepared nurses advance themselves by learning new technologies of practice and mastering the foundational sciences content basic to understanding the technology by types of nursing cases. They may devise new techniques.

Work combinations of professionally qualified nurses include the following:
- Nursing practice and **scholarly endeavor** in nursing science and related sciences
- Scholarly endeavors in nursing sciences and related sciences and nursing research
- Theory formulation and development and scholarly endeavor in nursing and related sciences
- Development and validation of nursing technologies and techniques combined with the first two combinations listed here
- Teaching nursing and scholarly endeavor in nursing sciences and related sciences and nursing practice

Nurses' combinations of occupational choices reflect their interests, talents, and values, as well as the form of their educational preparation for nursing, their associations with nurses in particular occupational fields, their advanced nursing education, and their occupational experiences leading to understanding of nursing as a professional field.

It should be understood that in combinations the occupational fields support one another. Nurses who choose particular combinations must develop themselves in accord with foundational knowledge, skills, and orientations specific to each. As shown in Fig. 4-1, nursing knowledge (developed and validated as theoretically and practically practical nursing science as well as applied nursing sciences) is common to the six nursing occupational fields. Nursing science (practical science and applied science) informs the six occupational fields so that together they contribute to the existence and the advance of nursing as a profession. Although persons who engage in teaching nursing belong to two professions—the profession of nursing and the profession of education—they may align themselves more closely with one profession than the other. Ideally, however, they maintain a balance, understanding that they are engaged in education for the occupation and profession of nursing.

Nursing Practitioners as Scholars

To function effectively and to advance themselves in nursing practice, nurses must develop themselves as scholars or as students of nursing and nursing-related fields. Nurses qualified to function in some range of nursing practice situations must know authoritative sources in nursing and in fields that articulate with nursing within the frame of reference of types of nursing cases. Clinical nursing specialists are necessarily advanced scholars in nursing and the other fields that partially define their specialty.

Nurses competent for the leadership and governing role in nursing patients with the nursing diagnoses expressed for the type of case described in Chapter 12 would know both the nursing and the related medical literature with respect to nursing persons with complete self-care deficit resulting from cerebrovascular accidents, including foundations in neurophysiology, the physiology of voluntary muscles, and fluid and electrolyte balance.

To move as a nursing scholar or a student, it is necessary to identify within a field or a science the *areas* of knowledge to be investigated in relation to concrete practice problems about which knowledge is sought. Authoritative sources— persons or reference works—should be identified. Advanced practitioners and reference works in particular fields should be identified, their locations determined, and the relevant journals in particular fields identified.

To remain abreast in areas of nursing practice, nurses must become conversant with periodical literature in nursing and in nursing-related fields. Related fields could be a specialty area of medicine, psychology, or physiology. For this reason, nursing practitioners should have a foundation(s) in the sciences of humans that are enabling for reading the literature in those fields and keeping up with changes in them.

Nurses prepared for nursing practice in technical nursing preparatory programs should seek and maintain contact with advanced practitioners in their particular areas of nursing. Concrete problems should be explored with them, and authoritative references determined and pursued. Appropriate journals in nursing and nursing-related fields should be identified, access to them secured, and plans for reading developed and maintained.

All nurses should expend effort in resolving nursing practice problems, in clarifying and synthesizing knowledge, and in formulating and expressing insights achieved about problem solution. Discussions with colleagues, atten- dance at lectures, and discussions with advanced practitioners who are also advanced scholars may be helpful or necessary to resolve or solve concrete nursing practice problems.

Research and Development

Nurses engaged in the practice of nursing for individuals and groups are confronted with concrete practical problems of people that give rise to the occurrence of health-associated self-care and dependent-care deficits. Nurses in situations of nursing practice identify the absence of and the need for effective technologies for nursing diagnosis and for bringing about new conditions and correlations in practice situations. Refer to the listing of types of technologies in Chapter 8. An example of this nursing role follows.

The observation was made in a nursing clinic that some patients were not making progress in managing their conditions of diabetes mellitus, whereas other patients participating in the same kind of supportive-developmental nursing system became effective self-care agents. The question arose as the *why* certain patients were not making progress. These patients came to clinic, they appeared to participate and cooperate, but they were not effective in self-care. Asking the question *why* led to an investigation by the clinical nursing specialist of patients' behavior as they worked with the clinic nurse. The tentative diagnosis was made that these patients thought concretely and could not handle the content about regulatory care as it was being presented. This led to preliminary research toward answering two questions: Do these patients think concretely? How can nurses identify persons who think concretely? The goal of the investigations was to develop a diagnostic technology in the form of an assessment tool specific to one component of self-care agency grouped within the five sets of foundational capabilities and dispositions (see Table 11-2), namely, the capability of *operative knowing* (pp. 219-229).[4] This capability is shown within the substantive conceptual structure self-care agency in Figure 11-3. In this example, nursing research and the development and validation of a diagnostic technology were linked together.

Other examples of practitioners' involvement in research arise from the questions patients ask about how to care for themselves and nurses' failures to find answers from nursing or medical specialists or from authoritative references. Nurses also engage in research to determine what patients do and do not do in meeting certain health-deviation self-care requisites.

The modes of thinking and the processes required for engagement in clinical research and in the development and validation of technologies differ from the mode of thinking and the processes of nursing practice. Nurses in practice must help themselves understand and appreciate these differences in order to make judgments about feasible occupational combinations and about what they can do at particular times. All nurses in practice see combinations of phenomena that they do not understand but should understand for purposes for effective nursing. Ways and means to channel unsolved problems of nursing practice to appropriate nursing research and development centers should be instituted.

SUMMARY

Nurses develop within the profession of nursing as it exists during periods of nurses' education and training and their work in nursing. It is a social expectation that nurses move their profession to a developmental level that meets both the needs of nurses and the needs of members of society for effective and efficient nursing.

Forms of education for nursing were described within the frame of reference of education for the occupations and professions. The work of nurses in nursing administration and in nursing practice was addressed. The need for nursing practice models (Figure 8-3, stage IV development of nursing science) and the need for nursing population descriptions and models for the provision of nursing to populations (stage V development) were emphasized. The functions of nursing administration and nursing practitioners were specified. The continued need for nurses to understand and value professional education for nurses was noted. Some problems associated with moving nursing education within the model of education for the professions were indicated. The work combinations of nurses and nursing practice problems that demand nursing research and development were described.

The emphasis of the chapter is on what nurses can and should do in their communities and on the need for understanding of the kinds of education, training, and career development required to produce nursing for types of nursing cases. There is a lingering memory of the placement of vocationally prepared nurses, practical or vocational nurses, in mental health centers to guide and direct persons discharged from psychiatric institutions in their continuing care required because of psychic illnesses. This decision and similar decisions are unreasonable and lead to the judgment that they are made on the basis of ignorance or political expediency.

References

1. Roberts MM: *American nursing,* New York, 1954, Macmillan, pp 7-19.
2. Woodham-Smith C: *Florence Nightingale,* 1820-1910, New York, 1951, McGraw-Hill, pp 225-238.
3. Orem DE: Changes in professional nursing practice associated with nurses' use of Orem's general theory of nursing. Presented at Le Centre Hospitalier de Gatineau, Quebec, May 1987.
4. Nursing Development Conference Group, Orem DE, editor: *Concept formalization in nursing: process and product,* ed 2, Boston, 1979, Little, Brown.
5. Barnard CI: *The functions of the executive,* Cambridge, 1962, Harvard University Press, pp 72-75.
6. Walker DM: A nursing administration perspective on use of Orem's self-care deficit nursing theory, pp 252-263. In Parker ME, editor: *Patterns of nursing theories in practice,* New York, 1993, National League for Nursing Press.
7. Phenix PH: *Realms of meaning,* New York, 1964, McGraw-Hill, pp 193-211.
8. Peplau HE: *Interpersonal relations in nursing: a conceptual frame of reference for psychodynamic nursing,* New York, 1952, GP Putnam.
9. Orlando IJ: *The dynamic nurse-patient relationship,* New York, 1961, GP Putnam.
10. Travelbee J: *Interpersonal aspects of nursing,* ed 2, Philadelphia, 1971, FA Davis.

Elements of a
Nursing History

The content elements and format for taking a nursing history are developed in two sections with different goals. Section One is identified as a nursing history with two parts designed to explicate the self-care situation of a nurse's patient. Part 1 identifies changes in a patient's therapeutic self-care demand; Part 2 is concerned with the self-care agency of the patient. Section One of the nursing history was developed in 1985. Since that time it has been used and adjusted by Susan Taylor and graduate students in the School of Nursing, University of Missouri, Columbia. They also have used and adjusted Section Two.

Section Two of the history has the broader focus of explicating the conditions and pattern of living of a nurse's patient, including residence, features, activities, environmental conditions, and routine of self-care. This form was developed in cooperation with Evelyn Vardiman to gather information she needed to assist her patients in a day care center for persons with chronic mental illnesses. A proportion of the patients lived in the community, where they had to manage their own arrangements for and details of daily living, including housing and money management. Their problems of daily living and problems related to adequacy of their self-care and their difficulties in self-care were brought to the psychiatric day care center for consideration and action.

Nurses' use of nursing history forms should be guided by what information about patients is needed and when it is needed. Section One of the nursing history is useful to nurses in gathering initial information about highlights of a patient's self-care systems and developed powers of self-care agency. Section Two seeks detailed information about a patient's pattern of living, including details about how universal self-care requisites are met. Nurses may choose to use parts of each section.

NURSING HISTORY–SECTION ONE

Goal—Explication of the self-care situation of a nurse's patient (client)

A Nursing History–Part 1: Changes in the Therapeutic
Self-Care Demand

A. In relation to your present condition (name the condition and elicit
confirmation or adjustment from the patient), have you:

A.1 Used new regulatory measures in your daily or periodic self-care, for
example, restricting your activities, taking additional rest, eliminating
certain foods, taking prescribed or unprescribed medications? If so,
please name them.

How did you come to use these measures?

Did you know how to perform them or did you have to learn how?

If you had to learn, how did you go about this?

Are these measures still a part of your daily or continuing self-care?
All _____ Some _____ None _____

When did you discontinue the measures that are no longer a part of your
self-care regimen?

Why did you discontinue them? Give names of measures.

Of all the measures named, which ones do you judge to have been or to
be of value in your present situation?

A.2 In relation to your present condition, have you made specific observations about your own functioning, for example, when you experience
being tired, when your body temperature is elevated? If so, will you
name what you have observed that you see as relevant to your needs for
periodic or continuing self-care?

Did you (do you) follow a systematic plan for making these observations? If so, describe it. _____

Did you seek help in making observations? Did you seek help to learn
the meaning of what you observed? If yes, from whom did you seek
help? _____
_____

A.3 What, if any, parts of your routine of self-care have been changed by
your present conditions and circumstances? Routine of self-care has
been added to, Yes _____ No _____ .
Usual routine care measures are: unaffected _____ ; affected in this
way _____ ; virtually eliminated, Yes _____ No _____ .

A.4 In relation to your present condition, what do you suggest as in need of
special attention by nurses as they develop with you a program of
nursing care?

NURSING HISTORY–SECTION ONE

Goal—Explication of the self-care situations of a nurse's patient (client).

A Nursing History–Part 2: Self-Care Agency Focus

A. After or during childhood when did you come to bear or take on responsibility for your daily and periodic care to regulate your own functioning and development as related to your health and well-being?

Partial responsibility at age of _____ ; who bore or bears responsibility with you?

Full responsibility at age of _____ .

What sources of help, if any, did you use when you did not know what to do or how to manage your own care?

What sources of help do you currently use when you have self-care problems that you do not know how to handle?

B. Are there aspects of your self-care that you:

B.1 Attend to regularly? Yes _____ No _____
If yes, what are they?

B.2 have questions about? Yes _____ No _____
If yes, what are they?

B.3 tend to forget? Yes _____ No _____
If yes, what are they?

B.4 ignore? Yes _____ No _____
If yes, what are they? _____
Why do you ignore them? _____

C. In your contacts with physicians, have you been or are you able to talk to your physicians about self-care questions? Yes _____ No _____ . If yes, give an example of a self-care matter that you described to or discussed with one or more physicians.

What was the outcome in terms of your subsequent self-care?

If no, will you tell why you have not or do not discuss your self-care questions with your physician?

D. In the past have you had episodes of illness or disability when you were unable to provide your own daily self-care? Yes _____ No _____ . If yes:

D.1 Were you cared for? Yes _____ No _____
If yes, by whom? _____
What was your response to being cared for?

D.2 What was the extent of your inability to provide care for yourself? Could you perform some measures of care? Yes _____ No _____

D.3 With what conditions in yourself or your environment did you associate your inability to care for yourself?

E. How do you describe your past performance in providing self-care in order to regulate your own functioning? Consider completeness and effectiveness:

E.1 On a day-to-day basis.

E.2 When suffering illness or injury.

E.3 Performance over time

F. How would you describe yourself in relation to your present condition as being personally able to provide self-care that you consider essential for your health and well-being? Able _____ Not able _____

If able, why?

If not able, why?

F.1 Provided it is judged safe by your nurse(s), what parts of your routine daily self-care can you perform without placing yourself under stress?

No part? _____ These parts by name _____

_____

F.2 What parts of your routine of daily self-care do you judge that you will have difficulty in performing?

No part? _____ Will have difficulty with _____

_____

Do you judge yourself able to cooperate with and give needed guidance to persons who will help you with the difficult parts of your care? Yes _____ No _____

G. What are your present interests and concerns about:

G.1 meeting your known existent needs for day-to-day self-care?

G.2 recognizing and meeting emerging needs for self-care?

G.3 learning about and taking on a reasonable role in your own care according to your state of health?

G.4 becoming more knowledgeable about and skilled with respect to your own care?

    a. in making observations relevant to your care
    b. in making judgments and decisions about care
    c. in performing and observing results of specific care measures

NURSING HISTORY–SECTION TWO

Goal—To explicate the conditions and pattern of living of a nurse's patient, including residence features, activity mix, environmental conditions, routine of self-care.

A. Residence

 A.1 Do you live in a home with your family? Yes _____ No _____
   If yes, who lives in the home with you?

 A.2 If no, do you live alone? Yes _____ No _____
   If you do not live alone, with whom do you share your living space?

 A.3 Do you live in a house, apartment, room, other? Write in.

 A.4 Is where you now live your permanent residence or a temporary residence?

   How long have you lived in this place?

 A.5 Are you responsible for the costs and day-to-day upkeep of your place of residence?
   Yes _____ No _____
   If no, who bears this responsibility?

 A.6 What activities are routinely part of your daily living within your residence?

Food storage after purchasing	Yes _____	No _____
Meal preparation	Yes _____	No _____
Eating meals	Yes _____	No _____
Care and storage of clothing	Yes _____	No _____
Washing of clothing	Yes _____	No _____
Washing of linen (bed)	Yes _____	No _____
Care of bed(s) and bedding	Yes _____	No _____
Resting and sleeping	Yes _____	No _____
Hygienic care of self	Yes _____	No _____
Recreational activities and hobbies	Yes _____	No _____

   If yes, name _____

   _____

Work	Yes _____	No _____

   If yes, describe_____

   _____

Social engagements with		
one to two persons	Yes _____	No _____
more than two persons	Yes _____	No _____

A.7 Do you feel pressed for space in the place   Yes _____ No _____
where you live?
If others live with you, do they feel the same   Yes _____ No _____
as you feel?

A.8 Do you have concerns about your place of residence that are relevant to
your present condition and circumstances?   Yes _____ No _____
If yes, what are these concerns? _____
_____

B. Activity Mix

B.1 What is the nature of the actions in which you routinely engage each day?
School   Special Education _____
_____   Extended Education _____
_____
Work outside the home _____
Household routines _____
Care of dependents: Children by age _____
Adults by age and relationship _____
Community Projects _____

B.2 Has your routine related to the above changed because of present
conditions and circumstances?   Yes _____ No _____
If yes, in what way(s) has it changed? _____
_____

B.3 Have you or are you experiencing particular problems or difficulties
in accomplishing your usual routine of activities within or outside the
home?   Yes _____ No _____
If yes, would you tell about the problems that are of special concern
to you? _____
_____

C. Environment—What concerns, if any, do you have about environmental
factors?

C.1 Air quality, Yes _____ No _____ . If yes, describe _____
_____

C.2.a. Cleanliness of living areas, Yes _____ No _____ .
If yes, describe _____
_____

b. Freedom from vermin, Yes _____ No _____ .
If yes, describe _____
_____

c. Other, name and describe _____

_____

C.3 Adequacy of water for

Drinking   Quality Yes ____ No ____   Quantity Yes ____ No ____
Cooking   Quality Yes ____ No ____   Quantity Yes ____ No ____
Bathing   Quality Yes ____ No ____   Quantity Yes ____ No ____
Other uses, describe _____

_____

C.4.a. Adequacy of food supplies
       Quality, Yes ____ No ____   Quantity Yes ____ No ____
    b. Access to food supplies, Yes ____ No ____

C.5 Freedom from hazardous conditions stemming from:
    a. The numbers and relationships of individuals with whom you
       interact, Yes ____ No ____
    b. The health of persons with whom you associate, Yes ____ No ____
    c. The trustworthiness of these persons, Yes ____ No ____

D. Routine for Self-Care

D.1 Do you routinely or periodically use care measures to facilitate your
    intake of air, your breathing? Yes ____ No ____

    If yes, what are they?

    When do you use them?

    In what way do they help you?

    When did you start using them?

D.2 How much water do you drink during the 24 hours of a day?

    How much water do you usually drink at one time?

    When during the 24 hours do you drink water?

    Has your consumption of water changed? Yes ____ No ____

    When?

    How?

D.3.a. Think about what you consider an ordinary day and identify what and
       when you would eat.

    b. How does what you eat at other times differ from your described
       eating on an ordinary day?

c. Has what you eat and when you eat changed? Yes _____ No _____

When?

How?

d. Do you suffer from:
not having enough food? Yes _____ No _____
not having the right kind of food? Yes _____ No _____

D.4.a. Do you have any concerns or problems about bowel or bladder functioning?

b. If you use any special care measures related to the following, name the measures

passing of urine _____

_____

bowel elimination _____

_____

hygienic care after urination or defecation _____

_____

c. Describe the patterns of your bladder and bowel functioning in terms of frequency and time

d. Do you note the color and amount of urine you pass? Yes _____ No _____
If the color and amount of urine changed from the usual color and amount, would you be observant of the change?
Yes _____ No _____
Have you observed such changes? Yes _____ No _____
What are they?

e. Do you note the color, shape, and quantity of feces passed during bowel movements? Yes _____ No _____
Are you observant of changes? Yes _____ No _____
Have you observed changes? Yes _____ No _____
What are they?

D.5.a. What do you usually do to rest yourself when you experience a need for rest?

Under what circumstances do you experience a need for rest?

How frequent are these experiences?

When you feel that you need to rest, are you usually able to do so? Yes _____ No _____

b. Do you have regular hours for sleeping? Yes _____ No _____
If yes, what are they?

How do you feel when you get up after your usual hours of sleep?

Do you have a routine for preparing for sleep?
If so, what is it?

Do you know of conditions and circumstances under which it is difficult for you to have a restful sleep?

c. How many hours of the day do you estimate that you are
walking _____   doing mental work _____
standing _____   doing physical work
sitting _____   light _____
reclining _____   heavy _____
                            strenuous _____
                            engaged in physically active recreational activities _____
                            engaged in the use and movement of body or its parts for therapeutic purposes _____

d. When not actively engaged in work requiring concentration are you relaxed _____ or tense _____ ?

e. How frequently do you experience fear _____ ; anger _____ ; other emotions _____ ?

What is the duration of these emotional experiences?

How do you feel after such experiences?

f. What is your judgment about the balance you maintain between high energy consuming activities and experiences and restorative, restful activities and experiences including sleep?

D.6.a. How much time during a usual day do you spend alone?

During this time are you in proximity to other persons in the same general area _____ or are you quite isolated from other persons _____ ? How do you feel about being alone?

b. How many persons, of what ages and relations to you do you have contact with during a usual day? _____
_____

What is the length of your contacts?

What kinds of communication occur?

c. Do you judge that you require time alone for yourself? Yes _____
No _____
Do you judge that the time you have for yourself is
too much _____
not enough _____
just right _____

    d. Do you judge that your contacts with others are satisfying _____ or stressful _____ to you?
What adjustments, if any, in the kind or frequency of your social contacts do you see as beneficial to you?

E.1 Are there health hazards that you routinely take action to avoid? If so, name them and describe the avoidance measures you use. _____
_____

E.2 Are there health hazards that you ignore? If so, what are they?

What are your reasons for ignoring them?

F.1 Do you think about yourself in terms of the normalcy of your functioning? Yes _____ No _____
normalcy of your development? Yes _____ No _____

F.2 Do you seek and work out ways to ensure the maintenance or the bringing about of structural and functional normalcy? Yes _____ No _____
If yes, what are these means?

F.3 Do you seek and use means to promote your own development? Yes _____ No _____
If yes, what means have you used or are you using?

APPENDIX B

Features in the History of the Development of Self-Care Deficit Nursing Theory

My involvement in the stages of development of this general theory of nursing began in the year 1956. Some highlights are presented.

BEGINNING DEVELOPMENT

American nurses experienced increasing instability in practice situations during the period extending approximately from 1940 to 1960. An outstanding public health physician who worked intensively with nurses, physicians, hospital administrators and governing boards, specialists in public health, and others on state and national levels remarked that "nursing gets much of the blame for poor patient care" in hospitals, and nurses tend to accept the blame for conditions and problems that involve physicians, hospital technical services, and hospital administrators as well as nurses.[1]

This was a period when health care services, especially within hospitals, were affected by conditions that were destabilizing, to say the least. Changes included the following[2]:

- Changes in health care needs of people associated in part with the increasing numbers of individuals with chronic diseases and the decrease in acute communicable disease
- Revolutionary advances in knowledge and technique in medical diagnosis and treatment and in prevention and rehabilitation
- A threefold to fourfold increase in the number of individuals seeking hospital care
- An increase in the number of individuals providing care; an increase in total number and in number from specialized fields
- Changes in public attitudes toward health and increasing awareness of the advantages gained from effective health services for individuals and communities.

487

Nurses became concerned with questions about their proper work, about time available for nursing, and about their relationships to persons seeking and receiving nursing and to members of other health care disciplines. The subtitle to Nightingale's *Notes on Nursing: What It Is and What It Is Not* expressed the concern of many nurses during and beyond this period.

As long as stable conditions prevail in occupations or professions, members usually do not raise questions about their domain of practice. The unstable conditions in nursing practice demanded that nurses begin to deal with domain and boundary problems. However, nurses' endeavors to do so and to advance nursing as a practice field were hindered at times by lack of interest and understanding from persons outside nursing and at times by direct opposition from within nursing. Some recognized internal barriers to the advancement and development of nursing included the continuing focus of nurses on tasks and procedures, many of which were outmoded; demands of nurses that exceeded their preparation; the unstructured state of nursing knowledge; the inability of many nurses to formulate goals of care specific to nursing; and the inability of many nurses to communicate adequately about nursing with persons under nursing care and their families and with members of other health care disciplines, administrators, and officials of government.

Despite barriers, nurses' achievements during the period contributed to a forward, developmental movement that continued through the 1960s, 1970s, and 1980s. Virginia Henderson's organized, succinct, yet comprehensive statements about nursing's contributions to individuals, sick or well, with an expression of the reason why people need nursing, was published in 1955 (p. 4).[3] Hildegard Peplau expressed her conceptualization of nursing as a "significant, therapeutic interpersonal process" in her 1952 work *Interpersonal Relations in Nursing* (p. 16).[4] During the 1950s my own interest in and insights about the domain and boundaries of nursing began to take on more of a proper nursing focus in distinction to the more global preventive health care focus that previously had characterized them. A beginning formalization of my insights about nursing as a field of practice was expressed in 1956 and followed by a more precise expression in 1959.

From 1949 to 1957 as a nurse consultant with the Division of Hospital and Institutional Services of the Indiana State Board of Health, I had an intensive experience in working with the director and the professional staff of the division, with nurses in Indiana hospitals, and with nurses in the Division of Public Health Nursing. In 1956 I completed a study of administrative positions in nursing in one Indiana hospital and appended to the report a chapter entitled "The Art of Nursing."[5] Included in this discussion of nursing as art is the definition of nursing that appears in Chapter 2 of this text.

In 1958 and 1959, as a consultant in the Office of Education, U.S. Department of Health, Education, and Welfare, I participated in a project to upgrade practical (vocational) nurse training and to identify ways to include in practical nurse curricula an explicit nursing component. Such a component would give nursing meaning to the tasks around which the knowledge and experience components of training programs were organized. All vocational programs extract content from one or more disciplines. Therefore, in curriculum development (vocational), it is essential that one know how disciplines are structured or organized to extract content of various types without distortion and error. Knowing the relatively unstructured state of available knowledge about nursing practice, I was aware that I must have as a working tool at least a gross conceptualization of elements within the domain of nursing and of the relationships among them. This, I thought, would enable me to make some inferences about the structure of nursing as a field of knowledge necessary for nursing practice.

I proceeded not by reviewing and analyzing components of available statements about nursing, my own and others, but by reflecting on my experiences in nursing. I stated a proposition: *Not all people under health care, for example, from physicians, are under nursing care nor does it follow that they should be.* I then asked: *What condition exists in a person when that person or a family member or the attending physician or a nurse makes the judgment that the person should be under nursing care?* The answer to the question came spontaneously with images of situations in which such judgments were made and the idea that a nurse is "another self," in a figurative sense, for the person under nursing care.

My insights into the *human condition* associated with *requirements for nursing* were formulated as a concept and expressed as follows: the inability of a person to provide continuously for self the amount and quality of required self-care because of the situation of personal health. Self-care was conceptualized as the personal care that human beings require each day and that may be modified by health state, environmental conditions, the effects of medical care, and other factors. The expressed proper human object of nursing also specified that in child nursing situations, the parent or guardian is no longer able to provide the amount and quality of continuing care required by the child because of the child's health situation. This 1958 expression of nursing's proper object conforms to that expressed in my 1956 statement about nursing and in substance with that in Virginia Henderson's 1955 statement about nursing.

My understanding of the human condition that gives rise to requirements for nursing was both an ending and a beginning. It ended my search for an answer to the question: What is nursing? It brought me to a new developmental stage with respect to knowing and understanding nursing. There was an intellectual readiness to make explicit the elements and relationships that give form and meaning to nursing as a field of practice and a field of knowledge.

A CONCEPT AND A CONCEPTUAL FRAMEWORK

My work of theorizing about nursing had its formal beginning in 1958 with my formalization of the proper object of nursing considered as a field of knowledge and a field of practice. My efforts were joined with efforts of members of the Nursing Development Conference Group in 1965.

A Concept of Nursing System

As a result of combined efforts, a theoretic concept of *nursing system* was formulated, expressed, and revised in 1970.* My colleagues and I considered this theoretic position about nursing as a forward step in the development of a model adequate to guide nursing research and further the structuring of nursing as a body of knowledge. Before the expression of the concept of nursing system, its conceptual elements along with the concept self-care had been formalized and then validated in nursing practice situations. The theoretic concept of nursing system expressed group members' insights about the creative end product of the work of nurses and the dynamics of its production.

The term *system* with reference to the 1970 conceptualization of what nurses make is used in its broadest sense. *System* refers to persons or actions or things with relationships between and among them behaving together as a whole with changes in any one of the entities affecting the whole that is the system. A nursing system, however, is viewed as a particular type of system, a self-organizing system. Such systems exist "only when and for the duration that there are self-connecting links between the behavior or state of independent parts or subjects, the connection occurring at some point of conditionality between them (p. 125)."[6]

This view of nursing as a self-organizing system emphasizes that nursing is deliberately produced within time and place frames of reference, that it is produced through discrete deliberate actions or sequences of action, and that its existence depends on bringing about and sustaining relationships between persons and among actions that they select, decide to execute, and execute. Nursing has no concrete existence except through persons in relationships of nurse and patient and through what they choose and proceed to do or not do within the relationship. A *nursing system* is something constructed through actions of nurses and nurses' patients. It is a product that should be beneficial to persons with patient status in nursing practice situations when the time frame for production fits the time of occurrence of requirements for nursing.

The expressed conceptualization of nursing system can be viewed as an explanatory definition of nursing because it sets forth relationships and what nurses do when they nurse others. It can also be viewed as a general model. Meanings of terms used to express conceptual elements within the conceptual model of nursing system are summarized (Fig. B-1). Four terms are patient oriented; two are nurse oriented.

Legitimate patients of nurses are persons whose self-care agency or dependent-care agency, because of their own or their dependents' health states or health care requirements, is not adequate or will become inadequate for knowing or meeting their own or their dependents' therapeutic self-care demands.

Self-care is learned, goal-oriented activity of individuals. It is behavior that exists in concrete life situations directed by persons to self or to the environment

---

*See "Conceptualization of Nursing System," Chapter 7, p. 156, for this 1970 statement.

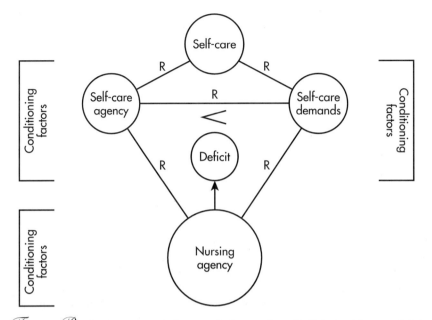

Figure B-1 A conceptual framework for nursing. *R*, Relationships; <, deficit relationship, current or projected.

to regulate factors that affect their own development and functioning in the interests of life, health, or well-being. *Dependent-care* is such activity performed by responsible adults for socially dependent individuals.

Legitimate nurses are persons who have the sets of qualities symbolized by the term *nursing agency* to the degree that they have the capability and the willingness to exercise it in knowing and meeting the existent and emerging nursing requirements of persons with health-associated self-care or dependent-care deficits.

Nursing agency is a complex power of persons educated and trained as nurses that is enabling when exercised for knowing and helping others know their therapeutic self-care demands, for helping others meet or in meeting their therapeutic self-care demands, and in helping others regulate the exercise or development of their self-care agency or their dependent-care agency.

Therapeutic self-care demand signifies a humanly constructed entity. It stands for a summation of measures of self-care required at moments in time and for some time duration by individuals in some location to meet self-care requisites particularized for individuals in relation to their conditions and circumstances. Care measures arise from the selection and application of specific methods or technologies to meet universal, developmental, or health-deviation self-care requisites.

Self-care agency is the complex developed capability that enables adults and maturing adolescents to discern factors that must be controlled or managed in order to regulate their own functioning and development, to decide what can and should be done with respect to regulation, to lay out the components of their therapeutic self-care demands (self-care requisites, technologies, care measures), and finally to perform the care measures designed to meet their self-care requisites over time. Dependent-care agency is the complex developed capability of responsible adults to do the foregoing for dependents.

A Conceptual Framework

Subsequent to expression of the 1970 theoretic concept of nursing systems, its dominant themes or conceptual elements were represented as a conceptual structure, a circle of terms and relationships (see Fig. B-1). This was done to emphasize the relationships of the theoretic concepts among themselves and to the production of self-care. Figure B-1 also shows the theoretic conceptualization of nurse and patient properties as being related to factors internal or external to persons who are nurses or nurses' patients that under some circumstances condition the qualitative or quantitative values of patient and nurse properties. These are named *conditioning factors.*

Elements expressed in the concept of nursing system and in the conceptual framework emerged from my own work and that of the Nursing Development Conference Group. All the conceptual elements were formalized and validated as static concepts by 1970. Since then, some refinement of expression and further development of substantive structure and continued validation have occurred, but no change of conceptual elements has been made. Each concept continues to undergo development through the identification and organization of secondary concepts that constitute its substantive structure. For example, the conceptualization of three types of self-care requisites—universal, developmental, and health-deviation—are secondary concepts within the broad concept therapeutic self-care demand, and each of these secondary concepts has a structure that must be explicated.

The explication of the structure of secondary concepts leads to identification of the component phenomena, the concrete features of conceptualized entities, and combinations of entities.

Secondary concepts establish a framework for integrating facts and segments of theory "from other disciplines and provide some direction to the selection of useful research methodologies (p. 130)"[6] for study of concrete life situations. For example, the secondary concept universal self-care requisites provides for articulation of facts and points of theory from physiology, bioclimatology, psychology, public health sciences, and other disciplines. The substantive (secondary) structure of the concept of self-care agency has been a fruitful base for research oriented to self-care agency in a variety of populations. This also is true for therapeutic self-care demand.

THE SIX EDITIONS OF *NURSING: CONCEPTS OF PRACTICE*

The five editions of *Nursing: Concepts of Practice* preceding this sixth edition presented theoretically practical content about nursing. This content was generated by the continued formalization and expression of the conceptual elements of the self-care deficit theory of nursing and its contributory theories of self-care, self-care deficit, and nursing system. The books also report with increasing detail the development of the essential practice features of nursing. The largely neglected practice feature of *nursing design* was introduced with a developed process structure in the fourth edition.

The integration of the conceptual constructs of the named theories with the essential practice features of nursing—for example, nursing diagnoses, nursing prescription, nursing design, and nursing treatment—is a consistent feature of the texts. This integration serves to give direction to the knowing, the thinking, and the judgment making of practicing nurses and nursing scholars. The integration or the weaving together of theoretically practical nursing knowledge from valid general theories of nursing with the operations necessary for the production of nursing in society is an essential step in moving a nursing theory from its status as theory to its functional place in the practical operations of nursing. The integrating capacities of each nursing practice operation should be understood and recognized. The sixth edition of the text continues these developments.

The idea of "stages of understanding nursing" (see Fig. 8-3) introduced in earlier editions provided a foundation for exploring and formalizing in this edition the form and the subject matter of the theoretically practical nursing sciences (see Chapter 8). Stages of understanding nursing express the intellectual demand on nurses to develop and formalize understandings about the proper object of nursing based on the reasons why humankind requires nursing; how nursing can be realistically modeled to conceptually reflect nursing as a requirement of humankind; the conceptual elements of a realistic, valid, general model of nursing and the expressed nature and possible ranges of variation of its conceptual elements; the use of the conceptual elements of a theory in identifying and describing instances in which persons require and can be helped through nursing (nursing cases); and finally about the development of models to guide the provision of nursing for individuals and groups.

The six theoretically practical nursing sciences named in the sixth edition are based on the *nature of the way or form* in which nurses provide care to persons who require nursing (nursing practice sciences) and the kinds of knowledge required by nurses to understand these forms of care (foundational nursing sciences). The named nursing practice sciences wholly compensatory, partly compensatory, and supportive-developmental nursing science, which indicate the *form* in which nursing is provided, are analogous to the practice sciences of medicine, such as internal medicine and surgery. The formalization and naming of the three nursing practice sciences was based on understanding the nature of nursing systems. This understanding was supported by the theory of nursing system (Chapter 7), the Nursing Development Conference Group's conceptual model of a nursing system, and the three general types of nursing systems (Chapter 13). The named foundational sciences that support the nursing practice sciences are the science of self-care, the science of the development and exercise of self-care agency, and the science of human assistance for persons with health-associated self-care deficits. The three foundational sciences support and are necessary for understanding and developing each one of the three nursing practice sciences.

The use of these ideas should facilitate the formalization and structuring of the subject matter of the nursing sciences, which have been unnamed and unstructured. Nursing's subject matter in widely scattered locations and in an unstructured state is not readily available to practitioners for their use and not conducive to the development of nursing scholars. These conditions place nursing researchers, as well as students in doctoral nursing programs, in the precarious position of not knowing where problems and findings fit or what is being added to what in their pursuit of hierarchic advancement in knowing nursing.

CONTINUED DEVELOPMENT OF THEORETIC ELEMENTS

In the 1990s both individual nurses and groups of nurses have worked to further develop or make adjustments in the conceptual elements of self-care deficit nursing theory and its contributory theories. One example of group work is that of the Orem Study Group,* whose members graciously responded to my request and that of Susan Taylor to involve themselves in further development of self-care deficit nursing theory. Three study groups were formed to address the theoretic interests of group members.

One study group studied the matter of *propositions* in relation to *theories,* as well as the conceptual construct *self-care agency.* A second group worked to develop the concept of *dependent-care* and its referents in social groups and to structure content that is descriptive and explanatory of this form of care. The third group worked with the concept *self-care requisite,* focusing on its relationship to the continued production of self-care systems in societies and on the structure of the process of formalizing and expressing *self-care requisites.* This work led to the idea of the appropriateness of formalizing a science of self-care and to identification of its areas of content and its subject matter, recognizing it as a science foundational to understanding nursing.

The work of the Orem Study Group in the 1990s demonstrated, as did the Nursing Development Conference Group in the 1960s and 1970s, that development of the main and substantive conceptual constructs of a general

---

*Group members: Gerd Bekel, Mary Denyes, George Evers, Elizabeth Geden, Marcella Hart, Donna Hartweg, Marjorie Isenberg, Bonnie Neuman, Dorothea Orem, Kathie Renpenning, and Susan Taylor.

theory of nursing requires concerted attention, creative thinking, ensuring the foundations for and the soundness of one's reasoning and judgment, the demonstration of relationships, and determination of the *relevance* of one's work to understanding nursing, both its nature and its production in social groups.

A PHILOSOPHIC INQUIRY

In 1997 a philosophic inquiry of "Orem's Self-Care Deficit Nursing Theory" was made available for the consideration of scholars of *self-care deficit nursing theory* and others (A brief summary of this work can be found on p. vii). This doctoral inquiry by Barbara E. Banfield[7] addresses the philosophic foundations for my work, expressed or implicit views of humankind, and the compatibility of self-care deficit nursing theory with various research paradigms. The results of Banfield's philosophic inquiry, including her discusison of its contribution to nursing knowledge, are important developments in the nursing profession at the beginning of the 21st century.

References

1. O'Malley M: personal communication, 1952.
2. O'Malley M, et al: What do we mean, improvement of patient care, and how do we implement it? Presented at Tri-State Assembly, Division of Hospital and Institutional Services, Indiana State Board of Health, April 9, 1958.
3. Harmer B: *Textbook of the principles and practice of nursing,* revised by Virginia Henderson, ed 4, New York, 1955, Macmillan, p. 4.
4. Peplau HE: *Interpersonal relations in nursing,* New York, 1952, Putnam, p. 16.
5. Orem DE: *Hospital nursing service: an analysis,* Division of Hospital and Institutional Services, Indiana State Board of Health, Indianapolis, 1956, p. 85.
6. Nursing Development Conference Group, Orem DE, editor: *Concept formalization in nursing: process and product,* ed 2, Boston, 1979, Little, Brown and Co., p. 125, 130.
7. Banfield BE: A philosophical inquiry of Orem's self-care deficit nursing theory, doctoral dissertation, Graduate School, Wayne State University, 1997.

APPENDIX C

Obstacles to and Other Factors That Affect Meeting Universal Self-Care Requisites

In the 1970s I participated in a survey of a nursing home population to identify (1) reasons for admission to the home and (2) factors that would condition the kind and amount of nursing required. One finding of the survey was that every resident in the nursing home had one or more health disorders, the effects and results of which established the conditions under which each universal self-care requisite had to be met and affected the choice of methods or technologies that could be used in meeting the requisite. The nursing question posed was: How can these requisites be met under prevailing conditions by a nurse, a dependent-care agent, or a self-care agent?

This question led to an investigation of the possible ranges of conditions that could affect the importance and the actual meeting of universal self-care requisites, including the need for specialized methods or technologies to overcome obstacles—the circumstances under which action to meet them must be undertaken. Preliminary survey lists of factors were developed to establish conditions and circumstances under which meeting each universal requisite would be of special importance or that would in some way limit how and to what degree they could be met. Preliminary survey lists for three requisites—maintain a sufficient intake of air, water, and food—were expanded through exhaustive surveys of standard and authoritative reference works, followed by validation of and revision of listings. Janet L. Fitzwater and I accomplished this work, with collaboration of Evelyn Vardiman in developing the project on the requisites for maintaining sufficient intake of water and food. This work extended from 1977 to 1983.

The listings of factors that can condition the meeting of each universal self-care requisite are presented. There is greater detail for requisites focused on intakes of air, water, and food because of the more detailed investigations of factors for these requisites. Universal requisites differ according to the concrete entities with which they deal, thus the form of expressing factors that affect the need to and the ways of meeting them differ. The requisites focused on air, water, and food are concerned with the *movement of these entities from the environment into the individual.* The requisite on excrements is concerned with *movement of materials from individuals to their environment.* The requisites related to activity and rest and solitude and social interaction are concerned with *balance establishment and maintenance.* Preventing hazards is concerned with *avoidance or elimination.* Being normal or promotion of normalcy is concerned with *living within human norms and one's human potential,* and this includes maintaining functioning within these norms to the degree possible under existing conditions and circumstances.

MAINTAINING A SUFFICIENT INTAKE OF AIR

Factors that interfere with meeting this requisite are organized by broad types (groups), subtypes (Roman numerals), characterizing features of factors (A, B, C, . . .), and conditions associated with characterized factors (1, 2, 3a, b, c, . . .).

Group One–Environmental Interference, the Availability and Composition of Air

I. Composition and oxygen partial pressure of atmospheric air not in accord with physiologic requisites
   A. Low oxygen partial pressure in atmospheric air
      1. At heights of approximately 12,000 feet resulting in arterial hypoxia in all persons
      2. In air in confined spaces resulting in arterial hypoxia
   B. Increase in carbon dioxide beyond 10 to 20 percent in inspired air, resulting in decreased respiratory minute volume and convulsive seizures
   C. Presence of irritant gases that stimulate nasal branches of the fifth cranial nerve, causing abrupt temporary inhibition of respiration

II. Availability of air
   A. Environments where air has been infiltrated by substances, such as smoke, or displaced by heavier-than-air gases
   B. Mechanical cutting off of available air by external blocking of air passages

Group Two–Interferences with the Process of Pulmonary Ventilation

I. Interferences with air flow
   A. Obstruction of air passages by foreign objects and materials
      1. Presence of deliberately placed or inspired foreign objects in nose, nasopharynx, larynx, trachea, bronchi
      2. Presence of blood in air passages resultant, for example, from
         a. Bleeding from nose or nasopharynx
         b. Bleeding from the trachea, for example, bleeding caused by a

low-lying tracheostomy tube, which erodes the innominate artery

   c. Lung hemorrhage

3. Presence of food or fluid or vomitus in larynx or trachea associated with

   a. Failure of the glottis to close during swallowing or gagging resulting from paralysis of the adductor fibers of the vagi

   b. Passage of food and fluid from esophagus to trachea through a fistulous connection

B. Abnormalities that interfere with air flow and increase airway resistance

  1. Obstruction of upper respiratory passages by

    a. Swelling of mucosa of mouth, nose, pharynx, or larynx with exudate, occlusion of airway, and difficult breathing associated, for example, with respiratory infections, hay fever, or other allergic reactions

    b. Polyps, nodules, enlarged adenoids and tonsils

    c. Deformities such as deviated nasal septum, laryngeal atresia

    d. Abscess formations such as peritonsillar abscess, sublingual abscesses, retropharyngeal abscesses

    e. Laryngostenosis, tracheal stenosis

  2. Dysfunctions that interfere with air flow

    a. Inability of the glottis to open because of paralysis of the abductor fibers of the vagi

    b. Laryngospasm

    c. Depression or suppression of the cough reflex and sneeze reflex, resulting in failure to clear air passages

    d. Diffuse narrowing of the bronchial tree that interferes with air flow and increases airway resistance (generalized obstructive lung disease)

      (1) Reversible as in bronchial asthma or in infections with excessive secretions

      (2) Irreversible as with fibrosis following infections, chronic bronchitis

II. Factors associated with changes in lung compliance and vital capacity of lung

A. Gross structural and positional factors restricting lung compliance and vital capacity

  1. Total thoracic cage motion limitations as in kyphoscoliosis

  2. Immobility of costovertebral joints, as in spondylitis

  3. Assumed positions of the body that interfere with lung expansion

B. Pressure factors associated with decreased lung compliance

  1. Change from natural negative intrapleural pressure to positive intrapleural pressure with pneumothorax

    a. Open pneumothorax with atelectasis

    b. Closed pneumothorax with atelectasis

2. Increased pressure on unaffected lung in tension pneumothorax resulting from deviation of the mediastinum toward the unaffected lung
3. Increased intra-abdominal pressure with restriction of movement of the diaphragm

C. Alterations of lung tissue affecting lung compliance or vital capacity
   1. Increase in rigidity of the lung parenchyma with decreased lung compliance, for example, that associated with pulmonary hypertension
   2. Reduction of number of available lung units with decreased lung compliance, associated, for example, with lesions of lung tissue resulting from biologic and chemical agents
   3. Decreases in lung compliance ranging to atelectasis associated with deficiencies of surfactant in the lining of the alveoli
      a. Premature infants
      b. Newborns who are not premature
      c. Adults with adult respiratory distress syndrome
      d. Individuals who undergo pulmonary-circulatory interruptions, as in use of heart-lung machines
   4. Decrease in elasticity of lung parenchyma with increased compliance and decreased vital capacity, as in obstructive pulmonary emphysema

D. Voluntary restriction of chest expansion during respiration because of associated pain, as in pleurisy and fractured ribs

E. Muscular and neuromuscular factors associated with decreased lung compliance or vital capacity
   1. Paralysis of muscles of inspiration, especially the diaphragm
   2. Paralysis of accessory muscles of respiration
   3. Spasm of respiratory muscles with temporary cessation of breathing, as in generalized convulsions
   4. Fibrotic muscles
   5. Specific neuromuscular disorders
      a. Progressive muscular dystrophy
      b. Myotonic dystrophy

III. Interferences with optimal alveolar ventilation with or without diffusion impairment

A. Nonfunctional alveoli associated with intracellular accumulations obstructing the air sacs (alveoli)
   1. Pulmonary edema
   2. Intra-alveolar bleeding
   3. Interstitial pneumonia
   4. Proteinosis
   5. Microlithiasis

B. Decrease in number of alveoli and total alveolar surface area resulting from destruction of septa of alveoli as in emphysema

C. Loss of alveoli and pulmonary capillaries resulting from removal of, destruction of, or pathologic changes in lung tissue

    1. Pneumonectomy, lobectomy

    2. Pulmonary infarction

    3. Fibrosis of lung; diffuse scarring of lung resulting from pulmonary hypertension (restrictive pulmonary diseases)

IV. Interferences with maintenance of gaseous equilibrium between alveolar air and pulmonary blood

  A. Alveolar hypoventilation, general or regional, associated with, for example, conditions that decrease expansibility of the lung

  B. Thickening of the alveolar and capillary membranes that separate blood and alveolar air (more restrictive of O_2 than CO_2 diffusion)

  C. Low ratio of pulmonary blood flow to ventilation as in

    1. Cardiac failure and dyspnea

    2. Vasospasm, thrombosis, embolus

    3. Congenital cardiovascular anomalies affecting pulmonary circulation

    4. Acquired cardiovascular dysfunction disorders (e.g., ischemia of heart muscle)

    5. Cardiac asthma

  D. Lowered oxygen capacity of pulmonary blood flow associated with

    1. Low hemoglobin content of blood as in anemias of all types

    2. Hemoglobin combined with something other than O_2 (e.g., carbon monoxide)

    3. Altered hemoglobin that cannot combine with O_2, for example, methemoglobin as in poisoning with chlorates, nitrates, acetanilid, ferrocyanides

V. Factors affecting the central neural and neurochemical regulatory mechanisms of respiration

  A. Interferences with the automatic rhythmic activity of the medullary respiratory center with its inspiratory and expiratory centers

    1. Interferences with neuronal functioning within the centers associated with

      a. Depression of the medullary respiratory center relative to high concentrations of CO_2 or to anoxia

      b. Tissue changes in the center associated with tumors, inflammatory disease, vascular accidents, edema

      c. Inadequate blood to respiratory center

    2. Interferences with normal periodic inhibition of activity in inspiratory center so that expiration can occur

  B. Interferences with chemical regulatory receptors (as in the carotid and aortic bodies) and mechanisms that adjust ventilation to keep alveolar CO_2 partial pressure constant and raise O_2 partial pressure when it falls to dangerous levels

Group Three—Changes From Normal Respiration Associated with Selected Physiologic and Psychologic States

I. States characterized in part by temporary cessation of breathing, for example
   A. Generalized convulsions with continued spasm of the respiratory muscles giving way to clonic movements of these muscles (breathing ceases and is followed by air entering the lungs in short, convulsive gasps)
   B. Breath-holding spells in young children in which crying and screaming are followed by apnea for as long as a minute

II. Absence of respiration
   A. Apnea in apparently healthy infants, characterized by (1) an episode of apnea during sleep with change in color and (2) unresponsiveness to gentle stimulation; mouth-to-mouth resuscitation or prolonged vigorous shaking is necessary to restore breathing
   B. Apnea in sick preterm hospitalized infants subjected to low levels of somatic and vestibular stimulation (as from touching and rocking) or associated with temperature instability in infant or environment
   C. Apnea in the first 24 hours of life secondary to sepsis
   D. Apnea associated with cardiorespiratory diseases, such as hyaline membrane disease, patent ductus arteriosus
   E. Apnea resulting from metabolic causes, such as hypocalcemia, hypoglycemia

III. States characterized in part by experiences of respiratory distress or by changes in depth and frequency of breathing, for example
   A. Anxiety states with persons experiencing difficulty in breathing, tightness in the throat, a feeling of smothering or suffocating sometimes with pronounced hyperventilation (symptoms of fear, anger)
   B. Hysteria and emotional disturbances with persons experiencing distressing dyspnea, sensations of smothering, needs for more oxygen, tightness of chest muscles
   C. Pulmonary or cardiac pathologic states with the experiencing of dyspnea by the individual
      1. On exertion
      2. At rest
   D. Periodic breathing in preterm infants
   E. Dyspnea and cyanosis in newborn associated with hypoplasia of mandible and glossoptosis

IV. States characterized in part by decreased respiratory rate with decreased pulmonary ventilation and vital capacity
   A. Cachexia
   B. Malnutrition

V. States with a marked increase in the work of breathing, for example, physiologic states characteristic of

    A. Injury
    B. Acute illness
This listing should be used as an exploratory tool that should be subjected to continuing validation and updating as new scientific findings emerge. It provides a basis for organization of nursing approaches already identified and validated. The question for investigation is: What can and should nurses do to help patients maintain an adequate intake of air when X condition is present? What should individuals be helped to do for themselves?

MAINTAINING A SUFFICIENT INTAKE OF WATER AND FOOD

Factors that interfere with meeting this requisite are organized by broad types (groups), subtypes (Roman numerals), and categories of factors (A, B, . . .) and named factors within the categories (1, 2, 3a, b, c, . . .).

Group One—Interferences with Taking and Holding Water and Food in the Mouth

 I. Conditions and circumstances that interfere with having access to water and food
      A. Conditions of communication
         1. Limited ability or inability to communicate needs or desires for water and food, for example, early developmental stage, low levels of cognitive development, limited or loss of awareness, speech defects or disturbances of speech pattern, aphasia
         2. Modes of communication not understood by persons who can procure water and food, for example, speech in a foreign language, sign language
         3. Failure to communicate needs for water and food to appropriate persons, for example, lack of knowledge about how to proceed, reluctance to ask for water or food, fear of persons who can procure water and food
      B. Conditions of access
         1. Inability to procure water and food for self
         2. Inaccessibility of provided water or food
         3. Water and food not available when needed or desired
 II. Characteristics of available water and food that provoke reluctance or refusal to take in or hold water or food in the mouth
      A. Water, food deviate from cultural norms
         1. Source of water not in accord with customary source
         2. Unfamiliar foods or unfamiliar preparation of food
         3. Food not in accord with religious or cultural prescriptions
      B. Water, food deviate from personal standards of acceptability
         1. Available food is disliked
         2. Water or food is displeasing to sight, smell, taste
         3. Texture of food is displeasing

4. Water or food is repugnant according to individual's standards of acceptability

C. Water, food are incompatible with structural or functional conditions of individuals or general health states

1. Incompatible with existent powers of mastication or deglutition
2. Incompatible physiologically, as in allergy
3. Not in accord with nutritional state or with digestive or metabolic powers

III. Internal and external conditions that interfere with attending to or suppress the desire for or the willingness to take in, receive, or hold water and food in the mouth

A. Interferences with attention

1. Loss of interest in drinking and eating
2. Sensory deprivation, sensory overload
3. High-level anxiety with narrowing of the perceptual field and agitation
4. Confusion, stupor, coma

B. Interferences with desire for or willingness to take in water or food

1. Human conditions that interfere with desire or willingness
   a. Satiety, anorexia
   b. Obtunded sense of thirst
   c. Nausea, vomiting, regurgitation of gas or small amounts of food from stomach
   d. Fear of choking
   e. Limited ability or inability to perceive color or texture or aroma of food or to taste food
   f. Visual or auditory hallucinations

2. Absence of psychic stimuli that promote salivation—sight of food, smell, sound of cooking, hearing descriptions of food

3. Behaviors that are not in accord with the reality of human requirements for water and food
   a. Negation of feelings of hunger with failure to eat or drink
   b. Refusal to eat when food is available
   c. Self-concept that negates the need for a sufficient intake of food
   d. Bulimia

4. Behaviors not in accord with the real characteristics of water and food, such as delusions about the characteristics of water or food, distorted perceptions of water and food, or olfactory hallucinations

5. Environmental conditions that can adversely affect the desire for water or food or willingness to eat or drink
   a. Social conditions—absence of preferred social situations for eating, strained relationships, aesthetically displeasing conditions

b. Biologic conditions—infestation with vermin, unsanitary conditions, aesthetically displeasing conditions

c. Physical conditions—offensive and disturbing noise level, undesirable climatic conditions, inadequate light levels, aesthetically displeasing conditions

IV. Conditions and circumstances that interfere with the natural processes of taking in and holding water and food in the mouth

A. Developmental and constitutional states, such as absence of suck or weak suck in infants

B. Anomalies of the mouth and face, including cleft lip, cleft palate, mandibulomaxillary discrepancies, developmental defects of the tongue or lips

C. Painful and obstructive conditions—inflammations and lesions, soft tissue swellings, intraoral tumors, tumors of face and neck

1. Stomatitis, gingivitis, glossitis, fissures of tongue

2. Tumors of mucous membranes, tongue, bony structures of mouth

3. Oral abscesses

4. Mumps (parotiditis)

D. Excessive flow of secretions from mouth and nose

1. Excessive flow of saliva as in Parkinson's disease, use of specific pharmacologic agents, increase in blood acidity

2. Excessive flow of nasopharyngeal secretions and lacrimal fluid, as in upper respiratory infections

E. Difficulty to inability to open or close the mouth

1. Temporomandibular joint disorders

2. Surgical procedures that temporarily prevent opening or closing the mouth, for example, wiring of teeth in occlusion

3. Neurologic conditions that affect, for example, ability to open mouth, maintenance of occlusion

F. Surgical procedures on the mouth, jaw, and tongue that involve excision and reconstruction restricting the taking in and holding of water and food in the mouth, for example, surgery of the lips, resections of maxillae or mandible, resection of hard or soft palate, hemiglossectomy or total glossectomy

G. Soft tissue changes in the mouth

1. Effects of dietary deficiencies and restricted or no oral water intake on the tissues and organs of the oral cavity

a. Sore mouth associated with degeneration of connective tissue of gums and periodontal ligaments and atrophy of tongue epithelium

b. Increased sensitivity of periodontal tissue to local irritants and trauma

c. Dehydration of tissues

2. Atrophy of oral mucosa in older people with resultant abnormal taste perception and burning sensation in mouth

H. Positions of the body that interfere with taking in and holding water and food in mouth, including Trendelenburg position and prone position

I. Unwillingness to open mouth to eat, based on false beliefs about consequences

Group Two—Interferences with Mastication

I. Conditions that interfere with the crushing and breaking up of food

A. Conditions of the teeth and jaws including

1. Malocclusion of jaws and teeth
2. Absence of teeth—incisors, molars
3. Temporomandibular joint disorders, such as ankylosis of joints—stiffening or fixation, dislocation of joint

B. Conditions of the masticatory muscles including

1. Weakness with fatigue of muscles after limited movement as in myasthenia gravis or the asthenia of metabolic disease
2. Weakness and atrophy of muscles associated with muscular dystrophy
3. Atrophy as in myotonia and long-standing myasthenia
4. Partial or total paralysis associated with lesions of the brainstem
5. Disturbances of motor functioning affecting coordination

C. Pain associated with mastication, as with soft tissue and bone lesions

D. Diminished amounts or absence of saliva hindering the moistening of foodstuffs and lubrication of the mucosa of the mouth

E. Habitual bolting of unchewed food

II. Conditions and circumstances that interfere with the mixing of food with saliva

A. Conditions and circumstances related to salivary flow and its composition

1. Diminished or arrested salivary secretion (asialism) associated with, for example,

   a. Body dehydration
   b. Not taking water and food by mouth
   c. Cessation of salivary function associated with inflammation of the salivary glands producing dry mouth (xerostoma)
   d. Vitamin A deficiency
   e. Use of atropine and other cholinergic blocking agents
   f. Fear, depression, anxiety, excitement

2. Blockage of salivary ducts by calculi, tumors, inflammatory conditions

B. Conditions of the muscles of the tongue and cheeks that interfere with placement of food between the dental arches and collection of food into a mass or bolus

1. Conditions of the tongue

   a. Microglossia, aglossia, macroglossia, and ankyloglossia
   b. Resection of part of tongue, removal of tongue

      c. Paralysis of half of tongue with atrophy that occurs with occlusion of vertebral artery

      d. Paralysis of extrinsic and intrinsic muscles of the tongue

  2. Conditions of the facial muscles, including weakness, atrophy, and paralysis

C. Bolting of unchewed food

Group Three—Interferences with Deglutition

I. Conditions and circumstances that interfere with the movement of chewed and moistened food or liquids from the mouth to the space between the base of the tongue and the posterior wall of the pharynx (oral, voluntary phase of swallowing)

  A. Inability to initiate or regulate voluntary action as in stupor and coma

  B. Interferences with the events of the oral phase of swallowing: closing of the lips and jaw; elevation of the tip of the tongue to the hard palate subsequent to the separation out of a bolus of food or the taking in of liquid; pushing the dorsum of the tongue upward and backward against the palate, moving the bolus of food or liquid into the pharynx; closing of the nasopharynx by the elevation of the soft palate

    1. Disturbances of motor functioning that interfere with

      a. Compressing the lips (orbicularis) and compressing the cheeks (buccinator)

      b. Elevation of the mandible—temporal muscle, masseter, and internal pterygoid muscle

    2. Anomalies of the lip, palate, and tongue

    3. Partial or total paralysis of the tongue; resection or removal of tongue

    4. Painful and obstructive conditions intraoral or of the face and neck

II. Conditions and circumstances that interfere with the arrival of food or liquid in the pharynx, movement through the pharynx and through the pharyngoesophageal sphincter into the esophagus (reflex pharyngeal phase of swallowing)

  A. Obstructive conditions and painful conditions of the pharynx

    1. Pharyngeal pouch associated with loss of support of the muscle fibers

    2. Obstructing tumor masses and foreign objects

    3. Abnormalities of the cricoid pharyngeal sphincter including spasm, delayed onset of relaxation, premature contractions with shortening of relaxation

    4. Inflammatory conditions and lesions of the soft tissues

  B. Disturbances of the neural mechanisms of the swallowing reflex

    1. Central lesions—pons, thalamus, frontal cortex, medulla

    2. Lesions of receptors in the mouth and pharynx and afferent fibers of the glossopharyngeal nerve and superior laryngeal branch of the vagus

    3. Lesions of the pharyngeal muscles

   C. Lesions that hinder the movement of the larynx cranialward and ventrally
   D. Lodging of food in the pharynx because of size of bolus or consistency of food
III. Conditions and circumstances that interfere with the passage of food and liquid through the esophagus and through the lower esophageal sphincter into the stomach (reflex esophageal phase of swallowing)
   A. Obstructive conditions including, for example
      1. Atresia
      2. Stenosis, congenital or secondary to disease or injury
      3. Esophageal webs
      4. Compressed esophagus with the opening to pharynx thrown out of axis by pharyngeal pouch
      5. Obstruction of lumen by foreign bodies, tumors
   B. Anomalies, including absence of esophagus, tracheoesophageal fistula, esophageal diverticula
   C. Painful conditions and conditions involving the integrity of the tissues of the esophagus
      1. Acute or chronic esophagitis associated with
         a. Compromised lower esophageal sphincter
            (1) Primary incompetence
            (2) Surgical removal or destruction, all leading to reflux
         b. Hiatal hernia; congenital short esophagus; columnar-lined lower esophagus
         c. Diseases such as scleroderma; neoplasms
         d. Pregnancy
         e. Secondary to factors including
            (1) Vomiting
            (2) Intubation
            (3) Anesthesia
            (4) Prolonged hiccups
            (5) Stress reaction
            (6) Recumbency that is forced, or associated with unconsciousness of long duration
            (7) Central nervous system lesions
            (8) Terminal phase of an illness
            (9) Use of alcohol secondary to irradiation and concurrent chemotherapy for persons with pulmonary small cell carcinoma
      2. Ulceration of the esophagus
      3. Esophageal varices
      4. Perforation of the esophagus
         a. As complication of esophagitis, peptic ulcers, neoplasms, presence of foreign bodies
         b. Spontaneous rupture during vomiting or coughing, or associated with gluttony

     5. Vertical lacerations of esophagus at gastroesophageal junction with severe hemorrhage

D. Disturbances of the neural mechanisms of the swallowing reflex: central lesions, lesions of receptors, neuromuscular lesions of esophagus and efferent nerve fibers

E. Motility changes and motor dysfunction associated with old age, use of alcohol, diminished or absent peristalsis when smooth muscle is replaced by dense fibrous tissue, as in scleroderma

F. Gastroesophageal reflux in newborn infant resulting from normal low resting pressure of the gastroesophageal sphincter

This listing of interferences should be subjected to refinement and continuing validation and should be kept in accord with scientific developments.

PROVIDING CARE ASSOCIATED WITH ELIMINATIVE PROCESSES AND EXCREMENTS

The factors that were identified as focusing attention on the meeting of this universal self-care requisite or on methods of meeting it were organized under categories of change, affective reactions, care performance, and environment.

Group One—Bowel Evacuation

I. Changes in bowel evacuation patterns, feces, and bowel integrity
    A. Change from individuals' patterns of evacuation—constipation, diarrhea
    B. Changes in the form, color, and other characteristics of feces
    C. Changes in bowel integrity—functional or structural changes
       1. Incontinence
       2. Obstruction of bowel—partial or complete
       3. Structural changes in bowel, for example, from infection, tumors, surgical intervention

II. Feelings and emotions associated with bowel evacuation
    A. Discomfort or pain
    B. Anxiety or fear associated with bowel elimination pattern or characteristics of feces

III. Care performance
    A. Required movements of body are difficult or impossible to execute
    B. Discomfort or pain associated with execution of required movements

IV. Environment
    A. Resources for receiving and disposing of feces are not readily available or adequate or safe
    B. Resources for aftercare of body parts for sanitary and aesthetic purposes are not available or adequate or safe
    C. The social and physical environment does not provide privacy for bowel evacuation or aftercare
    D. Prevailing practices about bowel evacuation and aftercare are not congruous with those of the individual

Group Two–Urination

I. Changes in pattern of urination, in urine, and in the integrity of organs
    A. Change from individual's normal pattern of urination
    B. Qualitative and quantitative changes in urine
    C. Changes in structural or functional integrity of organs
        1. Incontinence
        2. Paralysis of bladder
        3. Obstruction of urethra, bladder neck, ureter(s)
        4. Structural changes in ureters, bladder, urethra resultant from injury, pathology, or surgical interventions
II, III, IV. See under bowel; adjust for urination and urine.

Group Three–Perspiration

I. Change from usual pattern of sweating under specified conditions and circumstances
    A. Diminished or absent
    B. Increased
II. Reactions and feelings associated with
    A. Diminished or absent sweating
    B. Excessive sweating
III. Care performance
    A. Required movements of body are difficult or impossible to execute
    B. Discomfort or pain associated with execution of movement
IV. Environment—resources for care not available or adequate

Group Four–Menstruation

I. Change from normal pattern of menstruation or suppression
    A. Change in time and duration of bleeding or amount of bleeding
    B. Suppressed menstruation
II. Feeling and emotions associated with menstruation or its absence
    A. Discomfort or pain
    B. Anxiety or fear associated with changes in pattern of menstruation
III. Care performance
    A. Required movements of the body are difficult or impossible to execute
    B. Discomfort or pain associated with use of care measures or with required movements
IV. Environment
    A. Resources for care are not available, adequate, or safe
    B. Prevailing care practices are not congruous with those of the individual

MAINTAINING A BALANCE BETWEEN ACTIVITY AND REST

Factors were organized into two groups with subgroups. The main organizing groups were factors of human and environmental origin. Factors call attention to needs for special concern for meeting the requisite and the methods for use in meeting it.

Group One—Human Factors

I.   States that interfere with balancing activity and rest
   A. Debility and weakness
   B. Emotional states of apathy or excitement
   C. Wakefulness
   D. Narcosis, comatose states
   E. Overriding interests and concerns about some matter or affair of daily living
   F. Disability
   G. Inactivity or immobility prescribed for therapeutic purposes
II. Specific conditions that interfere with balancing activity and rest
   A. Dyspnea on exertion
   B. Uncontrolled pain
   C. Continuous discomfort
   D. Sensory overload; sensory deprivation
   E. Anxiety or fear associated with being
      1. At rest or active
      2. Alone or in contact with other persons

Group Two—Environmental Factors

I.   Social environment—what significant others want, permit, recommend, or demand
II. Resources and time are inadequate to
   A. Engage in productive work, recreation, preferred activities
   B. Change from one activity to other types of activities
   C. Change from being active to a resting state
   D. Obtain sufficient rest and sleep
   E. Maintain needed or desired physical conditions
III. Physical environment
   A. Climatic conditions that militate against activity or rest
   B. Noise that interferes with either rest and sleep or activity requiring concentration
   C. Unaccustomed noiselessness or personal need for it
   D. Personal preferences about light and darkness for rest and sleep
IV. The environmental situation
   A. Crisis situation in family or residence
   B. Disaster conditions resulting from earthquakes, hurricanes, floods, fires
   C. Disaster conditions from war

MAINTAINING A BALANCE BETWEEN SOLITUDE AND SOCIAL INTERACTION

Factors that signify need for attention to meeting this requisite and that affect methods of meeting it were organized under conditions of living and human and environmental conditions.

Group One—Conditions of Living

I. Isolation from other persons
    A. Minimal, infrequent contact to no contact because of location of residence
    B. Self-imposed isolation in a nonrestricted social environment
    C. Imposed isolation within the social group
II. Continuous demand for interactions with other persons throughout waking hours
III. Continuous involvement in provision of care associated with acute or chronic illness or injury

Group Two—Human Factors

I. Personal factors
    A. Characteristics of temperament and personality
    B. Chronological age and developmental stage
    C. Anxiety to fear of being alone or being with others
    D. Personal characteristics, including physical features, that elicit avoidance behaviors from others
II. Specific interferences
    A. Sensory impairments
    B. Inadequate communication skills
    C. Lack of skill and habit formation for being alone or with others
    D. Continuous seeking of contacts with others

Group Three—Environmental Factors

I. Persons for social contact and interaction are
    A. Pleasing, displeasing
    B. Preferred, not preferred
    C. Available, not available when needed
II. Physical environmental conditions and resources facilitate or hinder
    A. Social contacts and interactions
    B. Solitude

PREVENTING HAZARDS TO LIFE, FUNCTIONING, AND WELL-BEING

Factors that signify need to attend to meeting this requisite or affect methods for meeting it are organized in groups of human and environmental factors.

Group One—Human Factors

I. States
    A. Intense emotional states that restrict attention and awareness
    B. States of sleep and reverie
    C. Light to deep coma
    D. Debility and weakness

II. Specific interferences
  A. Disabilities that interfere with control of position and movement in space
  B. Limited awareness of self and environment in a specific time frame, regardless of cause
  C. Lack of knowledge of specific hazards or means to control or avoid them
  D. Modes of cognitive functioning that do not deal with abstractions and do not take into account what has not happened or has not been experienced
  E. Absence of reasonable concern about hazards
  F. Excessive concern about and fear of hazards

Group Two—Environmental Factors

I. Physical hazards
  A. Atmospheric and weather conditions
  B. Geologic hazards
  C. Physical hazards in the home, work situation, or recreational situations
II. Social conditions
  A. Dependents of individuals who are
    1. Indifferent to fulfillment of responsibilities to take care of their dependents
    2. Overprotective of dependents, not allowing freedom necessary for development
  B. Abandonment
  C. Exposure to personal abuse
    1. Psychologic
    2. Physical and psychologic
III. Resources—resources necessary for life and health are not available or adequate
IV. The community
  A. Does not act to prevent the occurrence of or control of known hazardous conditions
  B. Does not communicate information to members about existent hazards and measures to prevent or mitigate their effects
    1. Under usual conditions of living
    2. Under disaster conditions

PROMOTING NORMALCY

Factors when present that focus attention on the needs to meet this requisite or on methods for meeting it are organized under groups of human and environmental factors.

Group One—Human Factors

I. States
   A. Arousal states that result in restriction of knowledge or incorrect knowledge of self, environment, and situations of action
      1. Sleep and reverie
      2. Light to deep coma
      3. Intense emotional states that restrict attention and interfere with perception
   B. States of cognitive development (or modes of thought) in which persons do not deal with abstractions or that which has not been experienced
   C. States of physical disability that interfere with sensation and perception and ability to control position and movement in space
   D. Imposed states of restricted physical activity, resulting in a limited environment

II. Specific Factors
   A. Impairments of communication, reasoning, or memory
   B. Absence of or defects in bodily parts visible, not visible
   C. Anxiety to fear or anger associated with changes in self and in life-style
   D. Reluctance to refusal to attend to existent conditions in self or environment
   E. Overriding interests and concerns that rule out attention to conditions in self or environment that should be regulated
   F. Diminished powers to manage and care for self and to fulfill role responsibilities
   G. Unsatisfying conditions of living

Group Two—Environmental Factors

I. Social
   A. Exclusion from or rejection by family or intimate social group
   B. Exclusion from the larger society

II. Conditions and resources not supportive of personal developments and not adequate to maintain satisfying conditions of living

Glossary

Action The process of a person doing something, usually involving more than one step and occupying some time.

Agency The power to engage in action to achieve specific goals.

Agent The person who engages in a course of action or has the power to do so.

Agreement The act of two or more persons who unite in expressing complete accord about some matter.

Antecedent Knowledge A person's knowing elements, conditions, situations that were mastered and structured before use in practice situations.

Applied Science The structured development and use of an existent science to resolve points of theory or solve problems in another field of science.

Basic Conditioning Factors Personal conditions or environmental circumstances in a time-place matrix that affect the values or ways of meeting persons' existent self-care requisites; bring about new self-care requisites; or affect the development, operability, or adequacy of persons' capabilities to care for themselves or their dependents; conditions or events in a time-place matrix that affect the values of nurses' powers of nursing agency.

Care Watching over, providing for, and looking after a person or thing, performed by a responsible individual or group.

Caring An element of brotherly love that is interdependent with the elements of responsibility, respect, and knowledge demonstrated by persons who move out to, respond to, and give of themselves to others.

Case In nursing, a concrete instance of a person requiring and receiving nursing.

Case Load In nursing, the number of persons that a nurse provides with nursing individually or in multiperson units during the same time duration.

Case Management Operations In nursing practice the series of actions performed by a nursing practitioner to plan and control, that is, direct, check, and evaluate the professional practice operations of nursing diagnosis, prescription, and regulation to form an effective, dynamic system of service to nurses' patients.

Central Idea An expressed description of the model that accounts for the constitution and behavior of things whose interactions are explained by a theory.

Client A person who has arranged to receive and may be receiving a specific service from a person(s) who legitimately represents himself or herself as able and willing to provide the service for some duration of time.

Communicate To make common among humans intangible things such as thoughts, feelings, or information expressed in some tangible way, as through statements or diagrams.

Community A group sharing common characteristics or interests based in the intersubjective spontaneity of group members and an intelligently devised social order and perceived or perceiving itself as distinct in some respect from the larger society in which it exists.

Compensatory Making up for what is deficient.

Conceptualization The level of cognitional activity in which ideas from acts of understanding based on data of sense or data of consciousness are formulated and expressed as concepts to give an outward form to what is understood.

Concrete Concerned with actual things or instances; constituting an actual thing or instance.

Conditioning Factor A circumstance or a qualitative or quantitative feature of a factor(s) in a situation of action that affects the values or the operability of other situational factors.

Content In human experiences that which is experienced as distinguished from the act.

Contract A promissory agreement about specific matters between two or more competent parties creating a mutuality of agreements and obligations expressed in ascertainable terms.

Control The process of keeping things within the bounds of what is essential, correct, and proper.

Coordinated Combined in harmonious relations; unified for action.

Criterion A measure used in the making of a correct judgment about something that is accomplished.

Deliberate Action The process by which persons bring about, through what they do, foreseen conditions or states of affairs, moving from an intention of what is to be done to the bringing about of the foreseen condition or to the failure to do so.

Dependent-Care The practice of activities that responsible maturing and mature persons initiate and perform on behalf of socially dependent persons for some time on a continuing basis to meet their therapeutic self-care demands in order to maintain their lives and contribute to their health and well-being and regulate the exercise or development of their self-care agency.

Dependent-Care Agency The developed and developing capabilities of persons to know and meet the therapeutic self-care demands of persons socially dependent on them or to regulate the development or exercise of these persons' self-care agency.

Dependent-Care Agent A maturing adolescent or adult who accepts and fulfills the responsibility to know and meet the therapeutic self-care demand of relevant others who are socially dependent on them or to regulate the development or exercise of these persons' self-care agency.

Dependent-Care System Courses and sequences of action that are being or have been performed by dependent-care agents to meet the particularized self-care requisites of socially dependent persons for whom they are responsible.

Design A proposed way of making or doing something with a setting forth of the disposition of individual elements or details of elements in the process of production.

Design Unit In nursing practice, a distinct result-achieving component of a total pattern for the production of nursing for a patient.

Development A sequence of dynamic and increasingly differentiated arrangements and patterns toward realization of the hidden or latent possibilities of a thing.

Development (in Practice Fields) Study, investigation, and research leading to the formulation and formalization of technologies necessary for the work of a practice field; development includes establishing the validity and reliability of technologies under a range of concrete practice conditions.

Domain A field of activity or influence.

Empirical Derived from or guided by experience.

Factor One of the elements, circumstances, or conditions contributory to a particular situation or result.

Features Distinct parts, qualities, or characteristics of objects, persons, or situations.

Form The particular condition in which something appears, including its internal structure, disposition of details, boundary lines, and unity of the whole.

Foundational Nursing Science The study of the human and environmental factors in nursing practice situations that supply the fields of knowledge necessary for nurses to make essential observations and valid judgments and decisions in the practice fields of nursing.

Functions of Health Service Enterprise (a) Operations through which the specific health service(s) is provided, (b) operations to establish and manage the fulfillment of the defined purpose of the health service, and (c) operations to govern the whole enterprise and lead it to fulfill its purpose for existence in society.

Good That which is liked or fully approved with respect to what is under consideration.

Habit A way of thinking or acting acquired through repeated use of persons' powers or capabilities in a deliberate way of proceeding.

Health A descriptor of living things with respect to their structural and functional wholeness and soundness.

Help Providing for persons what they need to have, or to do or have done for them, by individuals who know what is needed and have the ability and willingness to provide a part or all of what is needed.

Hierarchy of Values Possible concrete objects of choice of individuals (excluding concrete objects of aversion) that are understood by them as being arranged in a particular order that influences choice and practical action.

Human Regulatory Function A descriptive name for the processes of self-care through which individuals act to continuously meet specific and known requirements for keeping features of their functioning and developing within human norms.

Insight An instance of persons apprehending in data the answers to a question for investigation proceeding from an accurate presentation of the problem, to cues, to images, to knowing.

Intellectual Virtues Habits or enduring dispositions that mentally dispose persons to act so that they make right judgments and choices in concrete situations with consideration of existent factors, conditions, and circumstances.

Interaction Reciprocal action or influence; persons' action or influence on each other.

Interdependence The mutual dependence of persons or of situational elements on one another for their proper operation in a situational context.

Intersubjectivity Person-to-person togetherness; mutual or reciprocal action or influence.

Judgment The mental act of asserting (affirming or denying) something on the basis of sufficiency of evidence and acts of reflective understanding.

Knowing Affirming what one correctly understands in one's own experience (after Lonergan).

Legitimacy Conformity to established rules, standards, and principles.

Managed Care A service provided for persons who are members of health insurance programs that offer what is referred to as comprehensive care, including continuing preventive health care from a primary care physician with referrals to medical specialists, hospitals, and other services, as required.

Meaning The idea that a word, statement, facial expression, bodily movement, or situation in a time-place matrix conveys to persons or is intended to convey; social and cultural changes are changes in meaning that are understood and accepted by members of communities.

Modality Form as contrasted with substance; in health care the method of employment of a therapeutic agent.

Model A postulated representation of an unobservable entity or process, with the elements used in the representation partly understood from their presence in another entity.

Moral Virtues Enduring habits that dispose persons to judge and to do what is good and avoid what is wrong or harmful to themselves or other persons in concrete situations of human living.

Nurse Person(s) educated and trained through technical or professional forms of education to meet nursing requirements of individuals and groups.

Nurse Variable In self-care deficit nursing theory, the nursing agency of nurses, that is their powers and capabilities to know and meet the nursing requirements of individuals and groups.

Nursing A direct human health service provided by a qualified person to help persons to continuously know and meet their own or their dependents therapeutic self-care demands and to regulate the exercise or development of their self-care or dependent-care agency whenever their limitations for action are associated with their own health states or that of their dependents.

Nursing Administration The body of persons who are responsible for and function in governing and executive positions in formally constituted organizations to ensure the provision of nursing to the whole of or a segment of the populations served by health service enterprises, the members of which have legitimate nursing requirements.

Nursing Agency The developed capabilities of persons educated as nurses that empower them to represent themselves as nurses and within the frame of a legitimate interpersonal relationship to act, to know, and to help persons in such relationships to meet their therapeutic self-care demands and to regulate the development or exercise of their self-care agency.

Nursing Design A professional function performed both before and after nursing diagnosis and prescription through which nurses, on the basis of reflective practical judgments about existent conditions, synthesize concrete situational elements into orderly relations to structure operational units. The purpose of nursing design is to provide guides for achieving needed and foreseen results in the production of nursing toward the achievement of nursing goals; the units taken together constitute the pattern to guide the production of nursing.

Nursing Diagnosis A deliberate process through which nurses in nursing practice situations carefully examine and analyze facts and judgments about persons who are their patients, and about properties and activities of these persons, to explain and state the nature and causes of their therapeutic self-care demands; the state of development, operability, and adequacy of their self-care agency; and the presence and extent of self-care deficits existent or projected.

Nursing Practice Nurses' responsibility for and regular engagement in nursing one or more persons (singly or in groups) in these persons' time-place localizations.

Nursing Practice Science The study of elements and factors, and relationships among them, that describes and explains the modalities of nursing cases (practice fields) and the rules and standards of practice that guide the diagnostic, prescriptive, and regulatory or treatment operations of nurses by categories of nursing cases.

Nursing Practitioner A person professionally educated and qualified to practice nursing who is engaged in its regular provision to persons individually or in multiperson units at the beginning or advanced scientific level of professional practice.

Nursing Prescription A deliberate action process through which nurses make practical judgments about what can and should be done to meet their patients' particularized self-care requisites and to regulate the exercise or development of their self-care agency under existent or projected changed conditions and circumstances.

Nursing Process A reference term used by nurses to subsume the professional operations of nursing practice, including work management operations.

Nursing Regulation or Treatment Nurses' use of valid and reliable measures to continuously meet their patients' particularized self-care requisites in order to keep their functioning and development within ranges compatible with life and with normal functioning and development; it also includes use of measures to ensure that patients' developed or potential powers of self-care agency are protected and the exercise or development of self-care agency regulated.

Nursing Requirements Existent needs of persons with health-associated self-care deficits for help and care to compensate for or overcome their deficits in order to know and continuously meet their therapeutic self-care demands and protect and regulate the exercise or development of their self-care agency; or the existent needs of persons with dependents for help because of the health state of their dependents so that the therapeutic self-care demands of their dependents can be met and their own dependent-care agency be developed.

Nursing Science A practical science with theoretically practical and practically practical components and a set of applied sciences.

Nursing Situations A combination of concrete circumstances involving both persons with health-related self-care or dependent-care deficits and nurses at some place in some time frame, with nurses acting to the advantage of the persons with self-care or dependent-care deficits.

Nursing Systems Series and sequences of deliberate practical actions of nurses performed at times in coordination with actions of their patients to know and meet components of their patients' therapeutic self-care demands and to protect and regulate the exercise or development of patients' self-care agency.

Object That toward which or because of which action is directed or taken.

Operation A particular process of a mental or practical nature necessary in some form of work or production.

Order A relation in a set of elements or members of a class (individuals, facts, objects of any kind) that arranges the elements of the set or the members of a class in a particular way.

Organization A structural arrangement of persons, things, or the actions of persons into orderly, unified relationships so that a forseen and desired purpose can be brought about through designed operations of the structured entity.

Organized Formed as or into a whole consisting of interdependent or coordinate parts toward ensuring harmonious or unified action.

Parameter A factor with variable values used as a referent to determine values of other entities.

Patient A person accepted for care and under care of health service professionals.

Patient Variables In self-care deficit nursing theory the therapeutic self-care demands and the self-care agency of persons under the care of nurses.

Pattern A combination of qualities or acts forming a consistent or characteristic arrangement.

Phases of Action In a result-achieving series of actions or a system of action, the major variations in the forms of actions that are performed, namely, to investigate the situation of action, actions to determine the result to be sought and the means to be used and action to produce the result sought.

Phenomenologic Pertaining to the study and description of observed or observable facts, occurrences, or circumstances in all areas of experience.

Plan The specification of the organization and timing of essential tasks to bring a design for something to be produced into actuality. Specifications relate to time and place of action and duration of actions, requisite environmental conditions and equipment and supplies, number of persons required at particular times and places, and control measures to be used.

Population All persons who have some characteristics in common, such as residence in the same geographic area or being served by the same health care institution or agency.

Postulate To set forth a proposition accepted as true as a basis for a specific chain of reasoning, a specific argument, or a specific system of thought.

Powers and Capabilities, Human Abilities and potentials that are associated with agency and activity and are manifestations of the nature of humankind; capabilities are powers that can be acquired or lost without affecting change in the fundamental nature of humankind (after Harré).

Practical Science The study of the principles and causes of things, including knowledge, that brings unity and meaning to the action domain of a practice field (speculatively practical knowledge) as well as knowledge that is preparatory for action in types of practice situations (practically practical knowledge).

Premise A proposition or one of several propositions supporting or helping to support a conclusion.

Prescriptive Operations In nursing practice, the action sequences engaged in by nurses to make practical judgments about and to specify in relation to qualitative and quantitative features of identified self-care requisites, the ways in which they can and should be met, and when and how to use the ways of meeting them; this is a prescription of the therapeutic self-care demand. Also included are nurses' prescriptions about what should be done to protect patients' capacities for self-care and ways and means to develop their powers of self-care agency or regulate their use.

Presuppositions Expressions of existent conditions or circumstances that are necessary to support judgments about the nature of and behavior of persons or things.

Process The series and sequences of actions or operations involved in the accomplishment of something moving from a beginning stage to the stage of the actual making or production or changing of something (the end or goal sought).

Production Performance of detailed operations to bring into being or make services or objects or arrangements of persons or things; production requires exertion of effort and the exercise of skill and creativity conjoined with knowledge of what is to be done and made and the means to be used.

Profession A type of pursuit that requires years of study and training before a person is ready to practice it as a life work and means of livelihood.

Professional-Technologic Operations In the health services, the processes of diagnosis, prescription, regulation or treatment, and case management performed by professional practitioners within their respective fields in their provision of health care to persons who seek or use their services.

Professionals In practice fields persons prepared through education, training, and experience to provide service in complex practice situations in which mastery and use of speculative knowledge and the technologies of the field are required, who also contribute to the extension and validation of knowledge, in the field.

Proper Object That which persons in a specific field of art or science study, observe, or endeavor to bring to some new condition or form.

Properties Characteristics or attributes of things.

Proposition Anything that is believed, disbelieved, doubted, or supposed communicated in sentences.

Prudence The habit that disposes persons to make right choices and decisions about what to do in concrete life situations in which relevant conditions may be extensive and complex.

Public Health A field of knowledge and a field of practice concerned with ways and means of enhancing and conserving the health of all members of a community and the community as a social entity.

Regulate To control, direct, or adjust in accordance with a principle or rule.

Regulatory Nursing System In nursing practice, a deliberate action process of ensuring that patients' calculated and prescribed therapeutic self-care demands are met, their powers of self-care agency are protected, and the exercise or development of self-care agency is regulated.

Relation A connection between a pair of reciprocally dependent things.

Research Careful, systematic study and investigation within a field of knowledge of unanswered questions and hypothesized answers to them.

Rules of Nursing Practice Principles that specify proper ways of thinking and acting and govern the conduct of nurses in nursing practice situations; rules may be general, applicable in all nursing situations, or specific to types of nursing cases. When principles or rules are institutionalized by a health service agency to be followed by all nurses, they are identified as regulations or policies.

Science The study of the behavior of things and materials, and the elucidation of their nature.

Self-Care The practice of activities that maturing and mature persons initiate and perform, within time frames, on their own behalf in the interests of maintaining life, healthful functioning, continuing personal development, and well-being, through meeting known requisites for functional and developmental regulations.

Self-Care Agency The complex acquired ability of mature and maturing persons to know and meet their continuing requirements for deliberate, purposive action to regulate their own human functioning and development.

Self-Care Capabilities Constituent developed abilities that together form the self-care agency of persons for effectively performing, within appropriate time frames, the investigative, judgment and decision-making, and regulatory or treatment operations necessary to keep their own functioning and development within norms compatible with life, health, and well-being. The performance of the three self-care operations rests on developed and exercised knowledge, skills, and motivations specific to self-care and on sets of foundational human capabilities and dispositions.

Self-Care Deficit A relation between persons' therapeutic self-care demands and their powers of self-care agency in which constituent developed self-care capabilities within self-care agency are not operable or not adequate for knowing and meeting some or all components of the existent or projected therapeutic self-care demand.

Self-Care Limitations Restricting human and environmental influences within time frames on persons' performance of the investigative, judgment and decision-making, and production operations of self-care.

Self-Care Requisite A formulated and expressed insight about actions to be performed that are known or hypothesized to be necessary in the regulation of an aspect(s) of human functioning and development continuously or under specified conditions and circumstances. A formulated self-care requisite names (1) the factor to be controlled or managed to keep an aspect(s) of human functioning and development within norms compatible with life, health, and personal well-being and (2) the nature of the required action. Formulated and expressed self-care requisites constitute the formalized purposes of self-care. They are the reasons for which self-care is undertaken; they express the intended or desired results—the goals of self-care.

Self-Care Systems Courses and sequences of action that are being or have been performed by individuals to meet their particular self-care requisites.

Self-Management Capabilities Abilities of individuals at various stages of human development to control their position and movement in space and to manage their own affairs.

Self-Organizing System Systems that exist only when and for the duration of time that there are self-connecting links between the behavior or state of independent parts or subjects, the connection occurring at some point of conditionality between them (after Ashby).

Service The providing of resources or courses of action required by persons or organizations.

Situation A state or condition that represents a combination of concrete circumstances arranged with reference to relations of circumstances to one another; this includes relations among properties and circumstances of persons involved that affect these persons to their advantage or disadvantage.

Social Dependency The condition of persons necessitating reliance on family, friends, or the larger community for support or aid.

Social Encounter The meeting of persons with one another or meeting of persons in groups.

Socialization The adjusting or making fit for cooperative, group living.

Societal Pertaining to large groups of persons associated together for various purposes or to these persons' activities or customs.

Standard A rule, pattern, or model for guidance in doing or making something so that what is done or made will be of a particular quality.

State A form of existence; the named combination of circumstances affecting a person or thing at a given time.

Status Role An expression that persons who fill specific positions in social units have relations to persons in other positions and bear responsibility for fulfilling prescriptions for organized action through which the position or status is filled.

Structure The arrangement of parts of a whole; something that is composed of parts.

System A set of objects together with relationships between the objects and between their attributes. The objects, the parts constituting the system, behave together as a whole.

Technology A practical means for bringing about or producing something.

Theory A model of a hypothetical construction that supplies an answer to the constitution and behavior of things whose interactions with each other are responsible for the manifested patterns of behavior (after Harré).

Therapeutic Contributory to support of life process; normal human functioning and development; prevention, cure, or control of disease and injury; prevention of disability; structural or functional compensation for disability; promotion of well-being.

Therapeutic Self-Care Demand The summation of care measures necessary at specific times or over a duration of time for meeting all of an individual's known self-care requisites, particularized for existent conditions and circumstances, using methods appropriate for (1) controlling or managing factors identified in the requisites, the values of which are regulatory of human functioning, for example, sufficiency of air, water, food; and (2) fulfilling the activity element of the requisite, for example, maintenance, promotion, prevention, and provision.

Thing A particular, concrete unity, identity, whole; grasped by considering the individuality and unity of data.

Treatment or Regulatory Operations In nursing practice, deliberate courses of action of nurses specified within individuals' therapeutic self-care demands that are performed to keep human functioning and development within norms compatible with life, health, and well-being; operations also include those actions selected by nurses for purposes of regulating patients' development or exercise of self-care capabilities and for overcoming or compensating for self-care limitations.

Unit of Action A number of actions that together can be regarded as a distinct meaningful part of a more comprehensive series of actions, through the performance of which a result is sought and achieved.

Unit of Service A term used to designate whether nurses provide nursing to persons as individuals or as members of multiperson units. In the first instance, the individual person is the focus or object of nurses' attention; in the second instance, the multiperson unit with its members is the primary focus or object of nurses' attention.

Value The good, the desired as the possible object of rational choice of individuals; values become known from questioning if this or that is truly good and not just apparently good, or whether this or that is worthwhile.

View An intellectual examination of a situation.

Well-Being A perceived condition of personal existence including persons' experiences of contentment, pleasure, and kinds of happiness, as well as spiritual experiences, movement to fulfill one's self-ideal, and continuing personal development.

Bibliography

Ackerman NW: *The psychodynamics of family life,* New York, 1958, Basic Books.

Allison SE: The meaning of rest: some views and behaviors characterizing rest as a state and a process, an exploratory nursing study, doctoral dissertation, Teachers' College, Columbia University, 1968.

Allison SE, McLaughlin K: *Nursing administration in the 21st century: a self-care theory approach,* Thousand Oaks, CA, 1998, Sage.

Allport GW: *Becoming: basic considerations for a psychology of personality,* New Haven, CT, 1955, Yale University Press.

Allport GW: *Personality and social encounter: selected essays,* Boston, 1960, Beacon Press.

Allport GW: *Pattern and growth in personality,* New York, 1965, Holt.

Andersen R, Anderson O: *A decade of health services: social survey trends in use and expenditure,* Chicago, 1967, University of Chicago Press.

Aquinas T: *Summa Theologiae, Prudence,* vol. 36, Gilby T, translator, Cambridge, MA, 1974, Blackfriars and New York, 1974, McGraw-Hill.

Argyris C, Putnam R, Smith DMc: *Action science,* San Francisco, 1985, Jossey-Bass.

Arnold MB: *Emotion and personality: psychological aspects,* vol I, New York, 1960, Columbia University Press.

Arnold MB: *Emotion and personality: neurological and physiological aspects,* vol II, New York, 1960, Columbia University Press.

Ashby WR: *An introduction to cybernetics,* London, 1964, Chapman & Hall.

Ausubel DP: *Some psychological aspects of the structure of knowledge,* Chicago, 1964, Rand MacNally.

Backscheider JE: The use of self as the essence of clinical supervision in ambulatory patient care, *Nursing Clinics of North America* 6:789, 1971.

Bailey NA: Toward a praxeological theory of conflict, *Orbis* 11:1018-1112, 1968.

Banfield B: A philosophical inquiry of Orem's self-care deficit nursing theory, doctoral dissertation, Graduate School, Wayne State University, 1997.

Barnard CI: *The functions of the executive,* Cambridge, 1962, Harvard University Press.

Black M: *Problems of analysis: philosophical essays,* Ithaca, NY, 1954, Cornell University Press.

Black M: *Models and metaphors,* Ithaca, NY, 1962, Cornell University Press.

Black M: Assessing patients' needs. In Yura H, Walsh MB, editors: *The nursing process,* Washington, DC, 1967, Catholic University of America Press.

Blocker CE, Plummer RH, Richardson RC Jr: *The two-year college: a social synthesis,* Englewood Cliffs, NJ, 1965, Prentice-Hall.

Bronowski J: *A sense of the future, essays in natural philosophy,* Ariotti PR, Bronowski R, editors, Cambridge, MA, 1977, MIT Press.

Brooks DL: Identification of selected nursing factors to determine the availability of learning experiences for students, master's thesis, School of Nursing, Catholic University of America, 1963.

Brown EL: *Nursing as a profession,* ed 2, New York, 1940, Russell Sage.

Brownlea A: Participation: myth, realities and prognosis, *Social Science in Medicine* 25:6, 1987.

Buckley W: *Sociology and modern systems theory,* Englewood Cliffs, NJ, 1967, Prentice-Hall.

Courtney R, Ballard E, Fauver S, Gariota M, Holland L: The partnership model: working with families and communities toward a new vision of health, *Public Health Nursing* 13:3, 1996.

525

Crowe FE, Doran RM, editors: *Collected works of Bernard Lonergan, Insight: a study of human understanding,* Toronto, 1992, University of Toronto Press.

De Montcheuil Y: Community. *In Guide for social action,* Chicago, 1954, Fides Publishers Association.

Dock LL, Stewart IM: *A short history of nursing,* ed 3, New York, 1931, GP Putnam's Sons.

Dougherty GV: *The metaphysics of order in the moral basis of social order according to Saint Thomas: philosophical studies,* vol. 63, Washington, DC, 1941, Catholic University of America Press.

Dubos R: Humanistic biology, *American Scholar* 34:179-198, 1965.

Dubos R: *Man adapting,* New Haven, CT, 1965, Yale University Press.

Entralgo PL: *Doctor and patient,* Partridge F, translator, New York, 1969, World University Library, McGraw-Hill.

Fawcett J: *Analysis and evaluation of conceptual models of nursing,* ed 3, Philadelphia, 1995, FA Davis.

Firth R: *Elements of social organization,* ed 3, Boston, 1961, Beacon Press.

Foucault M: *The birth of the clinic: an archaeology of medical perception,* Sheridan Smith AM, translator, New York, 1975, Vintage Books.

Fromm E: *The art of loving,* New York, 1962, Harper Colophon Books.

Fromm E: *The heart of man,* New York, 1968, Harper & Row.

Galdston I: *Medicine in transition,* Chicago, 1965, University of Chicago Press.

Gamm L: Advancing community health through community health partnerships, *Journal of Health Care Management* 43:1, 1998.

Gannon TJ: Emotional development and spiritual growth. In O'Brien M, Steimel R, editors: *Psychological aspects of spiritual development,* Washington, DC, 1964, Catholic University of America Press.

Geden E, Taylor SG: Theoretical and empirical description of adult couples collaborative self-care systems, *Nursing Science Quarterly* 12:4, 1999.

Gilby T: Appendix I, Structure of a human act. In Thomas Aquinas, *Summa theologiae: psychology of human acts,* vol 17, New York, 1970, McGraw-Hill.

Gilby T: Introduction and Appendix 2, 3, 4: In Thomas Aquinas, *Summa theologiae: prudence,* vol 36, New York, 1974, McGraw-Hill.

Guyton AC: *Textbook of medical physiology,* ed 8, Philadelphia, 1991, WB Saunders.

Hall LE: Another view of nursing care and quality. In Straub KM, Parker KS, editors: *Continuity of patient care: the role of nursing,* Washington, DC, 1966, Catholic University of America Press.

Hampton IA, et al: *Nursing of the sick,* 1893, New York, 1949, McGraw-Hill.

Harmer B: *Textbook of the principles and practice of nursing,* ed 5, revised by Henderson V, New York, 1955, Macmillan.

Harré R: *The principles of scientific thinking,* Chicago, 1970, University of Chicago Press.

Harrison TR, et al, editors: *Principles of internal medicine,* ed 5, New York, 1966, McGraw-Hill.

Hartnett LM: Development of a theoretical model for the identification of nursing requirements in a selected aspect of self-care, master's thesis, School of Nursing, Catholic University of America, 1968.

Hawley AH: *Environment, population, and ecosystem, in human ecology, a theoretical essay,* Chicago, 1986, University of Chicago Press.

Helson H: *Adaptation level theory: an experimental and systematic approach to behavior,* New York, 1964, Harper & Row.

Hemstrom M: Application as scholarship: a community client experience, *Public Health Nursing* 12:5, 1995.

Henderson V: *The nature of nursing: a definition and its implications for practice, research, and education,* New York, 1966, Macmillan.

Hildebrant E: Building community participation in health care: a model and example from South Africa, *Image: Journal of Nursing Scholarship* 28:2, 1996.

Horgan MV: Concepts about nursing in selected nursing literature 1950-1965, masters thesis, School of Nursing, Catholic University of America, 1967.

Houssay BA, et al: *Human physiology,* New York, 1955, McGraw-Hill.

Illich I: *Medical nemesis,* New York, 1976, Pantheon Books.

Jaco EG, editor: *Patients, physicians and illness: sourcebook in behavioral science and medicine,* Glencoe, IL, 1958, Free Press.

Johns EB, Sutton WC, Webster LE: *Health for effective living,* ed 3, New York, 1962, McGraw-Hill.

Katz RL: *Empathy: its nature and uses,* New York, 1963, Free Press.

Kirkpatrick FG: *Community: a trinity of models,* Washington, DC, 1986, Georgetown University Press.

Knutson AL: *The individual, society, and health behavior,* New York, 1965, Russell Sage.

Kotarbinski T: *Praxiology: an introduction to the sciences of efficient action,* 1st English ed, Wojtasiewicz O, translator, New York, 1965, Pergamon.

Labonte B: *Health promotion and empowerment practice frameworks,* Toronto, 1993, Centre for Health Promotion.

Leavell HR, et al: *Preventive medicine for the doctor in his community,* ed 3, New York, 1965, McGraw-Hill.

Lewin K: *Field theory in social science, selected theoretical papers,* Cartwright D, editor: New York, 1951, Harper Torchbooks.

Lonergan BJF: *Insight, a study of human understanding,* New York, 1958, Philosophical Library.

McHale J: Global ecology: toward the planetary society, *American Behavioral Science* 11:29-33, 1968.

Macmurray J: *The self as agent,* London, 1957, Faber and Faber.

Macmurray J: *Persons in relation,* New York, 1961, Harper and Brothers.

Maritain J: *Science and wisdom,* Hall B, translator, London, 1944, Centenary Press.

Maritain J: *The degrees of knowledge,* Phelan GQ, translator, New York, 1959, Charles Scribner's Sons.

Mechanic D: *Medical sociology: a selective view,* New York, 1968, Free Press.

Monnig MG: Identification and description of nursing opportunities for health teaching of patients with gastric surgery as a basis for curriculum development in nursing, master's thesis, Catholic University of America, 1965.

Nadel SF: *The theory of social structure,* Glencoe, IL, 1958, Free Press.

Nagel E: *The structure of science,* New York, 1961, Harcourt, Brace & World.

Neff WS: *Work and human behavior,* New York, 1968, Atherton.

Nightingale F: *Notes on nursing: what it is and what it is not,* London, 1959, Harrison & Sons.

Nursing Development Conference Group: *Concept formalization in nursing: process and product,* Boston, 1973, Little, Brown.

Nursing Development Conference Group: *Concept formalization in nursing: process and product,* ed 2, Orem DE, editor: Boston, 1979, Little, Brown.

Orem DE: *Hospital nursing service, an analysis,* Indianapolis, 1956, Division of Hospital and Institutional Services, Indiana State Board of Health.

Orem DE: *Guides for developing curricula for the education of practical nurses,* Washington, DC, 1959, US Government Printing Office.

Orem DE: Discussion of paper, another view of nursing care and quality. In Straub KM, Parker KS, editors: *Continuity of patient care: the role of nursing,* Washington, DC, 1966, Catholic University of America Press.

Orem DE: Levels of nursing education and practice, *Alumnae Magazine (Johns Hopkins School of Nursing)* 68:2-6, 1969.

Orem DE: *Nursing: concepts of practice,* ed 1, New York, 1971, McGraw-Hill.

Orem DE: *Motivating self-care: the reality, persons as self-care agents.* In Conference papers, hospitals in the community, a vision, Queensland, Australia, 1988, The Wesley Hospital.

Orem DE: *Nursing: concepts of practice,* ed 5, St. Louis, 1995, Mosby.

Orem DE: Views of human beings specific to nursing, *Nursing Science Quarterly* 10:1, 1997.

Orem DE, Taylor SG: Orem's general theory of nursing. In Winstead-Fry P, editor: *Case studies in nursing theory,* New York, 1986, National League for Nursing.

Orem DE, Vardiman EM: Orem's nursing theory and positive mental health, *Nursing Science Quarterly* 8:4, 1995.

Parker ME, editor: *Patterns of nursing theories in practice,* New York, 1993, National League for Nursing.

Parsons T: *The structure of social action,* New York, 1937, McGraw-Hill.

Parsons T: *The social system,* New York, 1951, Free Press.

Parsons T, Bales RF, Shils EA: *Working papers in the theory of action,* Glencoe, IL, 1953, Free Press.

Paul BD, editor: *Health, culture, and community: case studies of public reactions to health programs,* New York, 1955, Russell Sage.

Phenix PH: *Realms of meaning,* New York, 1964, McGraw-Hill.

Plattel MG: *Social philosophy,* Pittsburgh, 1965, Duquesne University Press.

McCool GA, editor, *A Rahner Reader,* New York, 1975, Crossroad Publishing.

Renard H: *The philosophy of being,* ed 2, Milwaukee, 1946, Bruce Publishing Company.

Richards LAJ: *Reminiscenses of Linda Richards, America's first trained nurse,* Boston, 1911, M Barrows.

Roach MS: *Caring: the human mode of being, implications for nursing,* Toronto, 1984, Faculty of Nursing, University of Toronto.

Roberts MM: *American nursing,* New York, 1954, Macmillan.

Sawyer L: Community participation: lip service, *Nursing Outlook* 43:1, 1995.

Sekgobela M: Community participation: the heart of community health, *Nursing RSA Verpleging* 1:9, 1986.

Selye H: *In vivo: The case for supramolecular biology,* New York, 1967, Liveright.

Sigerist HE: *Civilization and disease,* Chicago, 1962, University of Chicago Press.

Siler-Wells GL: *Directing change and changing direction: a new health policy agenda for Canada,* Ottawa, 1988, Canadian Public Health Association.

Simon HA: *Sciences of the artificial,* Cambridge, MA, 1969, MIT Press.

Solomon DN: Sociological perspectives on occupations. In Becker HS, et al, editors: *Institutions and the person,* Chicago, 1968, Aldine.

Somers HM, Somers AR: *Medicare and the hospitals: issues and prospects,* Washington, DC, 1967, Brookings Institution.

Sommerhoff G: *Analytical biology,* London, 1950, Oxford University Press.

Sorokin PA: *Social and cultural dynamics,* Boston, 1957, Extending Horizons Books.

Spalding EK, Notter LE: *Professional nursing,* Philadelphia, 1970, Lippincott.

Stewart DA: *Preface to empathy,* New York, 1956, Philosophical Library.

Stuart IM, Austin AL: *A history of nursing,* ed 5, New York, 1962, GP Putnam's Sons.

Stuart ME: An analysis of the concept of family. In Whall A, Fawcett J, editors: *Family theory development in nursing: state of the science and art,* Philadelphia, 1991, FA Davis.

Sullivan LC, Carr J: Promoting healthy hearts, Canadian Nurse 86:4, 1990.

Taylor S: An interpretation of family within Orem's general theory of nursing, *Nursing Science Quarterly* 4:4, 1989.

Taylor S, McLaughlin K: Orem's general theory of nursing and community nursing, *Nursing Science Quarterly* 4:4, 1991.

Teilhard de Chardin P: The human rebound of evolution and its consequences. In *The Future of Man,* Denny N, translator, New York, 1964, Harper & Row.

Ullman M: Health deviations and behavior. In Orem DE, Parker KS, editors: *Nursing content in preservice nursing curriculums,* Washington, DC, 1964, Catholic University of America Press.

U.S. Surgeon General's Consultant Group on Nursing: *Toward quality in nursing: needs and goals,* Washington, DC, 1963, US Department of Health, Education, and Welfare.

Van Kaam A: *The art of existential counseling,* Wilkes-Barre, PA, 1966, Dimension Books.

Vernon MD: *The psychology of perception,* Baltimore, 1962, Penguin Books.

Von Bertalanffy L: *Robots, men, and minds: psychology in the modern world,* New York, 1967, Braziller.

Wallace WA: *From a realist point of view: essays on the philosophy of science,* Washington, DC, 1979, University Press of America.

Wallace WA: *The modeling of nature, philosophy of science and philosophy of nature in synthesis,* Washington, DC, 1996, Catholic University of America Press.

Weiss P: *You, I, and the others, Carbondale and Edwardsville,* 1980, Southern Illinois University Press.

Whall A: Family systems theory: relationship to nursing conceptual models. In Fitzpatrick J, et al, editors: *Nursing models and their psychiatric mental health applications,* Bowie, MD, 1982, Brady.

Whipple DV: *Dynamics of development: euthenic pediatrics,* New York, 1966, McGraw-Hill.

Whitehead AN: *Adventures of ideas,* New York, 1964, New American Library.

Wiedenbach E: *Clinical nursing, a helping art,* New York, 1964, Springer.

Wiener N: *Cybernetics,* ed 2, Cambridge, MA, 1961, MIT Press.

Willig S: *Nurse's guide to the law,* New York, 1970, McGraw-Hill.

Woodham-Smith C: *Florence Nightingale, 1820-1910,* New York, 1951, McGraw-Hill.

Woolsey AR: *A century of nursing, with hints toward the organization of a training school, and Florence Nightingale's historic letter to the Bellevue School, September 18, 1872,* New York, 1950, Putnam.

World Health Organization: *Health promotion: development of discussion frameworks in the WHO regional office for Europe,* Geneva, 1988, World Health Organization.

Yovits MC, Cameron S, editors: *Self-organizing systems: proceedings of an interdisciplinary conference, May 5 and 6, 1959,* New York, 1960, Pergamon.

INDEX